Economic Analysis in Health Care

Economic Analysis in Health Care

Stephen Morris
Nancy Devlin
David Parkin

John Wiley & Sons, Ltd

Email (for orders and customer service enquiries): cs-books@wiley.co.uk

Visit our Home Page on www.wiley.com

Reprinted with corrections August 2007, April 2009

Reprinted November 2008, March 2010, December 2010

Other Wiley Editorial Offices

John Wiley & Sons Inc., 111 River Street, Hoboken, NJ 07030, USA

Jossey-Bass, 989 Market Street, San Francisco, CA 94103-1741, USA

Wiley-VCH Verlag GmbH, Boschstr. 12, D-69469 Weinheim, Germany

John Wiley & Sons Australia Ltd, 42 McDougall Street, Milton, Queensland 4064, Australia

John Wiley & Sons (Asia) Pte Ltd, 2 Clementi Loop #02-01, Jin Xing Distripark, Singapore 129809

John Wiley & Sons Canada Ltd, 6045 Freemont Blvd, Mississauga, ONT, L5R 4J3

Wiley also publishes its books in a variety of electronic formats. Some content that appears in print may not be available in electronic books.

Anniversary logo design: Richard J. Pacifico

Library of Congress Cataloging-in-Publication Data

Morris, Stephen.
  Economic analysis in health care / Stephen Morris, Nancy Devlin, David Parkin.
     p. ; cm.
  Includes bibliographical references and index.
  ISBN-13: 978-0-470-01685-5 (pbk. : alk. paper)
                                1. Medical care – Case studies. 2. Medical care –
Finance – Case studies.   3. Medical care – Finance – Cross-cultural studies.   I. Devlin, N. J. (Nancy J.)
II. Parkin, David.   III. Title.
  [DNLM: 1. Delivery of Health Care – economics.   2. Costs and Cost Analysis. W 84.1 M877e 2007]
  RA394.E2566 2007
  338.4'33621 – dc22
                                                                          2006100396

A catalogue record for this book is available from the British Library

ISBN 978-0-470-01685-5

FSC
www.fsc.org
MIX
Paper from
responsible sources
FSC® C013604

This book is for our lovely children: from Steve to Eve and Stella; from Nancy to Sophie, Molly and Hugh; from Dave to Susannah, Eleanor, Laura and Stephen

Contents

Preface

Each of us has, for many years, taught health economics courses to both masters and undergraduate students in the UK (and, in Nancy's case, New Zealand) – and our objective here was to write the sort of book we always wished was available for our students.

As health economics has grown as a subdiscipline, so too have the number of textbooks that are available. The many fine US textbooks in this subject are inevitably influenced by the particular system for funding and provision of health care in that country; the focus of these is not always appropriate for the principal concerns and issues in *other* health care systems. And while there are textbooks on health economics in the UK, for example, these generally either aim to provide an easy-to-understand, non-technical introduction to health economics for those with no economics background, or focus on one particular aspect of health economics, such as economic evaluation or health care financing. While some of these books are excellent, their objectives limit their usefulness as a teaching tool for a more general course in health economics.

This book is written to provide (we hope!) a useful balance of theoretical treatment and breadth of content for use in undergraduate modules in health economics for economics students, and for students taking a health economics module as part of their postgraduate training. Although we are writing from a UK perspective, we have attempted to give an international flavour to the book by drawing on examples, case studies and boxed highlights not just from the UK but from a wide range of countries including Canada, Finland, Ireland, Italy, New Zealand, Sweden, Thailand and the USA, plus multinational sources including the OECD, the United Nations, the WHO and the World Bank.

There are other things about this book that we hope will be of particular value to students. First, we have paid special attention to explaining key elements of theory in health economics – for example, the contributions of Arrow (1963) and a full account of the Grossman (1972) model, both of which we view as critical to any account of health economics. We have not shied away from presenting and explaining the technical aspects of the theory, but have endeavoured to do so in as user-friendly a manner as possible. Secondly, we have been careful to link the practice of economic evaluation to underlying concepts in production, costs and efficiency. This reflects our own view that, as the practice of economic evaluation has come to be dominated by increasingly sophisticated statistical and modelling techniques, the underlying economics concepts (and, incidentally, a remaining rich research territory) are sometimes overlooked.

We very much hope that this book will serve to provoke thought and stimulate a deep interest in health economics, in the same way as earlier writers, particularly Alan Williams, Victor Fuchs and Tony Culyer, served to inspire us in our careers.

Finally: both for you and for us, this book represents a starting point. In addition to what you read between these covers, we have a wide range of complementary teaching and learning resources – study questions, practical exercises, and animated slides, that we have developed over many years of lecturing, which will be made available online to lecturers and students using this text and will be continuously updated.

Stephen Morris, Nancy Devlin, David Parkin

Secondly, the health care sector of the economy is very large. In the USA, spending passed the US$ 1000 billion mark in 1997 and currently accounts for just over 15% of the US Gross Domestic Product (GDP). Forecasts by the Office of the Actuary at the Centers for Medicare and Medicaid Services (2005) suggest that spending on health care will account for US$ 3600 billion – nearly one-fifth of all US economic activity – by 2014. Researchers from the US National Bureau of Economic Research suggest that it is entirely plausible that health care spending will reach 33% of GDP by the middle of the century (Hall and Jones, 2004). In the UK, where health care is predominantly funded by general taxation, spending on health care comprises 17% of all government spending (Chote *et al.*, 2004) and health care is a major consideration in fiscal management of the economy. Indeed, health care is a major component of spending, investment and employment in every developed economy (Reinhardt *et al.*, 2002, 2004; Fuchs, 2005), so the economic performance of the health care system is crucially linked to the overall economic well-being of a country and its citizens.

Thirdly, decisions about how health care is funded, provided and distributed are strongly influenced by the economic environment and economic constraints. Global, national and local policy responses to health issues are increasingly being informed by economics ideas and methods of analysis. One good reason for understanding health economics, even if you do not intend ultimately to practise as an analyst yourself, is to be able to engage in policy debates as an informed critic. As Joan Robinson commented: 'the purpose of studying economics is not to acquire a set of ready-made answers to economic questions, but to learn how to avoid being deceived by economists' (Robinson, 1980, p. 17). Less cynically, for those working in the health services, familiarity with the theory and methods of economic analysis is becoming essential, both to understand the context of your practice and because evidence on productivity, efficiency and value for money are increasingly the norm in modern health care systems.

Health economics is the application of economic theory, models and empirical techniques to the analysis of decision making by individuals, health care providers and governments with respect to health and health care. It is a branch of economic science – but it is not merely the *application* of standard economic theory to health and health care as an interesting topic. Health economics is solidly based in economic theory but it also comprises a body of theory developed specifically to understand the behaviour of patients, doctors and hospitals, and analytical techniques developed to facilitate resource allocation decisions in health care. Health economics has evolved into a highly specialised field, drawing on related disciplines including epidemiology, statistics, psychology, sociology, operations research and mathematics in its approach. Alternatively, it may be regarded as an essential part of a set of analytical methods applied to health, which are usually labelled *health services research*.

This chapter provides a gentle introduction to some of the basic economics concepts that underpin the more detailed and rigorous treatment of health economics in the remainder of the book.

Chapter 1

Introduction to Economic Analysis in Health Care

1.1 LIFE, DEATH AND BIG BUSINESS: WHY HEALTH ECONOMICS IS IMPORTANT

You may come to this book knowing a great deal about economics, but not a great deal about health care, other than your personal experience of ill health and its treatment. Alternatively, you may come to this book with experience in the health care sector, but no training in economics. Whatever background you bring to it, we are confident that you will find the study of health economics fascinating. Learning to look at health and health care issues through the distinctive lens of the economist will forever change the way you think about them.

Understanding the economics of health care is important for a number of reasons. First, health is important to us as individuals and as a society, and health care is one, though not the only, way of modifying the incidence and impact of ill health and disease. The availability of health care can determine the quality of our lives and our prospects for survival. Economic analysis offers a unique and systematic intellectual framework for analysing important issues in health care, and for identifying solutions to common problems. Quite literally, then, the economics of health care is a matter of life and death.

1.2 HEALTH CARE AS AN ECONOMIC GOOD

Economics is a social science. Its central concern is the study of behaviour of economic agents – individuals, firms, governments and other organisations – when confronted with scarcity. Underpinning economic analysis are the general observations that:

- resources are limited; and
- potential uses of those resources are unbounded.

The focus of economic analysis is decisions and choices about the production and consumption of *economic goods*, defined as any good or service that is scarce relative to our wants for it.

Using this definition, health care is an economic good, in the following specific sense. The resources that are used to produce health care services, such as human resources, capital and raw materials, are finite: more of these resources can be devoted to the production and consumption of health care only by diverting them from some other use. Our wants for health care – what we would choose to consume, in the absence of constraints on our ability to pay for it as a nation or as a consumer – have no known bounds. No health care system, anywhere in the world, has achieved levels of spending sufficient to meet *all* its clients' wants for health care.

If we accept that health care is an economic good, the implications are quite profound. Choices must be made about what quantity and mix of health care to produce, how to produce it, who pays for it and how it is distributed. These basic economic questions are unavoidable. Health care is not available in endless supply, and the more health care we choose, the more of something else must be sacrificed. And because health care is so important to our welfare as human beings, these choices are particularly difficult and contentious ones to make.

The nature of choice, and the inevitable tradeoffs encountered in making these choices, are captured in what is probably the most fundamental notion in economics – *opportunity cost*. The opportunity cost of committing resources to produce a good or service is the benefits forgone from those same resources not being used in their next best alternative.

Each action taken by patients, by health care providers or by governments with respect to the use of health care involves the sacrifice of the benefits that would have been enjoyed by other, alternative uses of the resources used to provide that care. The concept of opportunity cost lies at the heart of *all* economic analysis: when economists refer to cost, we mean opportunity cost – not to an accounting procedure. For example, weighing up the costs and benefits of a decision to make beta-interferon available to all multiple sclerosis patients involves assessing the benefits to multiple sclerosis patients from that treatment, compared with the benefits that would have been possible by using those same resources to treat *other* patients, suffering other conditions. Box 1.1 illustrates the concept of opportunity cost in relation to a 2004 recommendation by the UK National Institute for Health and Clinical Excellence that the NHS should fund in-vitro fertilisation (IVF) services for infertility (NICE, 2004).

Focusing on opportunity cost provides a powerful way of sharpening thinking about decision making at all levels of the health care system. Table 1.1 represents these decisions as a series of choices, identifying the opportunity costs associated with each.

In a predominantly tax-funded health care system such as those in New Zealand and the UK, where the government fixes the budget at the start of each period, these choices are effectively a 'top-down' hierarchy of decisions, implemented in roughly the order shown. In other health care systems, such as Germany's social insurance system, or the complex mix of private insurance and federal- and state-funded pro-grammes in the USA, there is no hierarchy – for example, how much is spent on health care overall is partly determined 'bottom-up', by decisions of individual insurers and patients.

Regardless of how the health care system is organised, the key point is this: the produc-tion and consumption of health care incurs real, human costs, as well as creating real, human benefits.

Box 1.1 The opportunity cost of in-vitro fertilisation (IVF)

To provide one course of IVF treatment, the UK's National Health Service pays around £2700. If each patient received, on average, three courses of IVF, the benefit, for women less than 40 years of age, is an increase in the probability of a successful pregnancy, defined as a live birth, by 0.3. Is this good value for money?

Answering this question requires us explicitly to weigh up this benefit against the opportunity cost (Devlin and Parkin, 2003). The resources devoted to each IVF patient could instead by used to provide the following.

In the UK health care sector

One-third of a cochlear implant

One heart bypass operation

Eleven cataract removals

One hundred and fifty vaccinations for measles, mumps and rubella (MMR)

Elsewhere in the UK public sector

One-thousandth of a Challenger 2 military tank

Half a junior school teaching assistant for a year

Two thousand school dinners

From a limited budget, the most efficient mix of services to fund will be that which generates the greatest aggregate benefit. But efficiency is not the only criterion: equity – fairness in the distribution of health care and health outcomes – is also an important consideration in most health care systems.

Data Sources
Challenger 2 price estimates: http://www.armedforces.co.uk/army/listings/l0023.html
Department of Health (2005) *National Tariff 2005–6*, Annex A. http://www.dh.gov.uk
Devlin and Parkin (2003)
National Institute for Clinical Excellence (2004) *Costing clinical guidelines: fertility (England)* 23 February 2004. http://www.nice.org.uk

Table 1.1 Choice and opportunity cost in the allocation of health care resources

We face choices about:	If we decide to:	The opportunity cost is:
How much should we spend on health care as a country?	Increase public spending on health care by increasing taxes/social insurance contributions	Lower net incomes for consumers, so benefits of private consumption are forgone. Higher taxes for firms either lowers profits, reducing incentives to invest and creating incentives to cut costs, including labour costs, or results in increased prices where taxes can be 'passed on' to consumers
	Increase public spending on health care by spending less on other government services	The benefits forgone from lower education, social welfare or defence spending
	Increase public spending on health care by running a fiscal debt	Economy-wide consequences of public sector debt and borrowing
How much of the health care budget is allocated to each state/region/health care purchaser?	Increase the share of the total health care budget devoted to one geographical area/health care purchaser	The health and other benefits forgone from reduced health care services in other areas
What share of the purchaser's budget should we devote to each type of health care service or product?	Increase the resources devoted to one set of services or products	The health and other benefits forgone from reduced resources for other services and products
Which patients should get access to the treatments we have decided to fund?	Ensure patients with particular characteristics, for example those who have been waiting the longest, get access to services	The health and other benefits forgone as a result of those same services not being made available to other patients, with different characteristics
How much of our limited income as consumers should be spent on health-related versus non-health-related goods and services?	Spend more of our income on health-related goods and services	The utility forgone from our consumption of other goods and services

1.3 HEALTH AND HEALTH CARE

We have referred to the subject matter of this book as health economics, but we have so far mainly discussed health care. This is an important point: *health* economics is not shorthand for *health care* economics. Although health economists are interested in health care as a sector of the economy, it is recognised that the ultimate goal of health care is to improve health, and that other means by which health can be improved are of equal interest – as are the determinants of ill-health. Health economists may therefore be interested not just in the supply of treatment that hospitals provide but in the impact that this has on the health of patients and in the impact of housing, unemployment and lifestyles on the health of the population as a whole.

This is not to say that improving health is the only characteristic of health care that health economics takes into account. Many types of health care may impact on other aspects of a person's welfare – for example, providing reassurance or increased anxiety about their state of health, whether or not their health itself is changed. Some services offered by health professionals and health care organisations may be intended only to have such an impact, by simply providing information about health. And even when the main or sole purpose of health care is to improve health, the way in which it is provided may also be important – for example, the quality of meals that are provided during a stay in hospital may be important to people even if that aspect has no impact on health. But for most types of health care, their most important and interesting characteristic is that they are intended to alter health, not that they are services provided by the health care industry.

Given the importance of thinking about health itself, how is it to be conceptualised so that we can apply economic reasoning to it? The most powerful and important insight is that in addition to health care being an economic good, health itself can be thought of as a good, albeit one with special characteristics. It can be regarded as a 'fundamental commodity', one of the true objects of people's wants and for which other more tangible goods and services – such as health care – are simply means to create it. This theory originates from the work of Becker (1965) and Grossman (1972), but can be traced to eighteenth-century economists, principally Jeremy Bentham, who wrote of 'the relief of pain' as a 'basic pleasure' (Bentham, 1780). Economically relevant characteristics of health are that it can be manufactured by individuals and households; that it has an impact on people's welfare; that it is wanted and people are willing to pay for improvements in it; and that it is scarce relative to people's wants for it. Obviously, it is less tangible than conventional goods – though it may manifest itself in tangible ways such as episodes of sickness – and cannot be traded because it is intrinsic to people and cannot normally be transferred to others. Nevertheless, it is possible to derive important analytical insights by applying to it the tools of economic analysis such as demand and production theory, as will be demonstrated in Chapters 2 and 3. But in each case, as we discuss below, this application is not straightforward.

1.4 WANTS, DEMANDS AND NEEDS

If we accept that health is a 'fundamental commodity' we can analyse the demand for improvements in health in very similar ways to the analysis of demand for other goods and services. A key difference is that, because health is not tradeable, it is not possible to analyse it in the context of a market – improvements in health cannot be purchased directly. Instead, we focus on the production of health as the key means by which individuals express their demand for it, which may involve the purchase of goods such as health care, thereby indirectly purchasing health improvements. Health care therefore has a 'derived demand' from the demand for health. Of course, such analysis can be used for almost any goods or services but it is of particular importance in health because the consumption of health care is usually not in itself pleasurable – indeed it is often the opposite – but is undertaken simply to improve health.

In analysing the demand for most goods and services, economics distinguishes between a *want*, which is simply the desire by someone to consume something, and *effective demand*, which is a want backed up by the willingness and ability to pay for it. Although these concepts can easily be applied to the analysis of the demand for health care, there is a complication. There is a widespread view that what matters in health care is not wants or demands, but *needs*. 'Need' is a far less precise concept than demand and is open to a number of different definitions – see, for example, Bradshaw (1972). However, health economists generally interpret the need for health care as the *capacity to benefit* from it – that is, to obtain a valued improvement in health from it. It follows, therefore, that not all wants are needs and vice versa. For instance, many women are opting to give birth by caesarean section – it is one of the most commonly performed surgical procedure on women in the UK – and 42% of these procedures are elective (Jones, 2005). Clearly many women *want* caesareans, but largely for reasons which are not related to health; indeed, the procedure entails some risks. Further, some needs are not wants. For instance, a person may experience pain and discomfort relating to their teeth and recognise that they would benefit from seeking dental treatment, but they may not *want* to seek care.

As we will see, the implications of basing the allocation of health care resources on needs rather than demands are profound. They call into question some of the most deeply-held assumptions and convictions held in economics, such as the primacy of the consumer's viewpoint in assessing their own welfare and the reliability of market forces to create efficient outcomes.

1.5 THE PRODUCTION OF HEALTH AND HEALTH CARE

Like any other good or service, health care is produced, and an understanding of many important issues in health economics requires knowledge of production theory. It is important in the analysis of the costs and supply of health care, and will be discussed in more detail in Chapter 3. It is also a key input to the understanding and carrying out of economic evaluation, which is the subject of Part II of this book. It underlies some of the analysis of efficiency, which is, as has been noted, a key evaluative criterion. Moreover, as explained above, production is an important element of the theory of demand for health, so again some knowledge of concepts and tools of production analysis is required. It is therefore worthwhile considering briefly here the key elements and how they are applied in health economics.

Analysis of production is based on the concept of a *production function*. This is simply a relationship between the inputs to a productive process (resources such as personnel, equipment, buildings and raw materials) and the output of that process (for example, an amount of health care of a given quality). A production function focuses on analysing the relationship between quantities of inputs and quantities of outputs. It is not, however, a detailed description of the production process itself. Indeed, the production process is often regarded as 'black box' into which resources disappear and out of which emerge outputs, as illustrated in Figure 1.1. There may of course be other factors that affect the relationship between inputs and outputs – for example, market conditions – so the production function also takes account of 'mediating factors' as the figure shows.

Figure 1.1 Production function.

This model is valuable because it can be used to analyse many different issues in the same framework. This flexibility arises because we can measure inputs and outputs in different ways, and look at different aspects of the relationships between them. For example, we can measure inputs as quantities of physical resources or weight them according to prices or costs; similarly, outputs can be measured in physical quantities or in terms of prices, costs or other values. By varying all inputs by the same amount and looking at the impact on output, we can look at economies of scale: is it more efficient to have large or small hospitals? By looking at the impact on output of changing one input, we can look at productivity: if we add an extra nurse to a hospital, how much does it raise the number of treatments that the hospital provides? By looking at how different combinations of inputs can produce the same level of output, we can analyse substitution between factors: is it more efficient for nurses to replace doctors in undertaking certain tasks?

Application of this model to the production of health by individuals, which will be covered in detail in Chapter 2, uses very similar kinds of analysis. For example, what combination of prevention, self care and professional care would most efficiently produce a desired level of health?

1.6 DECIDING WHO GETS WHAT IN HEALTH CARE

As noted, to state that health care is an economic good is not to suggest that it is therefore the same as other consumer goods and services in every relevant respect. Indeed, a considerable part of past and current research in health economics is concerned with the questions of whether or not health care is 'different' and, if so, in what ways it differs and what the implications are for the manner in which society organises its production and consumption. Economics is concerned with *what* is produced, *how* it is produced and *for whom* it is produced – should these issues be decided differently for health care?

One way in which such decisions might be made is to allow market forces to determine who gets what. This is precisely the way in which production and consumption decisions about most economic goods and services – clothes, domestic insurance, MP3 players, industrial fork-lift trucks, books, wine, estate agencies, cinemas – are made. In the absence of government intervention, firms decide how much to produce and how to produce it, guided by the profit motive. Consumers decide how much to purchase and from where to purchase it, guided by their own view of their interests. Simple economic models of supply and demand predict how firms and consumers behave in such markets, and in some cases these will be relevant to health care. For example, in most countries, cosmetic surgery, such as liposuction, is bought and sold in private markets. A simple model, illustrated in Figure 1.2, would suggest that market forces will establish an equilibrium price (P), where the number of services demanded equals the number of services supplied (Q). The demand and supply curves in Figure 1.2 are explained in more detail in Chapters 2–4. Briefly, the demand curve slopes downward from left to right (P), indicating that as the price of liposuction falls the demand for it increases. The supply curve is upward sloping from left to right, indicating that as the price rises, the supply of liposuction also rises. In a private market such as this, not everyone who wants cosmetic surgery receives it; those who obtain such services are those who are both willing and able to pay for them. We can readily observe these effective demands. We do not observe wants that are *not* met because potential consumers are not either willing or able to turn them into effective demand.

However, in most countries and for most health care services and products, a reliance on unfettered market forces is rare. Typically, governments intervene in health care markets to a far greater degree than most other economic goods: regulating who may

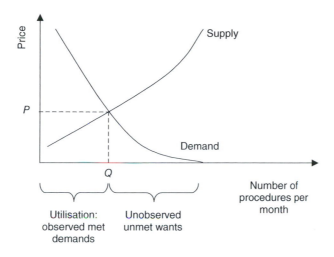

Figure 1.2 The demand for and supply of liposuction.

provide services; what providers can charge or what profits they may earn; subsidising health care either partially or fully, funded via various types of taxes; and, in some cases, directly providing health care, such as public hospitals. In the case of the UK National Health Service (NHS), the government dominates funding and provision of health care, so supply is essentially fixed in each time period by political decisions. Moreover, most health care is fully subsidised – nothing is charged at the point of consumption – so effective demand is higher than it would be if patients had to pay. Figure 1.3 shows a highly stylised economic model of the NHS, treating all health care services as measurable in some comparable unit on the horizontal axis. The demand curve is defined analogously to that in Figure 1.2. The supply curve is now vertical, indicating that supply is fixed at the level Q. Because there is no price system to reconcile supply and demand, demand exceeds supply. Who obtains health services is determined by factors other than price – for example, by waiting lists. A crucial difference is that in this case, because there is no distinction between wants, demands and needs, there are observed unmet needs.

Figures 1.2 and 1.3 show two extreme cases: a complete reliance on private markets and a complete reliance on public provision. In each case, not everyone who wants health care gets it – health care is rationed, either by price or by some other mechanism. In practice, most health care systems are a complex mix of private and public sector activities. Why are governments so often involved in health care? What is it that makes health care 'different'?

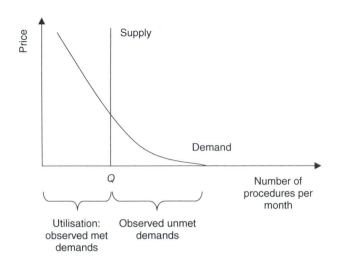

Figure 1.3 The demand for and supply of health care in the NHS.

1.7 IS HEALTH CARE DIFFERENT?

Arrow (1963) was the first to attempt a systematic analysis of this question; his seminal paper is still requisite reading for any serious student of health economics.

Arrow asserted that the principal characteristic of medical care is uncertainty. First, we do not know when we will become ill; or what health care we will require when ill health arises, or at what cost. Whereas the demand for most goods, for example food, is regular and predictable, ill health occurs randomly and its consequences can be severe. Secondly, there is uncertainty about how any given state of ill health will respond to health care. Recovery from a disease is as uncertain as its incidence.

Arrow noted the following key characteristics of consumer and provider behaviour in medical markets.

Patients Do Not Behave in the Same Way as Consumers

- They cannot 'test' the product before consuming it. Indeed, they often have difficulty gauging the quality of care even *after* experiencing it. Consumers of health care find it difficult to 'shop around' to get the best deal.

- It is difficult for patients to obtain information about what medical care is appropriate for their condition – medical knowledge is complex. As consumers, patients know considerably less than the seller, and place trust in the provider.

- There are interdependencies between consumers' actions: the health care seeking behaviour of one consumer in, for example, obtaining a vaccination against an infectious disease, affects the outcome – the likelihood of becoming infected – of others. In a more general sense, this interdependency extends to individuals caring about the health of others.

Doctors Do Not Behave in the Same Way as Other Firms

- Their entry into this 'industry' is restricted by medical licensing regulations.

- Advertising and overt competition are virtually absent in medical markets.

- Advice given by physicians is supposed to be completely divorced from self-interest – treatment is, or at least is claimed to be, dictated by clinical need, not by the financial interests of the provider.

- Providers with goals other than profit maximisation dominate provision. Profit maximisation is unlikely to be the sole or principal motivation of providers. Social and ethical factors are likely to be as important in determining their behaviour.

- Doctors sometimes charge different fees to different people: high fees to high-income people, and low fees to people with low incomes including, sometimes, charging no fees to very poor people.

The central tenet of Arrow's work is that *all* of the special economic features of medical care noted above stem from uncertainty regarding both the incidence of disease and the efficacy of treatment. Entry to the medical profession is limited to those who have met certain medical training requirements, because consumers cannot judge quality for themselves and need to be protected. And, because patients are poorly informed about what treatment is best for them, trust is the key feature in the doctor–patient relationship. If doctors were perceived to be behaving in a commercially aggressive manner, or their decisions to be influenced by pecuniary gain, this trust would quickly break down.

Finally, Arrow also noted that while the uncertainty element of ill health can be partly addressed through insurance markets, this too is problematic. Insurance markets 'work' where there is a given probability of the insured event arising; but for many conditions, demand is certain, because they are pre-existing chronic conditions. This means that there will be gaps in cover – many people will not be able to purchase health care insurance. Further, insurance works well where the person insured is unable to modify the probability of making a claim. In many cases, the demand for medical care will increase as a result of being insured, as consumers seek, and doctors provide, more and higher-quality care.

Arrow was careful not to claim that these characteristics are unique to medical care markets. For example, many professional markets share these characteristics. However, taken together, they suggest that health care is an extreme case. The behaviours of consumers and providers of medical care are very different from the norm of a competitive market in standard economic theory. This has two implications.

First, economic analysis of health and health care behaviours requires specialised theoretical approaches that acknowledge these 'differences'. Arrow's paper marked the intellectual beginnings of health economics. Since then, theoretical and empirical research on these issues – detailed in subsequent chapters – has considerably improved our understanding of medical markets.

Secondly, a reliance on unregulated private markets for medical care is unlikely to produce outcomes that are socially optimal. Private markets are efficient where consumers are well-informed and choose firms that deliver high-quality goods at competitive prices over poor-quality, high-price firms. In such markets, the consumer's strategy is represented by the phrase *caveat emptor* – let the buyer beware. In medical care, the roles of consumers and providers are very different, and the behaviours of each are affected by the incentives created by third-party payment for care by private or social insurance or by government.

1.8 DESCRIBING VERSUS EVALUATING THE USE OF HEALTH CARE RESOURCES

We have established that, although health care is an economic good, the ways in which consumers and producers of health care behave are often fundamentally different from those observed in other markets. Economic analysis plays a valuable role in *describing* these behaviours and *predicting* the outcomes of market interactions, in terms of prices, quantities traded and the distribution of services between people. However, economic analysis frequently goes beyond description and prediction and is concerned with *evaluating* how resources are used. Much of economics – including health economics – is concerned with whether or not one set of arrangements is preferable to another.

Analysis that is restricted to the description or prediction of behaviours and outcomes is labelled *positive economics*. Positive economics is concerned with investigating the relationship between economic variables. It is descriptive and predictive in nature, and can include both theoretical and empirical analysis. For example, we might describe the market for dental care in the UK as regulated private practices that provide services to patients who pay a price for care that is subsidised by the state. We might construct a theoretical model that predicts that as price rises, demand falls. We could then obtain data on prices, use of services and other relevant factors and use statistical analysis to test this theory. We might then conclude that an increase in the price of dental services by 10% will, controlling for other factors, lead to a reduction in the number of dental services demanded by about 6%. An example of evidence of this kind is the study by Manning and Phelps (1979). Such a study provides useful information for dentists and for those concerned with oral health policy. But the analysis, in itself, makes no judgement about the desirability of prices increasing, decreasing or staying the same – it simply tells us the consequence in each case.

In principle, facts are established in economics in the same way as in other sciences – as descriptions of theoretical relationships that are tested by real-world data. It is a characteristic of positive economics statements that they are in principle testable, whether they are derived by theoretical or empirical means. However, many statements by economists take the form of what are known as *stylised facts*. These are simplifications and generalisations of empirical findings, without precise scientific details. For example, the estimates given above of the response of demand for dental care to price changes would be regarded as valid only for the conditions under which the data were collected, such as the place and the time, and would have a quantified level of uncertainty attached to them such as a confidence interval. But if we were to observe a similar relationship in many other places and at many different times, we might state a stylised fact that the demand for dental care is not very responsive to changes in prices. Any theory of the demand for dental care would then have to be consistent with this finding.

The problem is that stylised facts are prone to misuse and to interpretation beyond the scientific goals of positive economics. As an example, Newhouse (1998) reported a survey of health economists in the USA and the UK, in which participants were asked whether they agreed with various propositions. One of these was that 'technological change is responsible for most of the medical care cost increase', which is a positive statement because it can be tested by reference to evidence. The vast majority (81%) of US economists answered this question 'correctly' – according to Newhouse's view of the evidence – by agreeing, but only around half (51%) of UK health economists agreed. The problem here is that the evidence may be very different in each country. In the USA, technological change is largely driven by market forces; in the UK, increases in health spending are politically determined, so responses to technology are a matter of choice, after weighing up costs and benefits on a case-by-case basis (Dolan, 1999). So this statement is context dependent and any view that it is a fact that can only be correct or incorrect, in a positive economics sense, is of doubtful validity.

Scientifically based positive economics provides useful information about how the world works. However, economics is also interested in what we ought to do with that information. For example, our study of the responsiveness of the demand for dental care to price might be used to determine what level of subsidy the government should provide to patients: should it be reduced, to deter excess demand, or increased to decrease unmet need? Such questions are typical of those that health economists are asked to investigate. Should we pay doctors on a fee-for-service basis, or by salaries?

Should the UK continue to fund health care through general taxation, or should it adopt a French-style social insurance system? Should the government continue fully to subsidise primary health care – or should GPs' patients be required to pay a fee? Should nurses be allowed full prescribing rights? Should Aricept™ be made available to people who have Alzheimer's disease?

In each case, scientifically based positive economics can be used to *describe* the outcomes, but a policy prescription ultimately relies on *value judgements* about their relative desirability. A value judgement is a weighing up of evidence based on the ethical and ideological values held by an individual or society. Analysis that relies at any point on value judgements is labelled *normative economics*. A normative statement can often be recognised by the inclusion of the word 'should' – for example, the NHS should not provide IVF because it provides small health benefits that are outweighed by its large costs. In summary, normative economics is concerned with the desirability of alternative economic outcomes; it is prescriptive in nature and rests on value judgements.

We noted above that an important implication of Arrow's observations about medical markets is that a reliance on private market interactions cannot be assumed to produce socially optimal outcomes. Although it does not make explicit recommendations, Arrow's paper is undertaken within a *normative* intellectual framework, observing, for example, that 'it is the general social consensus, clearly, that the *laissez-faire* solution for medicine is intolerable' (p. 967). The appropriate balance between private markets and public involvement is a central theme of health economics, and one that we will return to throughout this book.

Finally, it is important to note that the distinction between positive and normative economics is not always as clear-cut as our definitions above might suggest. One extreme view is that *all* economics research is normatively driven, in that the questions that are chosen to be the focus of positive economic investigation reflect a view on the relative importance of the topics and variables selected for analysis (Katouzian, 1980). Moreover, the interpretation of theory and data can be selected to fit a particular set of values. For example, the simple supply and demand model illustrated by Figures 1.2 and 1.3 could be used to make the points that the price mechanism is a different method of rationing from mechanisms such as waiting lists used in public services, rather than a means of avoiding having to ration; and that there may be an equal amount of unmet need using either system, but it is manifest in public provision and hidden in private provision. But it could equally have been used to make the point that publicly provided health care is not related to the value that consumers attach to health care, as expressed by their willingness to pay, and that this results in arbitrary shortages manifested as waiting lists. Given these ambiguities and complexities, one of the most valuable skills to possess as a health economist is the ability critically to scrutinise economic theory and empirical analysis – including the theory and analysis covered in this book! – to identify its both explicit and implicit normative content.

1.9 JUDGING THE USE OF HEALTH CARE RESOURCES

In economics, it is conventional to judge the use of resources using the criteria of *efficiency* and *equity*, which are dealt with in more detail in later chapters. These concepts arguably provide the main contribution of economics to decision making in health care. However, health economics inevitably has to deal with other criteria that may have analogies in other areas of economics but do not assume the same importance. The two most important are *effectiveness* and *ethics*.

The concept of efficiency is one of the most important in both positive and normative economics. Chapters 3 and 8 will give more precise and specific definitions of efficiency, but for our purposes a generic and non-technical definition, taken from Knapp (1984), is instructive: efficiency is 'the allocation of scarce resources that maximises the achievement of aims'.

The economic problem described earlier was that there are scarce resources and potentially unbounded uses for them. If our aim is to obtain the 'best' set of uses, defined in whatever way we like, then efficiency is simply the use of resources that maximises our achievement of it. For example, if our aim is to improve the health of the population given a fixed health care budget, an efficient allocation of resources will maximise the achievement of that aim.

In economic analysis more generally, efficiency issues largely concern the quantities provided of goods or services or the values attached to them. Whether or not the good or service actually 'works' is not usually a concern. However, health economics has to face that more fundamental issue: are health care services effective in improving health? Health economics analyses often assume that it is not possible for health services to be efficient unless they are effective, but the nature of health and health care means that effectiveness is not a clear-cut issue. In particular, economic evaluation of health care, which is covered in later chapters of this book, has to deal explicitly with the uncertainty surrounding the effectiveness of health care.

Efficiency is a relatively straightforward criterion compared with equity, for which it is far less clear how, for positive purposes, it should be measured and how, for normative purposes, it should be judged. It is far harder to give a general definition of equity, other than to distinguish it from efficiency and from other related concepts such as equality. Essentially, equity is a synonym for fairness; in this context, it means fairness in the distribution of health and health care between people. Equity is also relevant to assessments of the means by which health care is financed, principally the burden of finance, and whether the amount of money that people pay for health care is fair. Efficiency is largely concerned with the aim of maximising the value to society of health and health care, arising from production, consumption and distribution conditions, while equity is concerned with distribution as an object in itself. Equality means an equal distribution, but equity means a fair distribution, with the implication that it may not always be fair to be equal – giving equal amounts of health care to both healthy and sick people, for example.

The analysis of equity issues has both positive and normative aspects. It can be positive where the focus is on using economic analysis to measure or describe distributional characteristics, such as the way health, utilisation of health care, or health care spending are spread over individuals or groups of individuals in a society. Although equity is not the same as equality, positive economics usually analyses equity defined with respect to equality – for example, whether or not people have equal access to health care given equal needs for it, or whether people with equal use of health care services pay the same amount of money for that use irrespective of their ability to pay for it.

Normative analyses are to a great extent dependent on views about which equalities define fairness – for example, equal health outcomes for equal desert, or equal use of health services for equal willingness to pay for it. It should be said that there is far less agreement within economics about equity than about efficiency and that other disciplines such as philosophy have more to say about it. But it is always an important consideration in economics, and one of the special characteristics of health and health care is that people attach more importance to equity than for many other goods and services. Chapter 7 will look at these issues and their consequences in more detail.

As we have seen, normative economics requires us to acknowledge the role of values in making judgements. Usually these values are based on ideology, but in health and health care they are often based on ethics. In principle, ethical issues apply to the economic analysis of many goods and services, but in health and health care they are very important and health care professionals have developed normative criteria which, if implemented, would impact on the way in which health care resources are used. For example, the Stanford University Medical Center Committee on Ethics has promulgated a set of ethical principles: preserve life; alleviate suffering; do no harm; tell the truth; respect the patient's autonomy; and deal justly with patients. These principles are unexceptional when applied to an individual patient but, taken literally, they conflict with economic analysis when they are applied to the real world where there are many patients. If resources are scarce, preserving life for one person might have the opportunity cost of failing to alleviate suffering for another. A more sophisticated ethical code might resolve this conflict, but ethical issues are often raised not about economics principles but about the way in which economic issues are addressed. A particularly widespread view is that it is ethically wrong for people to profit from others' ill-health, though what is meant by profit is unclear, as it presumably does not include the salaries of doctors and nurses! This view leads to a general discomfort with market-based solutions to health care issues. Box 1.2 provides an example of the discomfort generated by proposals to allow trade in human organs.

Box 1.2 Why not allow a market in human organs?

In April 2005, 88 025 US citizens were waiting for organs, principally kidneys, for transplant operations that would dramatically improve their length and quality of life (UNOS, 2005). In the UK, approximately 6000 people are waiting for organs – and fewer than 3000 transplants are performed each year (UK Transplant, 2005). In nearly all countries there is a persistent shortfall between the number of organs available – the supply of organs and the number of potential recipients – the demand for them – which results in a substantial loss of life and health. Human organs, tissues and blood products are clearly economic goods.

Why do these shortages persist? One reason is that medical technology has increased the success rate of transplantation, reducing the rate of rejection and increasing the number and type of operations that can be performed. It is alleged that another reason is that the supply of organs relies exclusively on voluntary dona-tions: trade in organs is prohibited in the USA, as it is in all Western countries.

In 1999, an eBay trader in Florida attempted to sell one 'fully functioning kidney'. Bidding started at $25 000 and reached nearly $6 million before eBay removed the offer from its web-based auction (BBC, 1999). The outrage surrounding this event suggests a widespread view that buying and selling human organs is abhorrent.

Economists have for many years debated the case for allowing markets in blood – for a famous example see Cooper and Culyer (1968) and Titmuss (1972) – and in organs. Janet Radcliffe-Richards (1998, 2003), a bioethicist at University College, London, is among those who have recently questioned the rejection of proposals to legalise the trade in kidneys, concluding that there is little justifica-tion for the rejection of market solutions and that if the decision were based only on a careful weighing up of harms and benefits it is likely that it would be permitted. Of course, the supposition that legalising trade would improve the supply of good-quality organs is a positive economics question; moreover, it would have to be demonstrated that the health benefits from the extra supply outweigh the health benefits forgone owing to the additional resources used in collecting organs commercially. If that were the case, then the ethical counter to the argument against legalising trade is that even if it is true that trade in organs is abhorrent, the premature death and ill health resulting from an inad-equate supply of donated organs is also abhorrent.

Data sources

BBC News online network September 3 1999 http://news.bbc.co.uk

United Network for Organ Sharing (UNOS) provide daily updates on numbers of poten-tial organ recipients in the US: see www.unos.org

UK Transplant (2005) www.uktransplant.org.uk/ekt/statistics

SUMMARY

1. Health economics is the application of economic theory, models and empirical techniques to the analysis of decision making by individuals, health care providers and governments with respect to health and health care.

2. It is important because it offers a unique and systematic intellectual framework for analysing important issues in health care. This is useful because the health care sector consumes a great deal of resources, and because the organisation and delivery of health care are strongly influenced by the economic environment and economic constraints.

3. An economic good is any good or service that is scarce relative to our wants for it. Health care is an economic good.

4. A fundamental notion in economics is opportunity cost. The opportunity cost of committing resources to produce a good or service is the benefits forgone from those same resources not being used in their next best alternative. Consideration of opportunity cost means that the production and consumption of health care incurs real, human costs, as well as creating real, human benefits.

5. In order to understand the economics of health care it is important to understand the wants, needs and demand for health and health care by consumers, and the production of health and health care by producers.

6. Most health care systems are a complex mix of private and public sector activities. Government involvement in the finance and provision of health care is common. An important reason for this is the inherent uncertainty surrounding health and health care.

7. Economists often distinguish between positive and normative economics. Positive economics is concerned with investigating the relationship between economic variables. Normative economics is concerned with the desirability of alternative economic outcomes. Health economics has both positive and normative aspects.

8. In economics, it is conventional to judge the use of resources using the criteria of efficiency and equity. Efficiency can be simply defined as the allocation of scarce resources that maximises the achievement of aims. Equity is fairness in the distribution and finance of health and health care between people.

9. In health economics, we also have to take account of effectiveness and ethics. Effectiveness concerns whether or not health care 'works'; ethics essentially concerns strong value judgements widely held in health care.

Part

I

Health Care Markets

Chapter 2

The Demand for Health Care

2.1 DEMAND, PROFITS AND HEALTH POLICY TARGETS

As we saw in Chapter 1, there are many different ways in which health systems may be funded and organised. But in every type of system, an understanding of the demand for health care is fundamentally important. In private health care markets, firms have a keen interest in knowing the determinants of demand for their products and services so that they can forecast responses to changes in prices and consumers' circumstances, and the consequences for their revenues and profits. In public systems, information on population and patient demands enables policy makers to predict health care use, and to modify demand through measures such as charges or subsidies to meet health policy targets.

This chapter aims to familiarise you with economic theory regarding consumers' choices; to demonstrate how that theory informs empirical economic analysis; and to show the insights that economic research provides into the behaviour of consumers with respect to health and health care. Throughout, we use the term 'consumers' rather than 'patients', because this is consistent with the language of economic theory; moreover, 'patients' are a subset of people who demand health care, those who become customers of a health professional.

2.2 CONSUMER CHOICE THEORY

2.2.1 Preferences and Utility

Economists define the demand for any good or service, including health care, as the quantity that consumers are both willing and able to buy. Demand for a good therefore depends both on preferences – what consumers want and their ability to afford it. The law of demand evident in a downward-sloping demand curve, such as that shown in Figure 1.2 in Chapter 1, states that other things being equal, as price rises, demand falls, and vice versa. Underlying the relationship between price and quantity demanded described by the demand curve is a behavioural model of consumers' choices. Consumer choice theory explains *why* consumers behave or react in certain ways to changes in various factors. As we shall see, these models can provide rich insights into health-related choices and behaviours.

Consumer choice theory represents consumers' decisions as being driven by a single objective – the maximisation of *utility*, which means the level of satisfaction of their desires. Consumers obtain utility from the consumption of goods and services. The relationship between their level of utility, U, and their consumption of various quantities of these goods and services consumed, X, can be represented as a *utility function*:

$$U = U(X_1, X_2, \ldots, X_n) \tag{2.1}$$

The utility function is entirely subjective and idiosyncratic – the utility each consumer obtains from each unit of any one good and overall from any particular combination of goods depends entirely on their individual preferences – essentially, their likes and dislikes.

The consumer is, however, assumed to be *rational*, which essentially means that their behaviour is consistent with their aims. We assume that individuals behave as if they make decisions with the aim of maximising their well-being. This implies that their utility function obeys certain conventions. For example, the consumer must be able to compare any two 'bundles' (a term meaning a particular collection of different goods and services) and decide whether they prefer one to another or consider them equally desirable. Confronted with choosing between various possible bundles, the consumers' preferences between these must be complete – they must be capable of expressing a preference ordering over all possible bundles. Preferences must also be transitive – they must be logically consistent, such that if they prefer a bundle a to another bundle b, and b to a third possible bundle c, then a should also be preferred to c. Finally, it is assumed that consumers' wants are non-satiable: increasing their consumption of any one good will always increase their utility. More is always preferred to less.

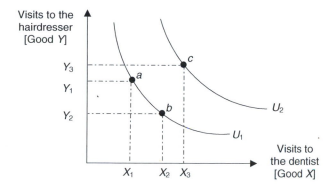

○ **Figure 2.1 Indifference curves.**

The way in which various bundles affect utility can be illustrated using *indifference curves*. For simplicity, imagine a world in which there are only two alternatives to choose between: visits to the dentist (Good X), and visits to the hairdresser (Good Y). In the same way that isobars show points of equal barometric pressure on a weather map, or contour lines show equal height of terrain in a geographical map, an indifference curve shows all the combinations of the consumption of two goods that yield the consumer equal satisfaction – in effect, they are indifferent between these bundles of goods. For example, points *a* and *b* in Figure 2.1 represent two quite different bundles of dentist's and hairdresser's services, but each generates the same utility to the consumer, U_1. Bundle *c*, which has a higher quantity of both services compared to bundle *a*, generates a higher level of utility, U_2. Indifference curves further from the origin generate higher levels of utility. Although only two indifference curves are drawn here, every conceivable combination of Goods X and Y can be placed on an indifference curve, enabling it to be compared with any other combination as yielding either higher, lower or identical utility.

The slope of the indifference curve is the *marginal rate of substitution* (MRS): it is the amount of Y that must be sacrificed if X is increased in order for utility to remain unchanged:

$$MRS_{XY} = -\frac{\delta Y}{\delta X} \tag{2.2}$$

Indifference curves are usually depicted as convex to the origin, reflecting the assumption that the MRS_{XY} falls as we move along an indifference curve from left to right, that is as the quantity of dental visits increases and visits to the hairdresser decrease. Why? This reflects an assumed nonlinearity in marginal utility – as the amount of visits to the dentist increases, each additional visit confers a smaller increase in total utility than the previous visit, that is, there is diminishing marginal utility of consumption;

and simultaneously, as consumption of visits to the hairdresser decreases, each further hairdressing visit sacrificed generates a higher loss of utility. For example, suppose that a consumer is currently consuming a bundle of services that comprises four visits to the hairdresser each year and no visits to the dentist. This consumer's preferences may be such that one visit to the hairdresser and one visit to the dentist is considered to be just as good as the existing bundle, that is the two bundles lie on the same indifference curve. To obtain one dentist's visit, the consumer can give up three visits to the hairdresser and remain just as happy as before: their $MRS_{XY} = 3$. Another way of thinking about this is that the amount of utility *gained* from consuming one visit to the dentist must be identical to the amount of utility *lost* from giving up three visits to the hairdresser. So, we can infer that the marginal utility of one dental visit must be three times that of a visit to the hairdresser. The MRS_{XY} can therefore be restated as the ratio of the marginal utilities, MU, for the two goods:

$$MRS_{XY} = \frac{MU_X}{MU_Y} \qquad (2.3)$$

Indifference curves cannot cross; nor, given our assumptions, can they have a positive slope: that would mean that, for one of the goods, an *increase* in consumption would actually lower utility and would have to be compensated with an *increase* in the consumption of the other good for utility to remain the same.

The notions of utility, preferences and indifference in consumer choice theory are sometimes regarded as entirely abstract constructs: if you cannot measure utility, what practical purpose do such concepts serve? Box 2.1 demonstrates one such use, in valuing health states; and Box 2.2 shows how utility functions for health care can be estimated empirically by observing the choices individuals make.

2.2.2 Budget Constraints and Maximisation

The decisions consumers make to maximise their utility are subject to a budget constraint: they are constrained both by their limited resources – the income they have available to spend – and the prices of the various goods and services between which they choose. The consumer receives an income (I) and faces a set of prices ($P_1, P_2, \ldots, P_n$) for each of the goods and services ($X_1, X_2, \ldots, X_n$). Consumers' behaviour can be modelled as a constrained maximisation problem: they maximise utility *subject to* their budget and prevailing prices. The budget constraint – defining what the consumer can actually afford to buy – is determined both by their income and the prices of the goods. In this simple example, we assume that consumers cannot borrow and therefore the sum of the amounts that they spend on each good – the amount bought multiplied by the prevailing price – cannot exceed their total income.

$$\sum_{i=1}^{n} P_i X_i \leq I \qquad (2.4)$$

Box 2.1 Using indifference curves to value quality of life

Imagine that you suffer from a chronic medical condition that causes you pain and limits your ability to go about your day-to-day life. If a treatment were made available that could completely eliminate these problems but had a side effect which reduced your length of life, would you accept treatment? The answer depends both on how you feel about your quality of life now, and how big the reduction in length of life might be. If the treatment improved your health and did not reduce length of life, your utility would increase, for example from U_1 to U_2 in the figure below. Using an iterative questioning process, we could gauge, for an improvement in health, what reduction in your length of life would leave you *just as well off* as before the treatment. The diagram shows that if quality of life improved by ΔH, length of life would need to reduce by ΔL in order for this person to remain on U_1 (Mehrez and Gafni, 1990; Buckingham and Devlin, 2006).

This procedure, known as a 'time trade-off', is widely used in health economics to gauge the value that individuals place on health and improvements in health. Values generated in this way are routinely used in economic evaluations in the UK, Canadian and Australian and New Zealand health care systems to make important decisions about whether new drugs, treatments and preventive services will be funded. Details of the way values are derived from the procedure, and how these are used in economic evaluation, are detailed in Part II of this book.

Box 2.2 Using utility functions to understand patients' choice of hospital in the NHS

In 2002, the UK Department of Health (DH) set up an experiment to see how National Health Service (NHS) patients would respond if offered, for the first time, a choice of the NHS hospital in which they would receive their surgical procedure. The participants in the scheme had all been waiting for six or more months to receive elective surgery from their local hospital in London. The aim was to see how hospital demand patterns would change and what factors would affect patients' choices.

Burge *et al.* (2005) investigated these questions using a discrete choice experiment (DCE) (Ryan and Farrar, 2000; DCEs are discussed in more detail in Chapter 10). First, the 'attributes' (characteristics) of hospitals that are important to patients were determined using focus groups and interviews with patients. These were: how long the patient would have to wait for their surgery; the reputation of the hospital, how far they would have to travel to get treated; and where/how their post-surgical care would be delivered. Price is irrelevant, since all NHS treatment, whichever hospital was chosen, is free of charge to the patient. Secondly, patients were asked to choose from different scenarios that described their local hospital and an alternative (hypothetical) hospital in terms of these attributes – for example, a short (or long) waiting time, having to travel a short (or long) distance, and so on. The characteristics are varied between scenarios and data recording the choices made are used to estimate patients' utility functions using econometric techniques.

The rationale for this approach is *random utility theory*. Simply put, this suggests that the analyst has incomplete information about the reasoning behind choices that are observed, and that this must be taken into account (see Manski, 1977). The utility that individual i associates with alternative a is given by

$$U_a^i = \beta_1 X_1 + \beta_2 X_2 + \beta_3 X_3 + \beta_4 X_4 + \varepsilon_a^i$$

where X_1–X_4 are hospital attributes (for example) waiting time, travel time, reputation, and follow-up care); β_1–β_4 are coefficients to be estimated, and ε is an error term to capture unobserved characteristics and measurement error. By dividing the β for any given attribute by the β for any other, the trade-offs that patients are prepared to make between attributes are made apparent – this is analogous to the idea of the *MRS* introduced above, except here the trade-offs are *between characteristics* of one good (or service) rather than *between alternative goods*.

Burge *et al.* (2005) found that while reduced waiting time is attractive to patients, it is not *all* that matters to them. For every additional hour of travel to a hospital, patients would require a reduction in waiting time of two months; to get treatment at a hospital with a reputation better than their local hospital, patients would be prepared to wait an extra 3–6 months for surgery. The results also showed how these preferences and choices were affected by patients' characteristics: for example, patients who were older and had lower education were more likely to choose their local hospital, even if they could get quicker treatment elsewhere; and those on low incomes were less concerned than richer patients about hospitals' reputations. This study's results are being used to inform the introduction of hospital choice throughout the NHS.

Assuming there are just two goods, the budget constraint can be depicted, as in Figure 2.2, in terms of the various bundles of goods X and Y which it is feasible for the consumer to purchase, given the constraints of their income and prevailing prices (P_X and P_Y). For example, suppose that the consumer's weekly income is £500, the price of dental visits is £100 and the price of hairdresser visits £20. The position of the budget line is determined by the consumer's income; the slope of the budget line is determined by the relative prices, P_X/P_Y. In Figure 2.2, an initial budget line is given by P_{X1}/P_{Y1}, that is, the slope is £100/£20 = 5. If the price of Good X were to fall from £100 to £80, *other things being equal*, the budget line would pivot outwards, and the new slope would be P_{X2}/P_{Y1}, that is £80/£20 = 4.

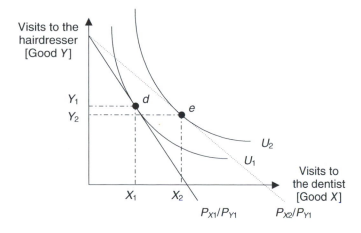

◯ **Figure 2.2 Maximising utility.**

The consumer maximises utility (Equation 2.1) subject to their budget constraint (Equation 2.4). Utility is maximised when the consumer chooses a bundle of goods for which the ratio of the goods' prices (the slope of the budget line) is equal to the ratio of the marginal utilities (the slope of the indifference curve).

$$MRS_{XY} = -\frac{\delta Y}{\delta X} = \frac{MU_X}{MU_Y} = \frac{P_X}{P_Y} \tag{2.5}$$

In Figure 2.2, where prices are P_{X1}/P_{Y1}, the consumer's utility-maximising choice is point d, consuming Y_1 and X_1. When the price of Good X falls, the consumer's new utility-maximising choice will be at point e. Another way of thinking about these points is that, in each case, given their preferences and prevailing prices, the utility-maximising consumer will divide their spending between the goods in such a way that $MU_X/P_X = MU_Y/P_Y$. In simple terms, the addition to utility per pound spent is equalised across all goods.

The assumptions of self-interest, rationality and utility maximisation that are central to economic models of consumer behaviour are frequently criticised on the grounds that they grossly oversimplify the factors that motivate human behaviour. For example, surely users of crack cocaine are not rational utility maximisers? Surprisingly, economic theory and evidence suggest this may not be so far fetched – see Box 2.3. Similarly, the assumptions appear to be incapable of explaining acts of charity and generosity to others, such as the donation of a kidney to a loved one. Here too economic theory can cope. 'Caring' can be incorporated into economics models simply by making an individuals' utility function depend not just on their own consumption, but also on the consumption of others. And where an individual's utility depends on the utility of others, redistribution or 'giving' can be modelled as utility-maximising behaviour (Hochman and Rodgers, 1969; Culyer, 1983). However, one important characteristic of consumer choice in health care – lack of information and asymmetry of information between the consumer and the supplier – has serious implications for the way health care markets might operate. We address this issue in Section 2.5 and in Chapter 5.

Nevertheless, it is worth emphasising that the purpose of economic models is to yield predictions that may be tested using data: the test of a good model is not whether its *assumptions* are realistic, but whether it is useful in explaining or predicting real-world behaviours (Friedman, 1953).

2.3 DEMAND FUNCTIONS

We earlier discussed the demand curve – the relationship between prices and the quantity of a good that consumers demand – but this is of course only one of many aspects of demand, and prices are only one among many factors that will affect it. In

Box 2.3 Rational addiction and price elasticity of demand

Consumer choice theory assumes consumers are rational utility maximisers. What about the consumption of heroin, cigarettes and other addictive products – surely addicts cannot be described as rational or capable or making decisions in their own self-interest? A landmark paper on the economics of addiction, by Becker and Murphy (1988), suggests exactly that: addicted individuals maximise utility consistently over time.

Their basic model rests on the idea that the utility of an individual at any point in time (t) depends on the consumption of two goods, x and y, where x is addictive and y is not, and also on a measure of the past consumption of x (but not y):

$$U(t) = u[y(t), x(t), S(t)]$$

Past consumption of x affects current utility through a process of 'learning by doing', as summarised by the stock of consumption capital (S). The marginal utility of x depends on past values for x, as measured by S.

The economists' definition of addiction is that a person is addicted to x if an increase in the current consumption of x leads to an increase in the future consumption of x. This is because past consumption of the good increases the marginal utility of present consumption. Individual choices are modelled as utility-maximising choices made over a whole life, given a set of preferences and expectations about future prices.

Among the predictions of this theory is that price elasticity of demand will be lower in the short term than in the long term. This hypothesis has been tested and confirmed in a large number of empirical studies; the model itself has also been extended in various ways: for example, explicit modelling of withdrawal; incorporating uncertainty; and allowing the possibility of regret over past choices.

economics more generally, prices are of great importance in their own right, which explains why the price/quantity relationship is at the centre of attention. However, in health care the role of prices is more subdued, and in some cases entirely missing, such as where the government fully subsidises a service or where it is fully covered by insurance. The demand curve is just one aspect of a more general concept – the *demand function*, which relates the level of consumer demand at a particular time and in a particular place to all of the factors that affect it. In this section, we will first look at what those factors are, then how we might in practice measure their effects, and finally what the evidence actually is of their effects on the demand for health care.

2.3.1 The Determinants of Demand

Health care includes a wide range of products and services, spanning health promotion, preventive interventions, diagnostic services, treatment, support services and palliation. Obviously, the nature of the relationship between demand and other factors will be quite different in each case, but the determinants of demand fall into some common categories. The most important of the factors affecting demand are generally held to be the price of the good, income, the prices of other goods, tastes and trends and population size and composition.

Price

If the price of a good falls, we generally expect more to be demanded, other things being equal – a finding consistent with consumer choice theory. Recall that in Figure 2.2, when the price of X is P_{X1}, X_1 is demanded; when price falls to P_{X2}, X_2 is demanded. Plotting these pairs of price and utility-maximising quantities on a diagram yields a downward-sloping demand curve.

This law of demand is relevant for most goods and services. For example, we might observe a downward-sloping curve for a consumer's demand for food supplements. This relies on them buying more food supplements when price falls. If all consumers responded to price changes in the same way, the market demand curve – the sum of all consumers' individual demand curves – would also be downward sloping.

It is sometimes argued that for some sorts of health care this analysis makes no sense. For example, it might be argued that it is unlikely that anyone will purchase more cancer chemotherapy simply because its price has fallen. Chemotherapy is not in itself a desirable good, so people will only wish to consume it if they have to, and in as small quantities as possible, whatever the price. It might also be argued that some health care is life-saving, so even if its price rose the quantity that anyone would demand would not necessarily fall.

These issues about individual consumers' demand for some types of health care arise because this is often a unique event, particularly in the treatment of acute illnesses and conditions, so that only a single intervention is consumed. For example, a service such as corrective laser eye surgery is something which any given person will only demand once, so their demand curve is *not* downward sloping – at every price up to the maximum amount that they are willing to pay, demand is constant at one, and above that it is constant at zero. However, because other consumers in the market are likely to have different willingness to pay, then the *market* demand curve will nevertheless be downward sloping with respect to price, because at lower prices there are more individuals who are consuming, rather than there being more consumption by all individuals. Similarly, even for life-saving treatments such as chemotherapy there will be some observable response to price, both at the market and the individual patient level, as there are usually other treatments, in this case surgery or radiotherapy, that are substitutes.

When thinking about the price of a good, it is natural to think in terms of a payment made by the consumer of the good to the provider of the good. But this is often only part of the total costs that the consumer must incur. As a simple example, if someone wishes to purchase a packet of aspirin, they may travel to a pharmacist, perhaps incurring transport costs, as well as paying for the drugs. In addition to these monetary outlays, there are also other costs such as the time spent travelling to and searching for the pharmacist, purchasing the drugs and returning home. Of course, this is the case for virtually all goods and services, but such costs are of particular importance in health care where there are subsidised user charges or even services free at the point of consumption. We can analyse the effects of such costs on consumer behaviour in the same way as prices, but must be careful to remember, when analysing provider behaviour, that the wider definition will not usually be appropriate.

The demand curve is of special importance in economics because it shows the impact of price which, as suggested, is seen as a key variable. It is also used to illustrate the effect on demand of other factors, with some special terminology used to distinguish changes in demand due to price changes from those due to changes in other factors. Figure 2.3 shows two demand curves, D_1 and D_2, that exist at different

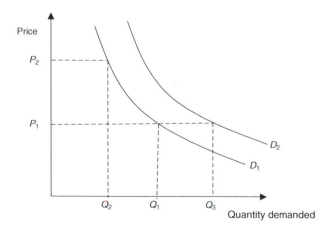

Figure 2.3 **Movements along and shifts in the demand curve.**

levels of the other factors. When the price of the good or service changes, there is a *movement along* the demand curve: for example, with the curve D_1, if price changes from P_1 to P_2 the quantity demanded falls from Q_1 to Q_2. When any of the other determinants of demand change, there is a *shift* in the demand curve: for example, if the size of the consumer population grows, the demand curve will shift rightwards from D_1 to D_2, and at the price P_1 the quantity demanded will increase from Q_1 to Q_3.

Income

Since demand is the quantity of a good that consumers are willing *and able* to buy in a specific time period, it is obvious that there must be a relationship between the demand for a good and individual's incomes. Again, this can be derived from consumer choice theory. Figure 2.4 shows what happens when income rises from I_1 to I_2; because prices have not changed, the budget line shifts outwards, retaining the same slope, and moves the utility-maximising point from d to e. In this case, the demand for good X rises as a result of the increase in income, but demand for good Y actually falls. The effect of income can be shown on a demand curve; for example, the shift in the demand curve shown in Figure 2.3 could be the result of an increase in income, assuming that the good is like good X. Another way to analyse this is to plot demand against income, other things held equal; this is known as an *Engel curve*.

Goods like good X are known as *normal* goods, because it is assumed that most goods are of this type. Goods like good Y are known as *inferior*. Examples include tooth extractions which, as a consumer's income rises, are replaced by demand for

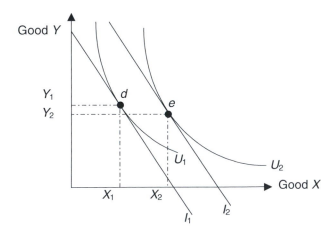

Figure 2.4 Changes in income.

conservative dental treatments such as root canal work. A normal good is further categorised as being a *necessity*, such as toothpaste, if the increase in demand is proportionately smaller than the increase in income, or as a *luxury*, such as cosmetic surgery and dental veneers, if the increase in demand is proportionately larger than the increase in income. This terminology arises because it is assumed that at low levels of income people only buy necessities; as their income increases they continue to buy the same amounts of these as before and spend their additional income on luxuries.

There has been contrasting evidence about the impact of income on the demand for health care, including the thought-provoking assertion that health care in aggregate is a luxury good. This has led to controversies and conflicting policy conclusions about the provision of health care. We discuss this in more detail in Section 2.7.

Prices of Other Goods

The demand for different goods is often interrelated since, as shown by the budget constraint, all goods compete for the limited income of the consumer. In Figure 2.2, we saw that the demand for good Y changed simply because the price of good X changed. Goods may be *substitutes* or *complements*. Other things held constant, if a fall in the price of one good causes a fall in the quantity demanded of another good then the goods are substitutes. An example of substitute goods is bariatric surgery and Anatrim™ for the treatment of obesity. If a fall in the price of one good increases the demand for another good, then these goods are complements. An example of complements is general medical practitioner (GP) visits and prescription medicines: prescription medicines are those that can only be obtained by prescription, so an increase in the price of attending the GP will, holding everything else constant, lower the number of GP visits, and will also lower the number of prescriptions.

Tastes and Trends

Tastes and trends may be extremely important in determining the demand for a good. A change in tastes in favour of a good, such as if a good becomes more fashionable, will cause an increase in demand. A change in tastes away from a good will cause a decrease in demand.

There are three ways in which tastes and trends might influence the demand for health care. First, trends in society surrounding healthy and unhealthy behaviours are likely to affect the overall health of the population, and thus ultimately the demands for health care. For example, in the 1950s smoking was seen as acceptable and desirable, with obvious consequences for long-term health and health care. Second, expectations and tastes regarding our health change through time, with consequences for the demand for health care. For example, in many countries in the 1940s, such as New

Zealand and Scotland, it was viewed as perfectly natural to have all one's teeth extracted in adulthood, whereas current generations expect to keep their adult teeth for life. The result is a fall in demand for dentures, and an increased demand for preventive and conservative dentistry. Finally, changes over time in tastes and trends towards specific types of health care might affect their demand. Examples include termination of pregnancy and the rise in demand for a wide range of cosmetic surgical procedures, such as face-lifts, tummy-tucks and breast enlargements.

Population Size and Composition

As the size of the population rises, market demand is also likely to rise. Similarly, if the population composition changes and there is change in the size of one particular subgroup of the population, for example women of child-bearing age, then this will affect the demand for goods and services traditionally consumed by this group, such as obstetric services.

This is likely to be an important determinant of market demand for health care. As the population size increases, so the total amount of morbidity will increase and demand for health care will grow. It is also likely that the composition of the population will change over time. For example, advances in medical technology and improvements in living standards mean that life expectancy is increasing and people live longer. Thus, the proportion of the population who are elderly will increase. In this case we would expect the demand for health care interventions typically consumed in the elderly population to also increase.

2.3.2 Estimating Demand Functions

Although utility cannot be directly observed, the quantities of goods or services which consumers demand, such as visits to the dentist, generally can. If we can also obtain data on the prices charged to or paid by consumers, and on other relevant factors such as consumers' incomes, then the relationship between demand and each of these factors can be modelled using econometric techniques, and a demand function can be estimated. For example, we could hypothesise that the demand for dental care will depend upon the following set of variables:

$$D = D(P, I, N, P_C, P_S, T, S) \qquad (2.6)$$

where P = price to the consumer, I = income, N = non-price access costs, P_C = prices of complements, P_S = price of substitutes, T = tastes and preferences and S = state of oral health. Estimating this equation would tell us which variables are or are not significant determinants of demand; what direction their influence has; the magnitude of their effect of demand; and what proportion of the variation in demand can be explained by the model.

Parkin and Yule (1988) estimated the demand for dental care in Scotland. Among other results, they reported the following function for the demand for dentures:

$$D_d = 157\ 505 - 10\ 960 \times P_d + 2141 \times P_o - 4432 \times I + 8867 \times A \qquad (2.7)$$

where D_d = annual demand for dentures, P_d = price of dentures, P_o = price of other dental services, I = income, and A = availability. This suggests that the demand for dentures is negatively related to the price of denture services, and is positively related to the price of other dental care services. This is plausible, since other types of dental care, such as complex endodontic treatment, are probably substitutes for the extraction of teeth and the fitting of dentures – so as the price of other dental care goes down, so too will the demand for dentures. Income has a negative effect on demand; interestingly, this suggests that as income increases, demand will fall. This means dentures may be regarded as an *inferior good*. This too is intuitively plausible: as consumers' incomes increase, we might expect fewer dentures to be demanded, as people instead choose other types of dental care. Finally, the authors included a variable for the number of dentists per 100 000 population, to capture possible effects of the availability of dentists on demand. This variable had a positive affect on demand, suggesting that the greater the supply of dentists that is available, the higher the demand for their services. The reasons why this might be are discussed in Section 2.5.

There is a considerable body of empirical evidence on the demand for health-related goods and services. An example related to the determinants of the demand for health insurance in the UK is provided in Box 2.4: the studies are interesting because they explicitly address the possibility that the public and private health care sectors interact.

2.3.3 Price and Income Elasticity of Demand

A useful way of summarising the relationships between price, income and other variables and the demand for health care is to express them as an *elasticity* measure. Elasticity measures the responsiveness of changes in one variable, for example quantities demanded or supplied, to changes in another variable, for example prices or income. The *price elasticity of demand* (PɛD) is the percentage change in quantity demanded divided by the percentage change in price. If the price of an ophthalmologist check-up in Singapore increases from \$200 to \$250, and the number of check-ups each week falls from 50 to 45, the percentage change in quantity is 10%, the percentage change in price is 25%, and the elasticity is 0.4. This elasticity is less than 1, indicating that, over the range of prices observed, demand is not particularly responsive to price – price rose and demand fell, but it fell *less* than proportionately. Elasticity is often measured over discrete ranges of price and quantity changes, but a more precise measure is given by calculating the elasticity at a given point on the demand curve, that is,

$$P\varepsilon D = (\delta Q / \delta P) \times \frac{P}{Q} \qquad (2.8)$$

Box 2.4 The demand for health insurance in the UK

Around 15% of the UK population has private medical insurance – despite access to comprehensive medical care services provided free at the point of demand through the NHS. Why would anyone buy private insurance? What are the determinants of demand for medical insurance policies? Besley *et al.* (1999) hypothesise that the demand for private insurance depends largely on the perceived quality of NHS services. They tested this using survey data that had been collected at five-year intervals between 1986 and 1991 and, for each participant, matched this with data on NHS services for their region. Demand was measured as a binary variable (1 if the individual purchased insurance, 0 if not) so the demand function that is estimated shows the effect of each variable on the *probability* of purchasing insurance. The results showed that the higher the number of people waiting over one year for treatment, the higher the demand for private insurance: an increase of 1 person per 1000 waiting for more than a year was associated with a 2% increase in the probability of an average person purchasing insurance. There was a strong positive relationship between the demand for insurance and the individual's income, education level and age.

Propper *et al.* (2001) also estimate a demand function for private health insurance in the UK, using data from 1978 to 1996. This paper also tests for the impact of public sector quality, but introduces extra variables for private sector quality, as well as variables to capture the influence of individuals' characteristics. Interestingly, they do not find a relationship between demand and NHS waiting lists, although the apparent difference between these results and Besley's may be because the latter's result relates specifically to the number of 'long waits' whereas Propper *et al.* included only the *total* number waiting – a variable that was, similarly, not significant in Besley's study. Propper *et al.* find evidence of quite complex links between the public and private sectors; for example, higher spending on the NHS appears to lower the demand for private insurance (with a lagged effect), and the availability of private sector facilities, such as hospitals and senior doctors, had a strong effect on the demand for insurance. Curiously, neither study includes the effect of the price of insurance – the insurance premium – on demand.

where P/Q is a given price divided by the quantity demanded at that price and $\delta Q/\delta P$ is the slope of the demand curve at that point.

Elasticity provides a useful means of comparing the responsiveness of consumer demand to price and other variables between different periods in time, in which the purchasing power of money may be different, between different countries, where the currency is different, and between different goods or services, where the units in which quantity is measured are different.

Further, the magnitude of price elasticity, that is whether it is <1, = 1 or >1, has direct implications for consumer spending and firms' revenues. For example, the Parkin and Yule (1988) study reported the price elasticity of demand for dentures to be 0.28. This suggests that an increase in the price charged by a dentist will reduce demand for dentures, but, because demand falls *less* than proportionately, both consumer spending and the dentist's revenue will increase as a result. The extra revenue from consumers who continue to buy dentures will outweigh the loss of revenue from those who no longer do so. Conversely, if the price elasticity were >1, an increase in price would reduce demand *more* than proportionately, and both quantity demanded and revenue will fall. In the special case where the price elasticity of demand equals 1, changes in price and quantity exactly balance each other and revenue does not change when prices change.

Income elasticity of demand is defined in a similar way, derived from the Engel curve. The point income elasticity is the percentage change in quantity demanded divided by the percentage change in income:

$$I\varepsilon D = (\delta Q / \delta I) \times \frac{I}{Q} \qquad (2.9)$$

where I/Q is any given income divided by the quantity demanded at that income, other things (such as price) being held equal, and $\delta Q/\delta I$ is the slope of the Engel curve at that point.

The income elasticity is related to the change in the proportion of income spent on a good, and its size therefore determines whether the good can be labelled as inferior, necessity or luxury. Specifically, if $I\varepsilon D < 0$ the good is inferior, if $0 < I\varepsilon D < 1$ it is a necessity, and if $I\varepsilon D > 1$ it is a luxury.

Measurement of demand for a good and incomes enables us to estimate the income elasticity and draw conclusions about the kind of good that it is – as we shall see in Section 2.7, controversially in the case of health care.

The most well-known and comprehensive findings on the demand for health care were produced by the RAND Corporation's Health Insurance Experiment in the US (Manning *et al.*, 1987). Families from six areas of the USA were assigned to one of 14 types of health insurance plans. The study is unparalleled in health economics not just because of its sheer scale – the sample comprised over 5800 individuals – but also because it is a rare example in economics of a controlled experiment. By assigning study participants to different health insurance plans, the effect of insurance cover, and thus prices to consumers, on the demand for health care could be observed, and other relevant factors controlled for. The study concluded that, overall, the price elasticity of demand for medical care was 0.22; that is, demand does respond to price, but is not particularly elastic. Although there are important differences between types of medical care, the evidence on price elasticity of demand for health care, both in this experiment and in other settings, generally estimates the price elasticity of demand to lie between 0.1 and 0.7. Thus, demand is responsive to price differences, but the elasticity is usually <1. A similar consensus is apparent on the effect of income: the income elasticity of demand tends to be positive but less than 1, suggesting that health care is a necessity. Non-price access costs – transport, time costs and so on – are also often important determinants of demand, with an effect on demand as great as that of price.

Much of the evidence on the responsiveness of demand to price comes from observing consumers' demand under various insurance/co-insurance or subsidy/part-charge arrangements, since changes in these arrangements provide natural experiments in which the changes in demand to changing out-of-pocket prices may be observed. The incentives to consumers arising from third-party health care financing are discussed in detail in Chapter 6.

2.4 MODELLING CHOICES ABOUT HEALTH

The consumer choice theory introduced in Section 2.2 provides the basis of a theoretical framework for understanding choices specifically relating to health and health care originally developed by Grossman (1972). Grossman's approach is often described as a human capital model, because it draws heavily on the human capital theory of Becker (1964). The principal contribution of Grossman's model is the distinction between health as an output – a 'fundamental commodity' which is the source of utility to people – and medical care as an input to the production of health. In Grossman's model, health is both demanded and produced by individuals. Health is demanded because it affects the total time available for the production of income and wealth, and because it is a source of utility in itself. Essentially, ill health reduces both our happiness and our ability to earn.

Health is modelled as being produced by individuals, using a variety of means: diet, lifestyle choices and medical care. How efficient individuals are in production depends on their knowledge and education. Medical care is but one input to the production of health. Each individual is modelled as starting life with a 'stock' of health, which has characteristics similar to capital: health depreciates through time with age, but can also be increased through investments of time, effort – such as going to the gym – and knowledge, or by seeking health care.

Grossman's model captures two important insights. First, that health care is but one means of generating improvements in health; indeed it is now widely accepted that medical care is not the major determinant of health. Second, individuals do not demand health care for its own sake: the utility received from the consumption of health care is generated not from health care per se but from the improvements in health that result. Thus the demand for health care is a *derived* demand.

Grossman's model has become an important tool used by economists to analyse health and health care decisions, and we therefore present it in some detail. First, in Section 2.4.1, we present a geometric model developed by Wagstaff (1986a, b). This is a helpful way of understanding the consumption aspects of Grossman's work, but it does not fully capture the investment aspect. Therefore, in Section 2.4.2 we also present the model in a more formal way, with an emphasis on health care as an investment.

2.4.1 Understanding Consumption of Health and Health Care

Figure 2.5 presents Grossman's ideas with respect to the demand for health and health care. There are three main elements. The first is a budget constraint, showing all

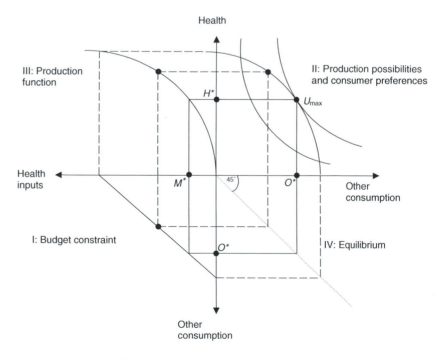

Figure 2.5 The demand for health.

the combinations of health inputs such as medical care (M) and other consumption (O) which it is feasible for the consumer to obtain, given their income and the prices of health care and other goods. This is shown in quadrant I. The second, shown in quadrant II, is an indifference curve representing the consumer's preferences by showing the combinations of health and consumption that yield the consumer an equal amount of utility. The consumer can *buy* health *care*, but they obtain utility, U, from *health*, H, and the consumption of goods/services, O. In order to understand the consumer's choices, we therefore need to know how the consumption of *health care* is 'turned into', that is gives rise to, improvements in *health*. This is the third element: quadrant III is a production function showing, for each level of health inputs, the amount of health which is produced. Quadrant IV contains only a 45° line: this is simply a device for mapping anything on the vertical axis in quadrant I onto the horizontal axis in quadrant III; both axes measure consumption of other goods and services.

All points on the budget line show a combination of health inputs and other consumption which is feasible for the consumer, given their income. We can show how any given level of health inputs which is feasible is converted into 'health' in quadrant III. This enables us to build up a 'frontier' in quadrant II and this shows the maximum health and consumption possible from each feasible combination of spending on health inputs and consumption.

Why does the frontier have its distinctive convex shape? The shape of the frontier is driven entirely by the nonlinearity in the production function in quadrant III. Additional spending on health inputs always increases health, but the increases become smaller and smaller. This phenomenon, known as diminishing marginal productivity, will be discussed in detail in Chapter 3.

All combinations of health and consumption on the frontier are feasible for the consumer to choose, but, given the preferences represented by their indifference curves, utility will be maximised at $U_{\max}$, with the consumer choosing H^* health and O^* consumption. In order to achieve the utility-maximising level of health H^*, this suggests that the consumer uses their income to purchase M^* medical care.

The model highlights that consumers choose a combination of health and other goods that maximise their utility, and the demand for health care is derived from that choice. The diagram can readily be used to predict the effect on consumers' decisions of a change in income, which causes the budget line to shift, an improvement in health care technology, which causes the production function to change shape or position, and so on. However, this geometric representation includes health (H) in a very simple way – whereas a key element of the Grossman model is a sophisticated analysis of health as a type of capital.

2.4.2 Understanding Investment in Health Care

We noted above that Grossman's theory is based on the idea of household production. The true objects of desire are 'fundamental commodities', which are created within households by using time and market goods. The total time that a person has available can be used either for direct production of these commodities or for work to obtain income to buy market goods. For example, in creating the fundamental commodity associated with eating, a household can have home-cooked, restaurant, take-away or pre-prepared meals. Each involves different combinations of the household's time (purchasing, preparation and eating) and market goods (full meals or the ingredients for them plus energy for cooking). Similarly, health can be produced by diverse activities and goods such as exercise, diet, medical care and surgery. The theory of health demand starts by assuming for simplicity that people derive utility from two goods: health (H) and a composite of all other fundamental commodities (O).

$$U = U(H, O) \qquad (2.10)$$

Both H and O are sums over time, weighted by the person's time preference; different people have different preferences for when they obtain benefits, some being more impatient than others (we explain this in more detail in Chapter 11). H is therefore a weighted sum of the number of healthy days that the person enjoys over their life. These healthy days derive from a person's *stock* of health (HS), so that the greater the health stock, the greater the number of healthy days the person will have. The health stock at a particular time (HS_t) is determined by the health stock in the previous period (HS_{t-1}) less any depreciation in health stock that has taken place over that period (d_t) plus any investment in health (I_t) that the person has undertaken:

$$HS_t = HS_{t-1} - d_t + I_t \qquad (2.11)$$

Health, in this way of thinking, is analogous to other types of capital, such as a machine. For example, one's health can depreciate over time owing to excessive alcohol use or the effects of ageing. But this can be offset by investments – in terms of both time and money – that will maintain or improve health, such as regular exercise to reduce weight and improve heart function or medical care to repair damaged health. Both O and I are produced within the household, and we can define a production function for each of them. Production of O and I uses market goods, medical care (M) and all other market goods (X) respectively, and time spent either in production of health (T_H) or in producing other goods (T_O). A third input to both is human capital, usually characterised as the level of education (E). The production functions are therefore:

$$I_t = I(M_t, T_{Ht}, E_t) \qquad (2.12)$$

$$O_t = O(X_t, T_{Ot}, E_t) \qquad (2.13)$$

It is assumed that a person will attempt to maximise their utility, but there are two constraints upon this, a time budget and an expenditure budget. The time budget (T) is obviously fixed at 365.25 days each year on average; and as well as the time spent producing, the person must also spend time working (T_W) and suffer some time spent sick (T_S):

$$T_t = T_{Ht} + T_{Ot} + T_{Wt} + T_{St} \tag{2.14}$$

The constraint on the expenditure budget is income, which depends on how much time is spent working and the wage rate (W). How much is spent depends on the costs of market goods M and X and their prices (P_M and P_X respectively). It is assumed that all income is spent:

$$P_M \times M + P_X \times X = T_W \times W \tag{2.15}$$

Both sides of this equation should be regarded as *present values* (see Chapter 11), because they refer to a person's lifetime income and expenditure. They are therefore discounted at the interest rate r.

Maximisation of the utility function, subject to these constraints and taking into account the production functions, leads to an equilibrium condition which can be interpreted as a person equalising the marginal benefits of health capital and its marginal cost. Marginal benefit consists of two parts, one relating to the enjoyment of health resulting from the investment (MB_H) and the other relating to the monetary investment returns that it produces (MB_M). These are commonly known as 'consumption' and 'investment' benefits, although these terms are not entirely apt. An element that is common to them is the marginal product of health (MP_H), measured as the number of healthy days generated by one unit of health stock. The two elements of benefit are the product of these healthy days and the *value* of a healthy day in consumption and investment, which, because they are equated with costs, are expressed in money values.

The consumption benefit is therefore the MP_H multiplied by the value of a healthy day in consumption. This value is measured by the undiscounted ratio of the marginal utility of healthy days (MU_H) to the marginal utility of financial wealth (MU_W):

$$MB_{Ht} = MP_{Ht} \times (1 + r)^t \times \frac{MU_{Ht}}{MU_{Wt}} \tag{2.16}$$

where $(1 + r)^t$ is a factor that ensures that the money value is not discounted.

Healthy days can also be used for working to create income, so that the 'investment' benefit is the marginal product of health multiplied by the wage rate:

$$MB_{Mt} = MB_{Ht} \times W_t \tag{2.17}$$

The marginal cost of health capital is the marginal cost of investment in health (MCI) multiplied by two factors: the real rate of interest, which represents the opportunity cost of investment, and the depreciation of health capital (d). The real rate of interest is the nominal rate (r) that could have been earned had the investment not been in health, less the change over the time period in the marginal cost of investment (ΔMCI), which can be interpreted as a capital gain, or a saving from investing now rather than in the future, assuming that marginal costs will increase over time. So, the equilibrium condition is

$$MB_{Ht} + MB_{Mt} = MCI_{t-1} \times [(r - \Delta MCI_{t-1}) + d_t)] \tag{2.18}$$

This equation is the key result of the Grossman model – although it derives from a complex model, it has an intuitively reasonable interpretation to it. The idea is that individuals invest in health up to the point where the marginal benefits from the investment, that is, the consumption benefit plus the investment benefit derived above, are equal to the marginal costs incurred by the investment. But as usual in economics it cannot be considered a good model until it is tested. We will therefore look at some of its predictions and their testing, and conclude with some criticisms that have been made of the Grossman approach.

2.4.3 Predictions of the Grossman Model

Equation (2.18) is very important for empirical testing of the Grossman theory. Unfortunately, it is not possible to estimate this as it stands owing to the complicated relationship between MB_H and MB_M, so testing has worked by looking at consumption benefits only, by setting $MB_M = 0$, or investment benefits only, by setting $MB_H = 0$. To demonstrate some of the predictions of the model, we will look at the second of these possibilities, using the concept of the *marginal efficiency of capital* (MEC). This arises from an assumed relationship between the cost of capital, ($C = (r - \Delta MCI) + d$), and the health stock, HS, which is illustrated in Figure 2.6. It is assumed that as the level of health stock increases it becomes more and more difficult to generate health by investing in it. In other words, investment is subject to *diminishing returns* (see Chapter 3), which explains the convex shape of the MEC curves.

This theory is useful because it provides a basis for hypotheses about the effect of important determinants of health on the demand for health and health care – propositions that can then be tested using data, which in turn enables more accurate predictions about health behaviour.

For example, the model yields hypotheses about age. Age is assumed to affect the depreciation of health capital; in particular it increases as people get older. Suppose that a person has the curve MEC_0 and an equilibrium at C_0, with health stock HS_0. In the next time period, they have a higher cost, C_1, owing to depreciation and

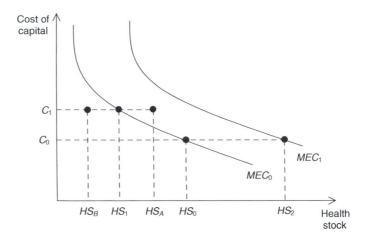

Figure 2.6 The marginal efficiency of health capital.

therefore a lower preferred health stock, HS_1. However, the demand for investment in health – and therefore the demand for health care inputs – depends on what effect the depreciation had on the health stock. If it fell from HS_0 to HS_A, the actual stock would be higher than the new preferred stock, HS_1, so there would be no investment in health. However, if it fell to HS_B, investment would be necessary to raise it to HS_1.

Similarly, we can examine the effect of a change in wage rates (W). W affects both sides of equation (2.18). On the benefits side, an increase in W will raise the value of the production of healthy days, since working time is now more valuable. On the cost side, the opportunity cost of the person's time also increases, and because investment in health requires a time input, the opportunity cost of such investment also increases. But since there are other inputs to investment that do not increase, the proportional change will be greater for benefits than for costs, so the returns to health will increase at all levels of the health stock. In Figure 2.6, this is represented by a shift of the MEC curve from MEC_0 to MEC_1, accompanied by an increase in preferred health stock from HS_0 to HS_2. The demand for investment in health will therefore increase.

Much attention has been given to the relationship between health and education. An increase in education will increase the efficiency of non-market production, which increases the MP of health inputs. This would shift the MEC curve outwards, and raise the optimal health stock. Once again, however, the predicted effect on the demand for health care is ambiguous.

These propositions have been the subject of a considerable empirical literature – for example, see Wagstaff (1986b, 1993). The model has been used to examine such diverse issues as the impact on health of environmental quality, measured by the level of pollution (Erbsland *et al.*, 1995), and the demand for malaria treatments in a developing country (Masiye and Rehnberg, 2005). Empirical evidence about the assumptions of the model have been mixed in terms of confirming or refuting them, but this should be seen as a contribution to its development and there is no doubt that this will be an increasingly important way in which economists examine health issues.

There are of course some problems with the way that the Grossman model is currently formulated, though these are the subject of a large ongoing research programme (Grossman, 2000). In the way that it is usually used, it rests on some rather strong assumptions. For example, it assumes that consumers have perfect information and perfect foresight about their health, the rate of depreciation of their health, and the effect of various health care and other consumption on their health. Taken to the extreme, it suggests that people make well-informed and rational decisions about the date of their death! The model therefore does not take into account uncertainty – for example, about the timing of adverse health events – which, as we noted in Chapter 1, is a defining characteristic of health. This uncertainty extends to consumers' relative lack of information about the effect of health care on health. This has important consequences for the way consumers and providers of health care interact in the health care market, an issue we take up in Section 2.6 below.

2.5 NEEDS, WANTS AND DEMANDS

The application of demand theory to health and health care gives valuable insights and one view could be that health is simply an interesting application of ordinary demand theory. But this is deceptive. In order to understand many aspects of health and health care it is necessary to look beyond straightforward economic concepts. In analysing the demand for health care, it is important to take account of the concept of *need*. This is true not only when considering individuals' consumption for health care, it is also the case that a characteristic of health policy in most countries is that the concept of need, rather than demand, dominates views about the aims of health services.

If you ask most people what determines their demand for health care, their answer will most likely be that 'people go to the doctor when they need it'. By contrast, the straightforward economics answer would be because they *want* to do so, which sounds peculiar because unless they have a psychological disorder (such as Munchausen's syndrome) no-one wants health care for its own sake (Evans, 1984). On the face of it, Grossman's theory provides a reconciliation of these two views, because people *want* health improvements and *demand* care that will produce them. However, need is more complicated than that. Need implies an imperative to have health care, because it will deal with a health problem; by contrast, demand simply implies the willingness and ability to pay for health care. Moreover, people have limited knowledge about such needs – about both the existence of health problems and the health care that will deal with them; by contrast, the usual assumption in economics is that in making demands people are the best judges of their own wants.

Economists prefer to define need as *capacity to benefit*, which means the capacity for a patient to benefit from health care. Even if someone is sick, they are not in need of health care unless they could benefit from it. This type of need must be distinguished from need that is related to a person's health state rather than health care, so that it is independent of whether that state can be improved through the provision of health care. Moreover, the generally preferred view of economists is that any definition of need relies on expert judgement of the likely benefits of treatment; alternative definitions refer to individuals' perceptions of their needs, which depend on their knowledge of health care, their knowledge of health, and their expectations about what is 'normal' with respect to health. Of course, experts do not always agree and their judgements may change over time, so even this more rigorous definition of need is not at all straightforward to apply.

Needs and demands can thus be regarded as two very different ways of viewing matters, but taken together they give useful insights. Two extreme positions might exist. Sometimes there might be demand where there is no need. People might be pessimistically mistaken about their health state or optimistically mistaken about the possibilities for improving it. In practice, the more important case is that there might be need where there is no demand, and if health services simply respond only to demand, this implies that there will be *unmet need*. Some of this unmet need will be due to deficiencies in information, which will be looked at in more detail in the next section of this chapter. This kind of analysis views the other source of unmet need as *barriers* to the use of health care. From an economics viewpoint these can be categorised as supply factors, which are the availability of services to meet needs, and demand factors, such as prices and individuals' incomes, which affect their ability to access services.

2.6 ASYMMETRY OF INFORMATION AND IMPERFECT AGENCY

As was emphasised in Chapter 1, a characteristic of health care markets is uncertainty: about diagnosis, about available treatments, and about their effectiveness (Arrow, 1963). Some of this uncertainty is 'irreducible' (Pauly, 1978) – neither the doctor nor the patient can know with certainty what the consequences of treatment will be. As suggested, this leads to the problem of unmet need. However, much of the uncertainty is one-sided: the consumer lacks the medical training and knowledge to make informed choices.

Information is itself an economic good: obtaining information, for example by engaging in consumer research to compare prices and qualities of alternative health care providers, or checking the relative cost and efficacy of alternative treatments, is worthwhile if the benefits exceed the costs. Where the costs of obtaining information are too high, if information is highly specialised or difficult to obtain, or the likely benefits too low, for example where it is for a one-off treatment, consumers may choose to remain 'rationally ignorant' and to delegate decision making to the supplier. As McGuire (2001) puts it, 'In a patient's contact with the doctor, the doctor's position is not "here is the price of my services, how many do you want?" It is more like "Here is what you should do".'

This relationship between doctor and patient is often presented as a principal–agent problem. The doctor is an *agent* acting on behalf of a *principal*, who is the patient, in making decisions about what health care to purchase. If doctors made these decisions in a manner fully consistent with patients' preferences, unaffected by the consequence for themselves, they would be acting as perfect agents – essentially, making the health care decisions that the patients themselves would do if they had access to the same information. Much of the economics literature has focused on the possibility that doctors either cannot or do not act as perfect agents. Specifically, the hypothesis of supplier-induced demand (SID) (Evans, 1974), sometimes referred to as physician- or provider-induced demand (PID), is that doctors 'engage in some persuasive activity to shift the patient's demand curve in or out according to the physician's self-interest' (McGuire, 2001).

There is an extensive theoretical and empirical literature on this subject. Early studies focused on testing the effects of increased availability (an increase in the doctor : patient ratio) on the *utilisation* of health care (the amount that is used by consumers). A problem with this literature is that many of the findings may be consistent with a non-inducement model of how utilisation is determined (Rice, 1998).

Recall from Figure 1.2 in Chapter 1 that a market may have an equilibrium price at which supply and demand are equal – this determines the level of utilisation. Suppose, as in Figure 2.7, that from an initial equilibrium price of P_1 and a utilisation level of Q_1, there is a change in supply conditions – for example, a change in medical licensing regulations results in an influx of doctors from overseas, such that the supply curve shifts from S_1 to S_2. The SID hypothesis suggests that each doctor will recommend more or more frequent treatment to their patients than before in order to increase demand. Suppose that they are successful in raising demand from D_1 to D_2. In the new equilibrium, quantity is higher ($Q_2 > Q_1$) and price is lower ($P_2 < P_1$). So, if we observed empirically that an increase in the supply of doctors coincided with increased numbers of doctor visits, does this prove that SID occurred? The answer is no, for three reasons.

First, that observation is consistent with the predictions for any competitive market: if supply increases from S_1 to S_2, with *no* shift in the demand curve, we would get an

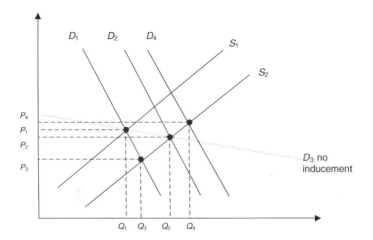

Figure 2.7 The problem of identifying supplier-induced demand.

equilibrium quantity of Q_3 which, like Q_2, is greater than Q_1, and price P_3, which, like P_2, is less than P_1.

Secondly, it is possible that the demand curve's shape is simply different to the way we thought. The equilibrium Q_2 and P_2, which we explained via an inducement effect, would be consistent with the equilibrium that would be observed if supply shifted from S_1 to S_2 and the demand curve was in fact D_3.

Thirdly, the increase in supply might result in a reduction in the costs of doctor visits such as searching for and waiting to see a doctor and travelling to the surgery, or might improve other aspects of quality, such as the length of each consultation. It may be these factors, which are themselves determinants of demand, that shift the demand curve from D_1 to D_2, rather than inducement. This third explanation could even explain cases where price actually *increases* following an increase in supply equilibrium, an empirical observation found by Fuchs (1978), for example a shift in the demand curve to D_4, resulting in a new equilibrium price of P_4, which is greater than P_1.

So, in general it seems that there is no way in which observed movements in prices and quantities can prove the existence of inducement. Of course, this also means that there is no way in which such data can disprove it.

A more general problem with this sort of approach is that it requires a *change* in supply in order to identify an inducement *response*. This does not tell us how much induce-ment was taking place before the change in supply conditions. If doctors can influence both prices and demand, how is equilibrium reached? Possibilities include that medical ethics may act to constrain physician behaviour; that physicians' utility depends both on their income and the well-being, or utility, of their patients; or that physician behaviour is aimed at achieving a 'target income', rather than maximising income. Ultimately, consumers act to constrain inducement: they may have less information, but the potential for consumer response restricts what even the most self-interested doctor can get away with. But a more fundamental problem is that supply and demand models essentially assume that supply and demand are independent, and they may simply not be a very good analytical tool if demand is partly determined by suppliers.

Some findings are clear: a comprehensive review of the evidence (McGuire, 2001) demonstrates that physicians do respond to financial incentives; they do appear to influence demand and to do so partly in response to self-interest. Box 2.5 gives an example of the evidence that is available on this issue. However, notwithstanding the considerable body of research, a definitive understanding of SID remains elusive. To understand whether patients are being induced to demand more services than they really want, we would need to know how much they would have demanded if they were as well informed as the physician; no such study has been conducted (Mooney, 1994; Rice, 1998).

2.7 AGGREGATE DEMAND FOR HEALTH CARE: THEORY AND EVIDENCE

Given the theory and evidence reviewed so far with respect to *individuals'* demand for health care, what factors would you expect to influence the demand of consumers *in aggregate* for health care, that is, the demand for health care by an entire country? Obvious answers might include the age structure of the population, levels of sickness and disease, the prevalence of smoking and obesity, and so on.

In fact, researchers have found that, using health care spending per person as a proxy measure for aggregate demand, most of the variation in health care demand between countries can be explained using just one variable: the country's income, generally measured as GDP per person. The strength of the relationship is evident even from a simple plot of GDP per person against health care spending per person such as Figure 2.8(a). This shows data for 168 countries in 2003, derived from the United Nations Development Programme's Human Development Report (HDR) (http://hdr.undp.org/hd). It is clear that the richer an economy, the more health care will be demanded.

An influential paper on this issue by Newhouse (1977), using a simple linear regression analysis on 13 countries, found that GDP per person of a country explains 92% of the variance in the level of spending between countries. Moreover, he calculated that the

Box 2.5 Supplier-induced demand by Irish general practitioners

In one of the earliest studies of its kind, Tussing and Wojtowycz (1986) investigated demand-inducing behaviour among Irish general practitioners (GPs). In the study, GPs in Ireland treat both public and private patients. They are remunerated by the state for public patients and by the patient, at a higher rate, for those treated privately. There is therefore financial incentive for GPs to treat more patients of all types, and private patients in particular. The authors undertook a nationwide survey of 1069 households in Ireland, collecting data on health care use and a range of covariates. In addition, they collected a measure of whether the demand for GP services was stimulated by the GP: with respect to each person's most recent GP consultation, they asked in the survey whether a subsequent return visit was arranged by the GP. They then ran a regression model that regressed whether or not a return visit was arranged by the GP against a set of controls for gender, age, distance of the GP from the patient's home, average income in the area, individual eligibility for free GP care, the proportion of the local population eligible for free GP care, and GP density (GP to population ratio).

The authors found that 23.5% of all most recent visits to the GP led to a return visit being arranged by the GP. The regression results indicated that, after controlling for the other covariates, a physician-stimulated visit was positively correlated with GP density and negatively correlated with the proportion of the local population eligible for free GP care and with average income. Hence, the authors observed in their data that, among other things, an increase in supply was associated with an increase in demand. They concluded that 'all three results . . . point to significant self-interested physician-induced demand by Irish GPs'. In fact, the results are also consistent with no inducement in a competitive market. For example:

- As shown in Figure 2.7, if supply increases and there is no shift in the demand curve, the equilibrium quantity will still rise.

- The increase in supply might result in a reduction in the time and travel costs incurred visiting the GP, and these may have caused demand to rise.

- The demand curve may look different from that hypothesised by the authors, and the increase in demand may in fact be entirely consistent with the actual shape of the demand curve for GP visits in Ireland.

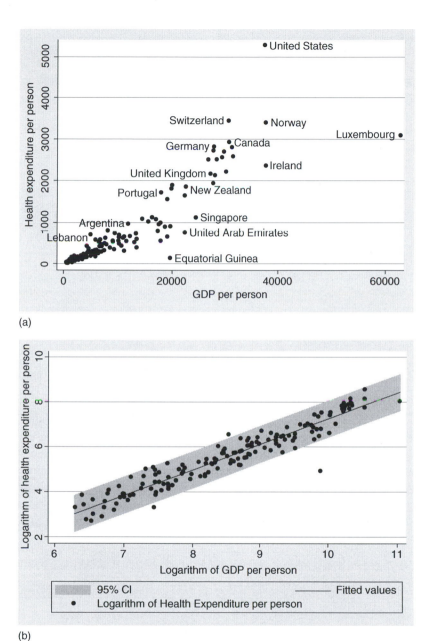

Figure 2.8 The relationship between income per person and health care spending per person in 2003. (a) Income and spending in US dollars. (b) Logarithmic plot of income and spending in US dollars. Source: Data from United Nations Development Programme, Human Development Report (http://hdr.undp.org/hd).

income elasticity of demand was greater than 1 at all levels of income, with an average value of 1.31. This led him to conclude that health care is, at a national level, a luxury good and that 'countries that spend more may well buy more caring, but little additional curing'. We can replicate his findings using the HDR data. On close inspection, the data in Figure 2.8(a) suggest that the relationship is not a straight line, but is curved upwards. Figure 2.8(b) displays the data transformed into logarithms, and this looks much more like a straight line relationship. The regression line on this is a good fit – in fact, it also explains 92% of the variance! The 95% confidence interval (CI) further shows that this is a phenomenon that applies universally to countries, as there are very few outliers. The income elasticity calculated from this regression line is 1.13, slightly less than Newhouse's value, but still significantly above 1.

Newhouse's original finding and conclusions were the catalyst for a vast literature re-examining the determinants of health care spending. Parkin *et al.* (1987) pointed out that Newhouse's use of exchange rates to make the currency conversions required to make between-country comparisons is not appropriate for goods and services, such as health care, which are not traded internationally. Re-estimating the income elasticity using purchasing power parity (PPP) conversions, they found income elasticity not to be statistically significantly different from 1, although subsequent empirical studies have not in general supported that finding.

More fundamentally, Parkin *et al.* (1987) and others have argued that the statistical relationship has a weak theoretical base, providing little guidance either to what explanatory variables should be included or to what the causal mechanisms are. Subsequent studies have explored more complex models, including variables to capture the age structure of the population, the extent of public sector provision of health care, urbanisation and number of doctors (Leu, 1986; Gerdtham *et al.*, 1998, 1992a, 1992b), tobacco and alcohol consumption, unemployment and various institutional characteristics of the health care system (Gerdtham *et al.*, 1998). The results from these studies, like our analysis of the HDR data, nevertheless continue to suggest that GDP per person explains most of the variation in health care spending, although the estimate of the income elasticity varies.

More recently, contributions to this literature have focused on econometric issues arising from the time series and panel data properties of the data sets used, testing for unit roots and co-integration. McGuire *et al.* (1993) were the first to examine these characteristics of the data; subsequently, Hansen and King (1996) looked at this in more detail and suggested that, given the time trends apparent in the data, previous estimates of income elasticity may be spurious. These results have variously either been confirmed (Blomqvist and Carter, 1997; Roberts, 1998) or contradicted (McCoskey and Selden, 1998). A review of this literature by Gerdtham and Jönsson (2001) suggests that the most likely reason for the differences in results is differences in methods; they conclude that further research is required to provide a definitive answer.

The original concern raised with respect to this issue remains. Is the observed relationship merely a statistical one or is there causation? Does the sheer strength of the apparent relationship between health care spending and income suggest an 'iron law' – and if so, does this imply that the health sector will end up taking an ever larger share of GDP in the world's economies? Is this something we should be concerned about – is it inefficient? – or is the unabated increase in health care spending an appropriate response to the preferences of increasingly wealthy economies? We should also note that the focus of these studies is on total and average health care spending and GDP per person. This may obscure important within-country differences both in *what* money is spent on, for example differences in the mix of inputs used in health care or the mix of outputs produced, and in the underlying *distribution* of health care and income between persons.

Finally, the suggestion that countries' additional spending is on caring rather than curing was probably intended by Newhouse to be deliberately provocative rather than a true deduction from the data. This is helpful in showing how the economists' technical term 'luxury good' does not always easily translate into ordinary language. In ordinary use, we might deduce that if extra health care is a luxury, that is because it has no effect on health, and only curative health care has an effect on health. In economics terms, however, there are no reasons why as incomes improve countries would not wish to buy, in increasing amounts, goods that improve their population's health or why curing services should not have a positive impact on health.

2.8 CONCLUSION

Economic models of demand and of consumer choice theory are clearly pertinent to issues of interest to providers and funders of health care. They also provide the fundamental basis for methods used to value health improvements and health services, as detailed in Part II of this book, which deals with the principles and methods of economic evaluation.

An important aspect of health economics, as an area of applied microeconomics, is the analysis of market failures and the extent to which deviations from the explicit and implicit assumptions of the competitive model – such as rationality and perfect information – impact on market and non-market equilibria and outcomes. We have touched on some of these themes, as they pertain to consumer decision making, in this chapter; these issues are considered in more detail in Chapter 5.

Having considered demand-side factors in this chapter, in the following chapter we describe the supply side – production and costs – in health care.

SUMMARY

1. Economists define the demand for any good or service, including health care, as the quantity that consumers are both willing and able to buy.

2. The demand curve, which graphically is shown by a curve that is downward sloping from left to right, shows that – other things being equal – as prices rise, demand falls.

3. Consumer choice theory explains why consumers behave or react in certain ways to changes in various factors in order to maximise their utility. This theory underpins the demand for goods and services. Consumers are assumed to be rational, which means they have complete preferences, that their preferences are transitive, and that their wants are non-satiable.

4. The way in which the consumption of different bundles of goods and services affects utility can be illustrated using indifference curves. These show all the combinations of two goods that yield the consumer equal satisfaction.

5. The slope of an indifference curve is the marginal rate of substitution. This is the amount of one good that must be sacrificed if consumption of another good is increased in order for utility to remain unchanged.

6. The decisions that consumers make in the pursuit of utility maximisation are constrained both by their limited resources and by the prices of the various goods and services between which they choose. Hence, the consumption problem facing consumers is to maximise their utility subject to a budget constraint. Under these conditions, utility is maximised when the consumer chooses a bundle of goods for which the ratio of the goods' prices – the slope of the budget line – is equal to the ratio of the marginal utilities – the slope of the indifference curve.

7. There are various factors affecting the demand for goods and services, including the price of the good, income, the prices of other goods, tastes and trends for the good, and population size and composition. Changes in the price of the good result in movements along the demand curve. Changes in any of the other determinants of demand result in a shift in the demand curve.

8. Elasticity measures the responsiveness of changes in one variable, for example the quantity demanded, to changes in another variable, for example price. Evidence suggests that the demand for health care is price inelastic, that is, demand is not particularly responsive to changes in the price of health care.

9. A theoretical framework for understanding choices specifically relating to health and health care was developed by Grossman. In the model, individuals invest in health up to the point where the marginal benefits from the investment, which include a consumption benefit plus an investment benefit, are equal to the marginal costs incurred by the investment.

10. When analysing the demand for health care, it is important to take account of the concept of need. Economists commonly define need as the capacity for a patient to benefit from health care.

11. Health care is characterised by asymmetry of information. In particular, doctors are usually better informed about health and health care than are patients. For this reason, a principal–agent relationship usually develops in which the doctor (the agent) makes available their specialist knowledge to the patient (the principal).

12. If doctors acted as perfect agents they would maximise the utility of the principal. The hypothesis of supplier-induced demand is that doctors act as imperfect agents – failing to maximise the patients' utility – in order to maximise their own utility. Unfortunately, supplier-induced demand is difficult to detect, since empirical findings may be consistent with a non-inducement hypothesis.

13. When considering the aggregate demand for health care (the demand for health care by an entire country), researchers have found that, using health care spending per person as a proxy measure for aggregate demand, most of the variation in health care demand between countries can be explained by the country's income.

Chapter 3

The Production and Costs of Health Care

3.1 INTRODUCTION

Applying economic theories of supply to health care requires us to consider carefully its particular characteristics as an economic good. Nevertheless, the same analytical framework can be applied to health care as for any other good or service. Supply theory analyses the behaviour of firms in the economic environment in which they operate, and in health care this can be applied equally to pharmaceutical companies selling in private markets and general medical practices serving the public sector. Supply of a good or service depends on its production: the amount that will be produced under different circumstances and the cost of production of different amounts. This chapter is concerned with how economic analyses of production and costs are applied to health care. It is of interest in its own right, particularly in its analysis of efficiency, but it also contributes to the theory of supply and market structure and behaviour, analysed in Chapter 4, to markets and market failure, discussed in Chapter 5, and to economic evaluation, the subject of Part II.

To emphasise the fact that conventional economics tools are used, we will sometimes use generic descriptive terms that may seem unfamiliar when applied to health care. For example, health care comprises an extremely diverse range of goods and services, including surgical procedures, screening programmes, pharmaceuticals and counselling services; we refer to all of these as 'products'. There are also many different types of health care provider, including hospitals, GP practices, pharmaceutical companies and ambulance services; we refer to these as 'firms'. The quantity of health care 'product' produced by a health care 'firm' is referred to as its 'output'.

However, we do need to be careful in defining what we mean by the output of health care, because use of an inappropriate definition may be misleading. There are two opposing views about the nature of health care output. It is often argued that the ultimate output of the health sector is health; we should regard what hospitals, for example, produce as changes in health. The other view is that health is really only produced by individuals, who may use the services that hospitals produce to do so. So, the output of health care is the amount of care provided and that can be regarded as an *intermediate* output that is used in the creation of the final output, which is health. In this chapter, we will regard both of these as valid measures of output; our case studies include examples of output both as changes in health and as numbers of treatments provided.

There are problems with each view of output. The view that output is changes in health could be misleading in cases where changes in health might not reflect the amount of health care provided, especially where there is uncertainty about whether or not treatments will be successful. Moreover, as discussed in Chapter 1, health is not a good that can be directly traded, so it is difficult to use this concept in analysing health care markets. However, regarding health care as a service in its own right carries the danger of ignoring the main purpose of health care, which is to affect health. It would be at best misleading if we were to judge one health care facility as being more productive than others when some of the health care that it provides does not affect health, or even is harmful.

The economic theory of production and costs is often presented using examples in which a firm produces a single product. However, an important aspect of health care production is that the more usual case is of a multi-product firm. Hospitals, for example, produce an enormous variety of health care products. We introduce each concept by looking at the simple case of single-product firms, but this is preliminary to analysing the more usual multi-product environment.

3.2 THE THEORY OF PRODUCTION

3.2.1 Production Functions

Chapter 1 introduced the important concept of a *production function*, the relationship between the inputs to and outputs of a firm's productive process as moderated by 'mediating factors' such as the environment in which the firm operates. These inputs are sometimes referred to as factors of production, factor inputs, or simply factors. These are commonly categorised into three broad types: labour; land or raw materials; and capital.

Consider the production of cataract removals in a surgical unit contained within an eye hospital. The inputs to production are resources such as the time of a surgeon, an anaesthetist and a nurse, which are all types of labour, and the use of an operating theatre and equipment plus materials such as drugs, dressings and disposables, which are all types of capital. There will also be inputs that are used in pre- and post-operative care of patients, including perhaps the use of a hospital bed. The production function analyses how these various inputs combine to produce output in terms of the number of operations. For example, to what extent can different inputs, such as surgeons and nurses, be substituted for each other? If we use more nurses, how many more operations will we be able to perform? How many more operations will we be able to perform if we use more or all of the inputs? This enables us to ask questions about efficiency: What is efficiency in production? How can we measure it?

For a firm producing a single output from n resource inputs, a production function may be expressed as

$$Q = Q(x_1, x_2, x_3, \ldots, x_n, \sigma, \varepsilon) \tag{3.1}$$

where Q is the quantity of output, $x_1, \ldots, x_n$ are the quantities of the inputs, σ represents *returns to scale*, which is described below, and ε represents the managerial and organisational efficiency of the production process. However, we will start by looking at the input–output relationship isolated from these other effects. This requires us to imagine that we know the input–output relationship under ideal conditions determined purely by the technology of production – the maximum output that the technology can produce with a particular combination and quantity of inputs. This is known as *technical efficiency*.

3.2.2 Isoquants

A technically efficient level of output can often be achieved using differing combinations of inputs. For example, the number of operations that can be carried out in a hospital depends on the number of medical and nursing staff that the hospital has and on other inputs. To some extent, it is possible to substitute between medical and nursing staff, because some tasks could be carried out by either type of staff. To demonstrate how this can be analysed, we will simplify the production model to include just two inputs; in this example, the number of doctors employed (x_1) and the number of nurses employed (x_2). For this two-input case, the production function for output level Q_0 is

$$Q_0 = q(x_1, x_2) \tag{3.2}$$

Figure 3.1 shows a traditional representation of the production function, an *isoquant*. An isoquant shows all of the technically efficient combinations of inputs (nurses and doctors) that can be used to produce a specified quantity of output (number of

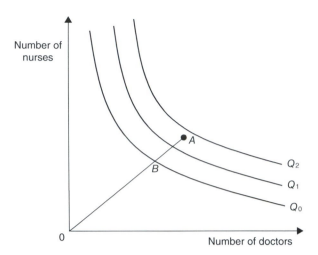

Figure 3.1 Production function and isoquant.

operations). The production function generates a different isoquant for each quantity of operations, so the figure actually shows an isoquant map, including isoquants for three different levels of output, Q_0, Q_1 and Q_2. Isoquants farther from the origin represent higher quantities of output.

A firm is *technically efficient* if it is producing at a point on the isoquant. Another way of viewing technical efficiency is that the firm cannot produce more of a good or service without using more of at least one resource input. This definition is related to the concept of *Pareto efficiency*, which will be considered in more detail in Chapters 5 and 8. Technical efficiency can be quantified in a number of ways, but one of the most useful is the *Farrell radial measure* (Farrell 1957). For example, a hospital might use the combination of nurses and doctors shown by point A in Figure 3.1 to produce output Q_0, and is therefore not technically efficient. Technically efficient hospitals may produce anywhere on the isoquant, so it is not possible to express inefficiency simply in terms of using too many doctors or too many nurses – hospitals producing at some points on the curve use either more doctors or more nurses, but of course use far fewer of the other type of labour. However, the line $0A$ – a ray – shows all points that use the same relative proportions of doctors and nurses. A technically efficient hospital that used the same ratio of doctors to nurses as hospital A would produce at point B. Hospital A's degree of technical efficiency is therefore measured by the ratio $0B/0A$.

3.2.3 Marginal Products

To examine how output varies with the inputs employed, it is useful to understand the concept of a *marginal product* (*MP*). The marginal product of an input is the change in output resulting from a change in the quantity of the input used, other things held constant. In the example above, if we increase the number of nurses but no other inputs, how many more operations could the hospital carry out? The *MP* is given by the partial derivative of the production function with respect to the factor. For factor x_n, the marginal product is

$$MPx_n = \frac{\partial Q}{\partial x_n} \qquad (3.3)$$

As more units of any one input, such as nurses, are added to the production process, holding constant the number of other inputs (doctors), the marginal product tells us the associated increase in output (operations). Where the use of nurses is initially quite low, the increase in output resulting from adding an additional nurse may be quite large. However, successive increases in the use of nursing inputs will eventually result in smaller and smaller increases in output. This is the *law of diminishing marginal returns*. This law is observable in many production processes: Box 3.1 gives an unusual example in health care.

3.2.4 Substitutability between Inputs

The slope of the isoquant is called the *marginal rate of technical substitution* (*MRTS*) of the inputs. It measures how substitutable the factors of production are. The *MRTS* decreases as we move along the isoquant, which is why it is convex to the origin, reflecting the fact that, in our example, it becomes increasingly difficult to substitute nurses for doctors and attain the same level of output. The *MRTS* is given by:

$$MRTSx_ix_k = -\frac{\partial x_k}{\partial x_i} \qquad (3.4)$$

and it can be shown that the *MRTS* is equal to the ratio of the marginal products of the factors:

$$MRTSx_ix_k = -\frac{\partial x_k}{\partial x_i} = \frac{(\partial Q/\partial x_i)}{(\partial Q/\partial x_k)} = \frac{MPx_i}{MPx_k} \qquad (3.5)$$

We can show that this is the case using our example of substituting nurse for doctor time. Suppose that the *MRTS* of doctors for nurses is −2, meaning that the number of operations provided will be the same if we substitute one doctor for two nurses. Employing one fewer nurse would decrease the number of operations possible by MP_{nurse}; so if the same number of operations is to be provided with two fewer nurses, the extra doctor would have to produce twice as much as this; therefore the MP_{doctor}/MP_{nurse} must be equal to −2, which is the $MRTS_{doctor,nurse}$.

Box 3.1 Diminishing returns to health expenditure

In 2003 the World Health Organisation (WHO) published the World Health Report 2003, which reports data for 192 WHO member states on health expenditure and life expectancy at the aggregate (national) level. The health expenditure calculations from the report are plotted against life expectancy estimates:

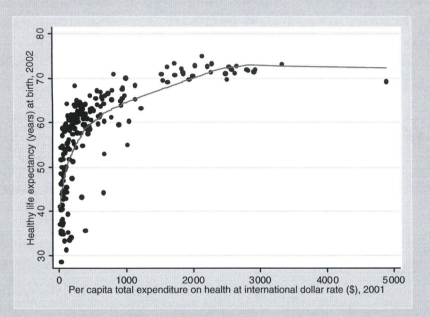

The total quantity of inputs that a country devotes to health care is proxied by total expenditure on health per capita in 2001, based on National Health Accounts converted to US dollars using purchasing power parities. The output of the country's health care system is proxied by health-adjusted life expectancy (HALE) at birth in 2002, based on current rates of population morbidity and mortality. It can be interpreted as the equivalent number of years in full health that a newborn can expect to live based on current rates of ill-health and mortality. The relationship between them is consistent with the view that health expenditure has diminishing returns. It is positive up to an expenditure level of around $2800 per capita. Additional expenditure beyond this level has a negligible incremental effect on life expectancy.

What does the assumption that the *MRTS* declines as we move from left to right along an isoquant imply about the *MP*s of the different inputs? It reflects an assumption that the *MP* of any factor diminishes as the intensity of its use increases – in this case, the greater the ratio of nurses to doctors, the smaller the *MP* of nurses and the larger the *MP* of doctors. It is often explained in economics textbooks as being a result of the law of diminishing marginal returns. However, that is incorrect, as that law is explicitly an assumption about the case where one factor is variable and all other factors are fixed. As we will demonstrate in Section 3.4, it is possible to have constant or even increasing marginal returns even with a concave isoquant. The specific shape given to isoquants constitutes a separate assumption about the nature of production, although clearly the rationales of the two assumptions are very similar.

See Box 3.2 for an application of *MP* and *MRTS* to the production of live births in Thailand.

3.2.5 Production Frontiers

The isoquant is a theoretical device, which can, however, in principle be estimated from real data on inputs and output. Another view of the production process using real data is a *production frontier*, illustrated in Figure 3.2. The figure is based on a scatter diagram of observed input combinations that produce a given output Q_0. For example, each dot might represent an observed number of doctors and nurses for different health care providers producing a given number of operations. The frontier Q_0Q_0 is defined as a set of boundary points consisting of all firms that are technically efficient. Any of the dots inside the boundary, such as point *A*, are technically inefficient. Again, the

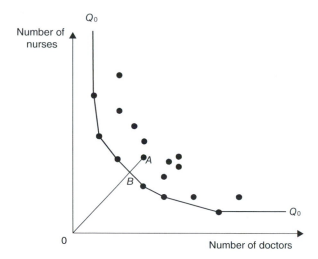

Figure 3.2 Production frontier.

Box 3.2 The production of live births in Thailand

Suraratdecha and Okunade (2005), using data from 1982 to 1997, constructed a production function for the health care system in Thailand, where 'the rapid growth in the use of limited resources and the escalating national health expenditure, raise the critical economic question of whether the use of health care resources [is] efficient'. The output measure was the number of live births per 1000 population, which was related to three labour inputs (doctors, nurses and pharmacists) and one capital input (the number of hospital beds). The data also took into account regions within Thailand, time as an indicator of technical progress, and the number of hospitals and medical practices as an indicator of the effects of the scale of production.

It was found that the numbers of nurses and of beds had a positive influence on output, but that numbers of doctors and pharmacists had a negative effect. The calculated marginal products (MPs) for nurses and beds are therefore positive, but not only were the MPs of doctors and pharmacists negative, they were larger in absolute terms. However, the MPs varied widely across regions: for example, the nursing MP varied from 6.52 in Bangkok to 36.01 in the Northeast, with a national average of 16.48. This pattern was the same for all of the inputs; however, over time the regional MPs converged towards the Bangkok levels.

There was evidence of technical progress, with increasing use of physicians and to a lesser extent of pharmacists over time, but lower use of nurses and beds. The analysis suggested strong economies of scale, with a 10% rise in health system capacity associated with a 26% rise in output, although this again varied by region. Estimates were made of the possibilities for substitution between inputs, which confirmed that the isoquants were of the theoretical shape, convex to the origin.

level of inefficiency can be measured by the Farrell ratio $0B/0A$. Such a frontier is sometimes called a *best practice* frontier, because it does not compare firms to a theoretical ideal but to the best observable performance within an industry.

3.3 MULTI-PRODUCT FIRMS

A hospital does not usually produce only one generic output of, for example, 'operations'; not only are there many different types of operation, hospitals provide medical and other types of care as well as surgery. Although there may be varying degrees of specialisation in the way in which these different types of care are produced, there will be some input factors that could be used for many different types of care, for example basic nursing.

The production function for a firm producing m outputs from n inputs can be expressed in implicit form as

$$H(q_1, q_2, q_3, \ldots, q_m, x_1, x_2, x_3, \ldots, x_n) = 0 \tag{3.6}$$

This means that for a given amount of inputs, different amounts of the various outputs can be produced. Figure 3.3 illustrates this as a *product transformation curve* (PTC), which is also sometimes referred to as the production possibility curve, frontier or boundary. This shows all the possible combinations of the two outputs that can be produced with a given amount of inputs. As with the isoquant, every point on the curve is assumed to be technically efficient. For the two-output one-input case, the PTC can be defined as

$$X_0 = h(q_1, q_2) \tag{3.7}$$

The slope of this is known as the *rate of product transformation* (RPT). It defines the degree of substitutability of the outputs, and is given by

$$RPT q_1 q_2 = -\frac{\partial q_2}{\partial q_1} \tag{3.8}$$

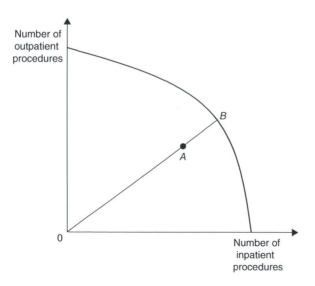

Figure 3.3 Production transformation curve.

The *RPT* decreases as we move downwards along the *PTC*, which shows that it becomes increasingly difficult to substitute q_2 for q_1 while maintaining the same level of input. It can be shown that the *RPT* is equal to the ratio of the marginal product of the input in production of q_2 to the *MP* of the input in production of q_1:

$$RPTq_1q_2 = -\frac{\partial q_2}{\partial q_1} = \frac{(\partial q_2 / \partial x)}{(\partial q_1 / \partial x)} = \frac{MPq_2x}{MPq_1x} \qquad (3.9)$$

The proof is analogous to that of why the *MRTS* for one output is equal to the ratio of *MP*s of two inputs. Suppose that the *RPT* of inpatient (q_1) for outpatient care (q_2) is −10, meaning that the number of inputs used will be the same if we substitute one inpatient for ten outpatient procedures. Reducing the number of inpatient procedures by one would release $1/MP_{IP}$ units of the inputs; providing ten more outpatient procedures would use $10/MP_{OP}$ units. If the amount of inputs is to remain the same, these must be equal, so the ratio of MP_{OP}/MP_{IP} must be equal to −10, which is the $MRTS_{IP,OP}$.

Again, it is possible to analyse this using the concept of frontiers and to measure efficiency using the Farrell measure described earlier. Figure 3.4 shows the equivalent production frontier. The *RPT* is not smoothly defined; it is constant between frontier points and changes only at those points. In both Figure 3.3 and Figure 3.4, point *A* represents an inefficient hospital, as it lies within the *PTC*. An efficient hospital that produced the same ratio of outputs would produce at point *B*. The ratio $0A/0B$ is a measure of the relative technical efficiency of hospital *A*. An example of this technique, applied to nursing home care, is shown in Box 3.3.

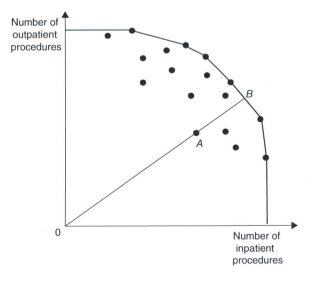

Figure 3.4 Production frontier: two outputs.

Box 3.3 A multi-product production function for nursing-home care in the United States

Nyman and Bricker (1989), using data for one year, constructed a production frontier for nursing homes in Wisconsin, USA, noting that 'nursing homes, with expenditures nearing 1% of GNP, represent an important industry – one whose importance is expected to grow as the population ages'. They had five outputs; these were numbers of patients according to the kind of care they required: skilled nursing facility (SNF), intermediate nursing tacility (INF), 'limited' care, 'personal' care and residential care. They included four inputs: these were hours of different types of labour: nurses, social workers, therapists and other staff.

From these data, Farrell technical efficiency scores were calculated for each nursing home. Those that defined the frontier had, of course, the highest possible efficiency score of 100%; the lowest score was 23% and the average was 89%. Factors that influenced these scores were analysed. For-profit homes had higher efficiency scores; for-profit nursing homes used 4.5% less labour per patient than did non-profit homes. Other factors that were associated with higher efficiency scores were a smaller proportion of SNF patients, lower wages and location in an urban area.

One problem with this kind of study is that it is important to make sure that the output measures used reflect important aspects of the service. In this case, the output is simply numbers of patients. Aspects of quality or what level of service patients received are not included. If, for example, staff in non-profit homes spent more time with patients, which led to an improvement in their well-being and satisfaction, the additional hours would in this kind of analysis simply be seen as inefficiency rather than a better service.

3.4 RETURNS TO SCALE, ADDITIVITY AND FIXED FACTORS

A question that is often posed is how big health care facilities should be. For example, is it better for general practitioners to have separate facilities, or should they have a group practice? This question involves a number of different issues, concerned with demand as much as supply, but one of them is the extent to which merged practices can provide more health care than individual practices. This is the issue of *returns to scale*. It is closely related to *economies of scale*, which we consider in greater detail below.

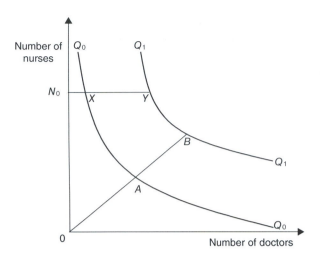

Figure 3.5 Isoquant map, returns to scale and returns to a fixed factor.

If, when all inputs are multiplied by any positive number λ output increases by λ^v, where v is a constant, the production function is *homogeneous*. For example, if we have twice as many doctors and nurses and all other inputs ($\lambda = 2$) and this results in four times as many operations, then the production function is homogeneous, with $v = 2$. Homogeneity is defined as:

$$q(\lambda x_1, \lambda x_2, \ldots, \lambda x_n) = \lambda^v q(\lambda x_1, \lambda x_2, \ldots, \lambda x_n, \lambda^v) = \lambda^v Q \qquad (3.10)$$

The constant v is the *degree of homogeneity* and is a measure of the returns to scale: if $v = 1$ there are constant returns to scale; if $v < 1$ there are decreasing returns to scale; and if $v > 1$ there are increasing returns to scale.

Figure 3.5 illustrates this using an isoquant map, in this case with two isoquants whose production is, respectively, Q_0 and Q_1 operations, where $Q_1 > Q_0$. If the numbers of doctors and nurses shown at point A, where production is Q_0, are both doubled, this would give the numbers represented by point B. If the isoquant passing through point B is for a production level of $Q_1 = 2{\times}Q_0$, then there are constant returns to scale. If Q_1 is more than double Q_0, there are increasing returns; if it is less than double, there are decreasing returns.

There are several sources of increasing returns to scale. One is the ability of large organisations to specialise, which applies to many inputs including the labour force, capital equipment and management. For example, a small hospital may have to employ general surgeons to deal with many areas of surgery, but a larger one may be able to employ specialist surgeons, who become proficient in performing specific types of surgery and are able to produce more output. Another is that there may be technical and managerial indivisibilities: for example, some inputs such as machinery and other types of equipment are only efficient to use at a higher scale of production; capacity may be of a fixed size and spare capacity can be exploited at higher levels of production. For example, it may be inefficient to locate a GP practice in a rural area where there are only a few patients. Many aspects of a firm's overall activities may not increase proportionately as output increases, such as selling and promotion. For example, expanding public health campaigns to stop smoking to twice the number of people may not incur twice the costs since the initial costs of devising the campaign are not incurred twice. Where there is uncertainty – as there is in many areas of health care – a larger scale takes advantage of the *law of large numbers*, which essentially means that predictions have a smaller confidence interval. For example, a maternity hospital might wish to ensure that it has sufficient delivery rooms available on 99% of occasions. If it has an average of two deliveries per day, it might require four delivery suites to achieve this, with an average overcapacity of 100%. If it has an average of eight deliveries per day, it might require only ten suites, with an average overcapacity of 25%.

The existence of decreasing returns to scale is contentious. It is often argued that they arise owing to managerial inefficiencies, because at higher levels of production managers can be overworked and the decision-making process becomes less efficient. An alternative view is that there are always increasing returns to scale in so many areas of production that they will always offset any management inefficiencies.

It is not quite so easy to define returns to scale for multi-product firms. For example, doubling the number of doctors and nurses in a hospital might enable twice the number of inpatient and outpatient procedures to be carried out, but that might not be the only efficient combination of outputs that could be achieved. It might be equally efficient, given the doubled level of inputs, to have three times as many inpatient procedures and only 50% more outpatient procedures. Identification and measurement of returns to scale in real multi-product industries such as health care is therefore particularly difficult.

Returns to scale derive from so-called 'long-run' factors, where all inputs are variable and can be flexibly assigned to different output combinations. Returns to scale for a hospital, for example, are relevant where all of the resources used by a hospital can be changed – buildings, equipment and consumables as well as the numbers of staff – to whatever numbers are required.

In the short run, though, it may be that the use of some resources is not so flexible. For example, there may be temporary shortages of certain types of labour or equipment or it may not be possible to expand the hospital site until new land is purchased and new buildings are constructed. In this case, we may be interested in what happens when some resource inputs are increased while others are fixed. As we noted in Section 3.2.1, it is usually assumed that this will be governed by the law of diminishing returns. However, although diminishing returns will definitely arise if the production function has constant or decreasing returns to scale, theoretically this will not occur if there are very strongly increasing returns to scale. Figure 3.5 demonstrates this. If the number of nurses is fixed at N_0 and there are constant returns to scale so that $Q_1 = 2 \times Q_0$, the number of doctors would have to increase from X to Y, which is clearly more than double; hence there are diminishing returns. However, returns to increased numbers of doctors would actually increase if Q_1 were greater than Q_0 by a multiplication factor greater than Y/X.

As well as economies of scale, another reason for mergers of health care facilities is that this enables different *types* of health care to be brought together in the same facility, especially specialist health care services. Sometimes this is due to factors such as convenience to patients, but it may also be that it is possible to produce more health care for a given set of inputs when it is produced in a shared facility than if it were produced separately. This might be because limited demand for each type of health care leads to spare capacity in some indivisible inputs, which could be used elsewhere. There are many potentially shareable inputs in health care, such as inpatient beds, outpatient facilities, operating theatres, intensive therapy units and general nursing, medical, administrative and support staff.

This issue is known as *additivity*, and is illustrated in Figure 3.6 using the concept of a production frontier. Suppose that a dentist can provide one filling or one scaling in 15 minutes, including examination of the patient. If one hour of dentist's time is divided between practices that specialise in these different procedures, it is possible to provide

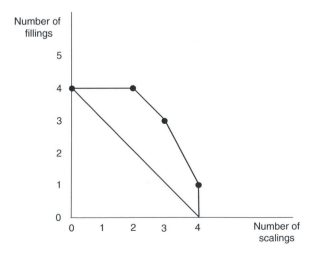

Figure 3.6 Additivity in production.

four fillings only, three fillings and one scaling, two fillings and two scalings, three scalings or one filling, or four scalings only. This is represented by the straight line – the rate of product transformation is one scaling for one filling. However, a general dental practitioner could, by combining examinations for the two procedures, provide the different combinations shown by the joint production frontier, for example three fillings and two scalings. This is known as *super-additivity*; output is greater with joint production than with separate production. It is also possible to have *sub-additivity*; where joint production output is lower than with separate production. In terms of the *PTC*, this can be expressed as follows:

If $h(q_1, q_2) = h(q_1) + h(q_2)$ joint production is additive.

If $h(q_1, q_2) > h(q_1) + h(q_2)$ joint production is super-additive.

If $h(q_1, q_2) < h(q_1) + h(q_2)$ joint production is sub-additive.

The presence of super-additivity means that, on efficiency grounds, primary health care facilities that offer a number of services and general hospitals may be justified. Specialised facilities are justified if there are many highly specialised inputs that are not suitable for sharing, or where a high level of demand means that there is no spare capacity of shareable inputs.

3.5 COSTS

So far, our analysis of how the level of output is determined has regarded the inputs as resources that exist in a physical sense. However, one of the key elements of economics is that it is concerned with values, and economists measure the value of resources by their cost – in particular, we use the concept of opportunity cost introduced in Chapter 1. Here, we investigate how costs vary as firms change the level of output that they produce. We are particularly interested in how firms can minimise costs, for two main reasons: first, it may be useful in explaining a firm's behaviour in a particular market; and secondly because it is an important element of efficiency that adds to the concept of technical efficiency that we have already examined.

3.5.1 Costs and Production

Costs of production obviously depend on the quantity and combination of resource inputs that are used. A particular input will have a cost attached to it; in general terms this can be regarded as the *unit cost* of an input, although it is often called the price of the input. The cost of employing a particular combination of inputs is defined by the equation

$$C = x_1 \times p_{x1} + x_2 \times p_{x2} + \ldots + x_n \times p_{xn} \qquad (3.11)$$

where $x_1, \ldots, x_n$ are the quantities of inputs and $p_{x1}, \ldots, p_{xn}$ are the unit costs of those inputs. This can be viewed in a different way. If this is evaluated for a particular level of cost, it defines all of the different combinations of the inputs that will cost a particular amount. For example, for the two-input model used earlier

$$C_0 = x_1 \times p_{x1} + x_2 \times p_{x2} \tag{3.12}$$

This is an *isocost line*, which is illustrated by the dotted line in Figure 3.7(a). It can also be viewed as a *budget constraint* similar to that introduced in Chapter 2, since it

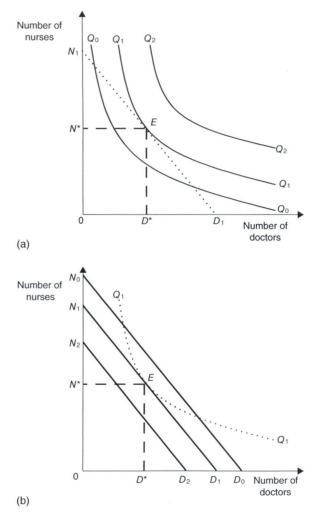

(a)

(b)

○ **Figure 3.7 (a) Maximising output subject to a cost constraint. (b) Minimising cost for a given output level.**

defines all the combinations of inputs that can be afforded for a given budget. In this case, N_1 is the number of nurses that could be employed if the entire budget was spent on them and D_1 is the same for the number of doctors.

The slope of the isocost line is the ratio of the unit costs of the two inputs:

$$\text{Slope} = \frac{p_{x1}}{p_{x2}} \qquad (3.13)$$

Figure 3.7(b) shows three isocost lines representing different cost outlays. The input prices are the same for all of them, which is why they all have the same slope. The farther they are from the origin, the greater the total cost.

The isocost line shows the relationship between *inputs* and cost. We can analyse the relationship between *output* and cost by linking it with the production function – the relationship between inputs and outputs. In doing so, we again make an assumption about efficiency. This type of efficiency has a number of different labels including *economic efficiency*, *cost-effectiveness* and *allocative efficiency in production* – the last of these will be explained below. There are two different ways of viewing it. It can be seen as minimising the cost of producing a particular level of output or, alternatively, as maximising output for a particular budget – in both cases subject to a set of fixed input prices and a particular production function. As we will show, the solutions to these two problems are equivalent.

Figure 3.7(a) illustrates the problem of maximising output for a given cost. The maximum output that can be produced given the constraint on cost is Q_1, where the isocost line is at a tangent to the highest attainable isoquant. The optimal combination of inputs is at point E, with N^* nurses and D^* doctors. Higher levels of output such as Q_2 are not affordable and other points on the isocost line all lie on a lower isoquant such as Q_0.

Figure 3.7(b) illustrates the problem of minimising cost to obtain a given output. The isoquant denoting the desired level of output is Q_1. The lowest attainable isocost line that enables this to be produced is $N_1 D_1$ and production should be at their point of tangency, E. It is not possible to obtain the desired level of output at a cost such as $N_2 D_2$ and other points on the isoquant all lie on a higher isocost line such as $N_0 D_0$.

As may be seen, these solutions are exactly the same. In both cases, at the point of tangency, the slope of the isoquant is equal to the slope of the isocost line:

$$MRTSx_1x_2 = \frac{MPx_1}{MPx_2} = \frac{p_{x1}}{p_{x2}} \qquad (3.14)$$

This may be rearranged to

$$\frac{MP_{x1}}{p_{x1}} = \frac{MP_{x2}}{p_{x2}} \qquad (3.15)$$

and, more generally, the efficient combination of inputs occurs when the following condition holds:

$$\frac{MP_{x1}}{p_{x1}} = \frac{MP_{x2}}{p_{x2}} = \frac{MP_{x3}}{p_{x3}} = \ldots = \frac{MP_{xn}}{p_{xn}} \qquad (3.16)$$

This ratio is of output measured in some physical units, for example the number of operations, to a price measured in some currency, for example pounds. The condition in equation (3.16) therefore means that when we have an efficient combination of inputs, the extra output per pound spent is the same for all inputs. If any input had a higher ratio than this, it would be efficient to employ more of it, that is, substitute it for other less productive inputs. Similarly, if any input had a lower ratio than this, it would be efficient to employ less of it.

Another way of viewing the efficiency achieved by producing output at the lowest possible cost is that, given the prices of inputs, it is not possible to produce more of any good or service without incurring greater costs. As with technical efficiency, this is a definition related to Pareto efficiency (see Chapter 8) and the terminology used in this context is *allocative efficiency in production*.

Figure 3.8 shows how allocative and technical efficiency can be quantified using a Farrell measure (Farrell 1957). An inefficient hospital with the input combination at point A

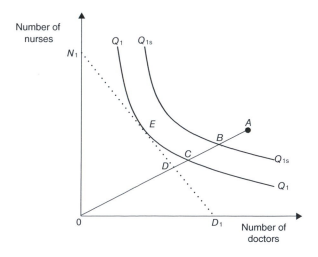

Figure 3.8 Technical, allocative and scale efficiency.

would be technically efficient at point C, as that is on the isoquant for Q_1. However, C is not the allocatively efficient point on the isoquant; that is point E. It would be allocatively efficient to use that input combination at point D, as that is on the isocost line N_1D_1. However, D is not the technically efficient point on that isocost line; again that is E. So we should really compare point A with point E; unfortunately, we cannot do that directly – we have to decompose overall efficiency into separate allocative and technical elements.

As before, technical efficiency can be measured as $0C/0A$, the deviation of the hospital from the technically efficient output. Allocative efficiency can be measured as $0D/0C$, the deviation of the technically efficient point from the allocatively efficient point. Overall efficiency can be measured as $0D/0A$, which is simply the product of allocative and technical efficiency, since $0D/0C \times 0C/0A = 0D/0A$. Note that this shows that technical efficiency is a *necessary* but not *sufficient* condition for allocative efficiency.

The final link in analysing the relationship between cost and output is to consider what will happen to the efficient input combination in response to changes in the desired output, represented by an isoquant, or to the budget, represented by the isocost line. There is an efficient input combination for every possible isocost curve and isoquant curve. The way in which efficient input combinations change as output increases is known as an *expansion path*, consisting of all of the tangency points.

3.5.2 Cost Functions

The production function in equation (3.1), which embodies both the isoquant and the expansion path, relates quantities of outputs with quantities of inputs; equation (3.11) relates quantities of inputs to cost. It is now possible to combine these to define a *cost function*, which relates quantities of outputs to cost:

$$C = C(Q, p_{x1}, p_{x2}, \ldots, p_{xn}) \tag{3.17}$$

This formulation emphasises that costs are also dependent on input prices, but for simplicity we will mainly used a shortened version of this:

$$C = C(Q) \tag{3.18}$$

It is also possible to define a multi-product cost function, equivalent to the multi-product production function defined in equation (3.6):

$$C = C(q_1, q_2, q_3, \ldots, q_m, p_{x1}, p_{x2}, \ldots, p_{xn}) \tag{3.19}$$

Two important measures derived from the cost function are *average cost* (AC) and *marginal cost* (MC). Average cost is simply total cost divided by quantity:

$$AC = \frac{C(Q)}{Q} \tag{3.20}$$

Marginal cost is the additional cost of an extra unit of output or for a continuous cost function:

$$MC = \frac{\partial C(Q)}{\partial(Q)} \qquad (3.21)$$

The difference between average and marginal cost is very important in applied health economics. Very often data are available on the average cost of health care services but not on their marginal cost, and using average costs as if they were marginal costs may be misleading. An example of this is the measurement of cost savings from schemes that allow some patients to be treated in the community without being admitted to hospital. Given data on total costs of inpatient stays, it is possible to calculate an average cost per patient, and it is tempting to conclude that avoiding an admission will reduce costs by that amount. However, it might be expected that the marginal cost of care varies with the level of 'output' – the number of admissions – and specifically that it is higher at lower output levels because this covers the most severe patients who are the most costly to treat. Less severe patients are those most likely to be suitable for treatment in the community, so the scheme will produce fewer cost savings than the average costs suggest.

An important point about multi-product cost functions is that it is not possible to define meaningfully what the average cost of a particular output is, because of shared inputs to their production that cannot be attributed only to them. However, it is possible to define the marginal cost of each output because this is calculated with the amount of all other outputs held constant. In practice, when multi-product organisations such as hospitals calculate costs for particular outputs, they use accounting rules to share out the costs of all inputs, whether directly attributable to an output or not, and calculate average not marginal costs. See Box 3.4 for an example of a study estimating a multi-product cost function.

The relationship between cost and output can also be expressed in terms of a frontier, which has exactly the same relationship to a cost function as a production frontier has to a production function; it is based on best practice from firms that achieve lower costs for the output produced. Box 3.5 shows an example of the use of cost frontiers.

3.5.3 Economies of Scale, Short-run Cost Functions and Economies of Scope

As with production functions, an important distinction is drawn between cost functions that assume that all inputs are variable and those that allow for some of the inputs to be fixed. As discussed, it is often assumed that if an input is fixed this is only a temporary state and that eventually it will be possible to vary it, whatever it is. As a result, there are somewhat different analyses of short-run cost functions, where some

Box 3.4 Factors affecting the cost of hospital services in the USA

Fournier and Mitchell (1992) estimated a multi-product cost function for 179 short-term general-care hospitals in Florida, USA from 1984 to 1986. The cost function included five different hospital outputs, hospital input prices and fixed inputs. They also looked at the effect of hospital ownership and competition on the cost function.

As the amount of output provided by the hospitals increases, the cost increases; the number of inpatient admissions, outpatient visits, emergency room visits and surgery minutes have a statistically significant and positive effect on costs, with inpatient admissions having the largest impact. Input prices were highly significant predictors of cost, with the salary of registered nurses being especially important. Capital stock had a significant positive impact on costs, which the authors interpret to mean that hospitals are employing too much fixed capital and equipment. The number of admitting physicians has a positive and significant effect on costs, which the authors interpret as evidence of either supplier-induced demand or the positive effect of a larger physician staff on quality, or both.

Investor-owned hospitals, and in particular those in a chain, had significantly lower costs than private non-profit hospitals and government-owned hospitals. Teaching status has a significant positive effect on cost.

The effect of competition depends on the type of health service. For maternity services, hospitals located in areas with a higher level of market concentration have higher costs. This suggests that maternity services operating in relatively competitive (with lower concentration) markets have lower costs. In contrast, higher concentration of admissions, surgery, radiation therapy and diagnostic imaging procedures has a significant and negative effect on hospital costs. The implication is that the costs associated with these services increase as the degree of market competition intensifies (becomes less concentrated). The authors suggest that this is consistent with the view that hospitals in more competitive markets are forced to engage in non-price competition, which tends to increase cost.

Box 3.5 A cost frontier for hospitals in Finland

Linna (1998) analysed the efficiency of 43 acute-care hospitals in Finland in 1988–1994, using two different methods of estimating a cost frontier. He noted that 'economic recession and the Government's budget deficit have placed increasing pressure on hospitals in Finland to contain costs. The state subsidy reform of 1993 was expected to enhance productive efficiency by introducing competitive elements into health care.'

The data used were for four types of output (inpatient and outpatient treatment, teaching and research), two price variables (wage rates and general local health care prices), three other factors affecting cost (teaching status, readmission rate and year of observation) and an indicator of scale (number of beds).

Among the conclusions were that cost efficiency improved over time; teaching and research raise costs, but teaching hospitals were no more or less efficient than other hospitals; and technological change was also improving efficiency. There was a 3–5% annual average increase in productivity, due in equal measure to improvement in cost efficiency and to technological change.

It was estimated that improving efficiency, presumably to the level of the most efficient hospitals, would reduce hospital costs by 1.0–1.2 billion Finnish marks each year. Finally, the improvement in productivity occurred before and after 1993, so it appeared that the subsidy reform had no effect on efficiency.

inputs are fixed, and long-run cost functions, where all inputs are variable. To be consistent with our treatment of production functions, we will consider long-run functions first.

Total costs, average costs and marginal costs are all related to the level of output. The relationships are illustrated in Figure 3.9 as cost curves, using the example of the cost of providing surgical care. The total cost curve is derived from the expansion path described earlier: efficient points of production at different levels of output, in this case the number of operations. Returns to scale (changes in the level of output as the scale of operations changes) are translated into *economies of scale* (changes in the cost of output). Constant returns to scale would produce a straight line total cost curve, meaning no economies of scale, because both average and marginal costs would be constant.

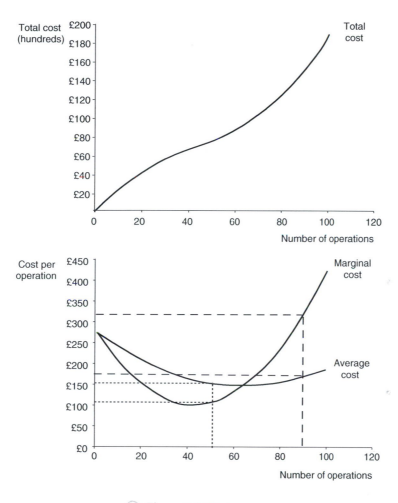

Figure 3.9 Cost curves.

It is usually assumed that economies of scale operate at low levels of output but that at some point there are no more to be gained and after that there may be diseconomies of scale. A long-run total cost curve must start at the origin, because it is assumed that firms can close down and incur no costs by producing nothing. After this it follows an inverse S-shape, reflecting the U-shape of the average cost curve. At low levels of output, average cost falls because of increasing returns to scale. However, returns to scale diminish, so average cost falls more slowly until all economies of scale are exploited; then there are constant returns to scale and average cost is constant. This is also known as the *minimum efficient scale*. In Figure 3.9, the minimum efficient scale is around 65 operations at a cost of £145 per operation. In this case, average cost starts to rise after this with more operations, implying decreasing returns to scale but, as has been discussed, this is a contentious concept, so it is often simply assumed that beyond the minimum efficient scale the average cost curve is constant.

The marginal cost curve also reflects this, and also has a U-shape. The MC curve crosses the AC curve at its minimum point – the minimum efficient scale. This is because if extra units of output cost less to produce than the average, their production must reduce average cost. If MC is less than AC (for example the dotted lines, where with 50 operations, $MC = £105$ and $AC = £150$), AC must be falling. Similarly, if extra units of output cost more to produce than the average, their production must increase average cost. So, if MC is greater than AC (for example the dashed line, where with 90 operations, $MC = £320$ and $AC = £170$), then AC must be rising. If AC is equal to MC, it is neither rising nor falling, which means that it is constant and at a minimum.

Economies of scale that derive from returns to scale involve changes in the physical quantity of factor inputs required. However, some economies of scale do not derive from increasing returns to scale. They are the result of paying lower prices for inputs because they are bought in large amounts; having lower costs of finance; and paying lower wages if the firm develops monopoly power in the labour market (see Chapter 4). Large hospitals, for example, are able to obtain large discounts by bulk buying not only of medical goods such as pharmaceuticals and disposables but also of goods used in their 'hotel' services.

The short-run cost function can be expressed as

$$C = C(Q) + F \tag{3.22}$$

where C is total cost, Q is output and F is fixed costs. Again, it is possible to define average and marginal costs. Short-run curves are drawn with similar shapes to the long-run versions, but for rather different reasons.

With zero output, total cost is not zero but at the level of fixed costs. It then follows an inverse S-shape, like the long-run curve, but does not reflect the expansion path, rather the law of diminishing returns. At low levels of production the marginal productivity of variable inputs increases, so the additional cost of producing extra units of output falls, and cost increases at a decreasing rate. But at some point, diminishing returns set in, the marginal productivity of the variable inputs fall, and extra units of output cost more to produce. This means that cost increases at an increasing rate. Using the example presented earlier of nurses employed on a ward, after diminishing returns have set in the marginal productivity of additional nurses falls. Therefore, the

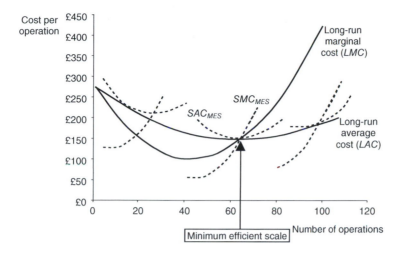

○ **Figure 3.10 Short-run and long-run cost curves.**

costs incurred employing each additional nurse achieve a lower return in terms of producing additional output and the marginal cost of producing additional output will rise.

Average cost again follows a U-shape, for two reasons. First, average cost initially falls as output rises simply because the fixed costs are being spread over greater and greater output. Eventually, this element may become so small that it is not a significant factor. Secondly, the pattern of increasing and diminishing returns causes average costs first to fall and then to rise. Marginal cost is of course unaffected by fixed costs, but its U-shape is again also due to changes in returns to fixed factors. Again, it is equal to average cost when average cost is at a minimum.

What is the relationship between the long-run and short-run curves? The short-run average cost curves, illustrated as dotted lines in Figure 3.10, can be seen as deviations from the long-run curve. A point on the long-run average cost curve (LAC) represents efficient production at a particular scale size. Short-run deviations from this cannot result in lower costs than the scale-efficient level of output, so the short-run curves are higher at every level of output above or below this, and are therefore at a tangent to the long-run curve. It is important to note that the long-run curve is therefore *not* composed of the minimum points of short-run curves. The long-run marginal cost curve (LMC) is similarly related to the short-run marginal cost curves. At the minimum efficient scale, long-run average cost is at a minimum, and is therefore equal to long-run marginal cost. The short-run average cost curve relevant to that scale, SAC_{MES}, has a point of tangency at its own minimum point, which is also equal to short-run marginal cost SMC_{MES}. Hence, the following condition holds at the minimum efficient scale:

$$SAC_{MES} = SMC_{MES} = LAC = LMC \tag{3.23}$$

Scale economies can also be quantified using Farrell measures. In Figure 3.8, the isoquant Q_{1s} represents efficient input combinations in the short run, while Q_1 represents the long-run or scale-efficient isoquant. Overall efficiency is measured, as before, by $0D/0A$. It can be decomposed into allocative efficiency, measured as before by $0D/0C$ and technical efficiency $0C/0A$; however, technical efficiency can also be decomposed into pure technical efficiency, measured as $0B/0A$, which is the deviation from the short-run isoquant, and scale efficiency, measured by $0C/0B$, which is the deviation of the short-run from the scale-efficient isoquant. These measures are related by $0B/0A \times 0C/0B \times 0D/0C = 0D/0A$.

It was suggested earlier that a multi-product firm, such as a general hospital, might be more efficient than single-product firm, such as a specialised hospital, because of the phenomenon of super-additivity. If that is so, then we would expect this to be reflected in lower costs for multi-product firms. This is called *economies of scope*. If there are economies of scope, then, for example, a general medical practice and a general dental practice would have higher combined costs than a health centre that undertook both medicine and dentistry.

Economies of scope may be defined using the concept of additivity in the cost function. An additive cost function means that the costs of joint production of outputs are the same as separate production of those outputs; in other words, there are no economies or diseconomies of scope. Similarly, a sub-additive cost function means that there are economies of scope and a super-additive cost function means that there are diseconomies of scope. More formally:

If $C(q_1, q_2) = C(q_1) + C(q_2)$ the costs of joint production are additive.

If $C(q_1, q_2) > C(q_1) + C(q_2)$ the costs of joint production are super-additive.

If $C(q_1, q_2) < C(q_1) + C(q_2)$ the costs of joint production are sub-additive.

Production functions and cost functions are closely related and the concept of additivity gives a good example of this. An important concept in understanding this close relationship is *duality theory*. An example of this described earlier was that maximising output for a given cost produces the same outcome as minimising cost for a given output. Using this theory, it can be shown that if costs are minimised in this way, then the additivity properties of the cost function are equivalent to those of the production function – sub-additivity of the cost function is equivalent to super-additivity of the production function and sub-additivity of the production function is equivalent to super-additivity of the cost function.

SUMMARY

1. The inputs into a production process are commonly categorised into three broad types: labour; land or raw materials; and capital.

2. A production function summarises the relationship between the inputs to and outputs from a firm's productive process. It describes how the various inputs combine to produce output, and can be used to quantify how output will change as more of the inputs are employed, how the inputs can be substituted for one another to produce the same level of output, and how efficient a particular production process is. An isoquant is a graphical representation of a production function, showing all the combinations of inputs that will produce a particular output. The production function generates a different isoquant for each level of output, and a firm is technically efficient if it is producing at a point on the isoquant.

3. The marginal product of an input is the change in output resulting from a change in the quantity of the input used, other things held constant.

4. The slope of the isoquant is called the marginal rate of technical substitution of the inputs, which measures how substitutable the factors of production are.

5. Health care providers often produce more than one type of output. In economic terms they are multi-product firms. The production function for a multi-product firm can be shown graphically by the product transformation curve, the slope of which is the rate of product transformation. This defines the degree of substitutability of the outputs.

6. If, when all inputs are multiplied by any positive number λ output increases by λ^v, where v is a constant, the production function is said to be homogenous. The constant v is the degree of homogeneity, and is a measure of the returns to scale from the production process. Increasing returns to scale in health care can explain why health care providers are often very large.

7. The concept of additivity can be used in health care to explain the merger of health care facilities. Super-additivity arises when it is possible to produce more health care for a given set of inputs when it is produced in a shared facility than if it were produced separately.

8. Costs of production depend on the quantity and combination of resource inputs that are employed, plus the unit costs of the inputs.

9. An isocost line defines all of the different combinations of the inputs that will cost a particular amount. The slope of the isocost line is the ratio of the unit costs of the two inputs.

10. Isocost lines can be combined with isoquants to determine the cost-minimising combination of inputs to produce a given level of output or the output-maximising combination of inputs for a given cost. These occur where the slope of the isoquant is equal to the slope of the isocost line, or where the marginal rate of technical substitution is equal to the ratio of the unit costs of the two inputs.

11. Cost functions relate the firm's costs to its level of output. Three useful ways of showing this relationship are total cost, average cost and marginal cost functions.

12. At low levels of output, average cost falls because of increasing returns to scale: there are economies of scale. However, returns to scale diminish, so average cost falls more slowly until all economies of scale are exploited; then there are constant returns to scale and average cost is constant. This point, which is the minimum point of the average cost function, is the minimum efficient scale. Beyond this point, average costs may start to rise, indicating decreasing returns to scale.

13. Economies of scope may be defined using the concept of additivity in the cost function. An additive cost function means that the costs of joint production of outputs are the same as separate production of those outputs; in other words, there are no economies or diseconomies of scope. Similarly, a sub-additive cost function means that there are economies of scope, and a super-additive cost function means that there are diseconomies of scope.

Chapter 4

The Supply of Health Care

4.1 FIRMS, MARKETS AND INDUSTRIES IN THE HEALTH CARE SECTOR OF THE ECONOMY

In earlier chapters we introduced a number of concepts that deserve further explanation. In Chapters 1 and 2, we referred to *markets* and introduced the analysis of health care markets as the interaction of the *supply* of and demand for health care. In Chapter 3, we analysed production of health care within *firms* and also referred to the health care *industry*. In this chapter, we analyse the supply side of the market and the role of firms and industries in markets. So it is useful to begin by defining what we mean by those terms.

A market is simply a place where those who wish to supply goods and those who demand them are brought together in order to effect an exchange. In economics, these suppliers and demanders are often called sellers and buyers, as the assumption is that the good will not be exchanged for free but for money or sometimes for other goods. A market need not be a single place – it would be hard to identify this for an internet pharmacy, for example. In health care, buyers include households, who buy health care services either directly out of their own pocket or indirectly via a third party payer, and health care providers such as hospitals, who employ health care professionals via a labour market, and buy other inputs such as pharmaceuticals. Sellers include hospitals, who provide health care directly, and medical equipment and pharmaceutical companies, who provide inputs to the health care production process.

A firm is an economic unit that produces and sells goods, such as medical equipment, or services, such as dental care or health insurance. As suggested, it may sell directly to consumers of health care (people) or to other firms such as health care providers. An industry is a collection of economic units that sell similar products – for example the pharmaceutical, insurance or hospital industries. A stricter economics definition, which is important in analysing models of how markets work, is that the goods or services are close substitutes, as defined in Chapter 2.

The supply side of a market is the industry. In the same way as analysis of demand is based heavily on theories of how individual consumers behave, the analysis of supply is dependent on theories of how firms behave – indeed, this topic is often called the *theory of the firm*. In this chapter we build on the analysis of production within firms dealt with in Chapter 3 and look in more detail at the operation of firms in the health care industry. The health care industry is large and heterogeneous, containing many different types of economic unit, which can be grouped into sectors depending on their area of specialisation. Table 4.1 is a taxonomy summarising the main components of the health care industry.

Analysis of supply in economics is often dominated by theories of the firm that are based on an assumption that their overriding aim is to maximise profits. This can be viewed in two ways. First, such theories may indeed be reasonable descriptions of the

Table 4.1   Components of the health care industry

	Finance sector	Input sector	Primary care sector	Hospital sector
Key features	Economic units involved in the flow of funds from households to health care providers in return for the coverage of health risk	Provide inputs into the provision of primary care and hospital care	Typically the first level of contact with health care services	Outpatient and inpatient services, where access is often via a referral from primary care services
Examples of types of firm	Health insurance companies, managed care organisations	Pharmaceutical companies, medical devices companies, suppliers of capital equipment	General practitioners, opticians, pharmacists, dentists, physiotherapists, chiropodists	Specialist services (for example cardiology, neurology)

aims of some firms and can therefore be used in a positive economics sense to generate predictions about the way that firms and markets operate. However, an important aspect of health care provision is that the more usual case is of firms that not only do not aim to maximise profits, but do not aim to earn any profits at all. The aim of most pharmaceutical companies and many insurance companies is to generate profits, and profit maximisation may be a reasonable assumption for them; Box 4.1 demonstrates how profitable health care can be. By contrast, most hospitals and nursing homes and some insurance companies do not aim to maximise profit. But theories based on profit maximisation have a second use, because they provide a useful set of performance benchmarks against which firms' actual performance can be compared. So, we will start by introducing theories based on profit maximisation, but stress that for much of health care other theories will be more appropriate.

Box 4.1 Profit maximisation in the health care industry

One area of the health care industry in which profit maximisation is commonly perceived to be an overriding aim is the pharmaceutical industry. The table below reports revenues and profits earned by the ten largest pharmaceutical companies in the USA in 2002:

Rank	Company	Revenue (US$ millions)	Profits (US$ millions)
1	Merck	51 790	7 150
2	Johnson and Johnson	36 298	6 597
3	Pfizer	35 281	9 126
4	Bristol-Myers Squibb	18 119	1 895
5	Abbott Laboratories	17 685	2 794
6	Pharmacia	16 929	597
7	Wyeth	14 584	4 447
8	Eli Lilly	11 078	2 708
9	Schering-Plough	10 180	1 974
10	Amgen	5 523	–1 392
Total		217 467	35 896

Source: Public Citizen (2003).

The figures indicate that a profit of 16.5 cents was made on every dollar of revenue, which is substantially higher than the Fortune 500 company median of 3.1 cents per dollar of revenue.

4.2 STRUCTURE, CONDUCT AND PERFORMANCE IN THE HEALTH CARE INDUSTRY

A useful framework within which to analyse supply is the *structure–conduct–performance paradigm*. The dominant features of market structure are how many firms are in the industry and how big each firm's market share is, though there are other issues such as how similar the goods or services that the firms produce are and whether it is easy or difficult for new firms to enter the market. Conduct refers to how firms behave, which is in part determined by market structure and mainly concerns whether they compete or collude, covering issues such as their goals, pricing policies, investment and marketing strategies. Performance mainly relates to how efficient firms and industries are, either from a private or social point of view.

One of the key issues of structure is the degree of competition in markets, since that may have a large influence on the way in which firms have to operate. For example, hospitals operating in a highly competitive environment – the structure – may conduct their activities differently from those with few or no competitors. The more competitive the environment, the more aggressively the hospital may behave, in terms of pricing and the quality of care, in order to attract patients and raise revenue. This conduct will in turn influence performance, which may be measured in a variety of dimensions such as the number of patients treated, revenue earned, or profitability.

We can obtain an indication of how competitive a market is by observing the number of firms in the market: the greater the number of firms, the more competitive the market is likely to be. However, this is not an ideal measure because it does not account for the concentration of services within the firms in the market. For example, there may be many firms in the market, but if the largest provides 90% of total output the level of competition may not be as great as a market that has only two firms, each of which has 50% of the market.

A useful measure of market concentration, and therefore competition, is the Hirschman–Herfindahl index (*HHI*). This is a measure of market concentration in areas served by providers, and is based on the market shares of all providers within a given market:

$$HHI = \sum_{i=1}^{n} s_i^2 \tag{4.1}$$

where s_i is the market share in percent of provider i and n is the number of providers in the market. *HHI* can take values ranging from close to zero (low concentration; much competition) to 10 000 (high concentration; no competition). If, for example, $n = 1$, there is a single provider in the market (a monopoly) with 100% of the market share. In this case $HHI = 10\,000$. Conversely, if n is very large, indicating many different competing providers, and if each of these has a market share that is very close to 0%, then HHI will be very close to zero. Box 4.2 illustrates the use of the HHI to measure the degree of competition for hospital services in New Zealand.

This link between the number of firms and the degree of competitive pressure is not straightforward, however, because a firm's behaviour, even if it is the only one in the market – a monopoly – may be influenced by potential competitors as much as existing ones. The *theory of contestable markets* says that what is crucial to the conduct of

---

Box 4.2 Market concentration of hospital services in New Zealand

In 1993 the health care system in New Zealand was reformed in an attempt to introduce competition into the health care market and to encourage providers to provide health care at least cost. A quasi-market for hospital services was created in which the roles of purchasers and providers were separated. This enabled the purchasers (regional health authorities, RHAs) to award contracts to providers (publicly owned Crown Health Enterprises, CHEs, and private providers) on a contestable basis, and forced providers to compete with each other for contracts on a competitive basis.

Ashton and Press (1997) measured the degree of market concentration for hospital services before and after the implementation of the reforms. They state that 'while there is no guarantee that competitive markets will have low levels of market concentration and vice versa it is expected that unconcentrated markets are potentially more competitive. Market concentration measures therefore some indication of the potential for competition in a market.'

Market concentration was measured using the Hirschman–Herfindahl Index (HHI) in two stages:

1. The HHI for each geographical area j, $HHIa_j$, was computed based on the market shares of all providers serving that area.

2. The degree of market concentration for each CHE was calculated as the weighted mean $HHIa_j$ across areas treated by each CHE ($HHIc_j$).

The authors report for 1992 the percentage of providers with values for $HHIc_j$ less than 1800. Markets with a small proportion of providers below this value are considered to be highly concentrated. A range of values was reported using various inclusion rules for market areas:

Procedure	% of providers
Cataract removal	5.88–64.71
Prostatectomy	5.56–27.78
Knee replacement	14.29–42.86
Hip replacement	31.82–45.45
Tonsillectomy	45.00–65.00
Coronary artery bypass graft	60.00–80.00
Angioplasty	71.43

It was concluded that in 1992 there was a high degree of concentration for all seven procedures. Market concentration was highest for cataract removals and prostatectomies and lowest for angioplasties and coronary artery bypass grafts. The authors also present results for 1994, which identified only small changes in $HHIc_j$, with no discernible trends. On the basis of their findings, the authors conclude that markets for publicly funded hospital services in New Zealand are highly concentrated, and there was little change in the degree of competitiveness in the market immediately following the introduction of the quasi-market for hospital services.

firms is not the actual degree of competition they face in the market, but the threat of competition. The threat of competition is greater when the costs of entry and exit into the market are lower. At the extreme the cost of entry and exit might be zero. In this case the market is said to be perfectly contestable. Under these circumstances, even a monopoly provider is forced to adopt the same pricing and output strategy as it would if faced with a very large number of competitors.

Contestable markets are likely to arise when there are no sunk costs incurred on entering a market. Sunk costs are costs that cannot be transferred to another use, and therefore they cannot be recouped if the firm leaves the market. The existence of sunk costs implies that exit from the market is not costless, which reduces the contestability of the market. If market entry and exit is costless, and if this can be accomplished speedily, then firms may engage in hit-and-run competition where they enter the market for short period to earn high profits quickly and then exit again. Box 4.3 considers the role of contestability in health care in the NHS in the UK.

There are, however, other factors as well as market structure that affect a firm's conduct and therefore performance. Ownership is important, because it may affect the firm's objectives. For example, state-owned hospitals may have very different aims and objectives, and conduct themselves very differently from privately owned hospitals, even those with objectives other than profit maximisation. There is a wide range of ownership arrangements in health care, probably greater than in any other sector of the

Box 4.3 Contestability in health care

An example of contestable markets in health care is in the market for hospital services where contracts between payers and hospital providers are negotiated locally. In the local area there may be a single monopoly hospital. Building a new hospital is clearly a very costly exercise, and exiting the market will also be costly because much of the capital equipment in a hospital cannot be transferred to other uses: there are substantial sunk costs. However, entry into any one particular geographically defined market may be achieved at relatively low cost for a hospital already in existence but located in another area. In this case there is an option for the local payer to contract with a non-local provider if necessary. The market is therefore contestable because there is a threat of competition from non-local providers.

The use of contestability in this way to retain some degree of competition in the market for hospital services in the NHS in the UK was highlighted by Ham (1996) in an editorial in the *British Medical Journal*. He argued that:

> The middle way between planning and competition is a path called contestability. This recognises that health care requires cooperation between purchasers and providers and the capacity to plan developments on a long-term basis. At the same time, it is based on the premise that performance may stagnate unless there are sufficient incentives to bring about continuous improvement. [. . .]

> [T]here is the stimulus to improve performance which exists when providers know that purchasers have alternative options. [. . .] It is, however, a quite different approach than competitive tendering for clinical services, which would expose providers to the rigours of the market on a regular basis.

> The essence of contestability is that planning and competition should be used together, with contracts moving only when other means of improving performance have failed. Put another way, in a contestable health service it is the possibility that contracts may move that creates an incentive within the system, rather than the actual movement of contracts.

economy. Examples are sole proprietors, such as single-handed GPs, dentists and pharmacists; partnerships, such as GP practice partnerships; privately owned or publicly quoted companies, such as those in the pharmaceutical and insurance industries; cooperatives, owned by consumers or workers; public sector ownership, the dominant form in many countries for hospitals; and medical charities.

The impact of ownership on a firm's objectives is moderated by another factor, which is that under many forms of ownership owners are not managers. So, in establishing what the goals of a firm might be, we must ask: whose objectives are we referring to? In Section 4.4, we will discuss some theories of the firm that explicitly recognise that owners and managers are two distinct groups with different aims and objectives. The answer to the question of whose objectives count is further complicated in the health care industry, where in addition to managers and owners there is a third group that can influence the objectives of the firm, namely health care professionals.

A further factor affecting the market structure, and also therefore a firm's conduct and performance, is market definition. This is important because it determines the number of competitors and whether they supply differentiated or unique services. Market definition identifies which buyers and which sellers are included in a market. To define a health care market we need to determine its boundaries, which are defined by the geographical area covered by the market and the range of health care services included in it. For example, suppose a GP practice is located in a small village. If the market is defined as inhabitants of the village only, then the GP practice has no competitors and enjoys a monopoly. However, if the market is defined more widely and included other villages in the surrounding area, each of which has their own GP practice, then the market is larger and more competitive.

We also need to consider the range of products included in a market. For example, in the pharmaceutical industry, what are the product boundaries in the market for cholesterol-modifying drugs? Suppose a firm is considering developing a new drug within the class of drugs known as statins. The new drug may have an effect similar to but different from those of the other statins already available. How should the market be defined, and what competitors would the company have for its new product if it decided to develop it? One option might be to say that since the new product is different, even if only slightly, from current products, that there are no competitors and the company will enjoy a monopoly. This would be unrealistic, however, and it might be more appropriate to define the market in terms of the other statins currently available (for example, simvastatin, pravastatin, rosuvastatin, fluvastatin, atorvastatin). A further option would be to define the market even more broadly to include other cholesterol-modifying products, such as the anion-exchange resins (colestipol, cholestyramine), the fibrates (bezafibrate, ciprofibrate, fenofibrate and gemfibrozil), and nicotinic acid. Once it has decided who its competitors are, the company can then calculate the expected profits from the new drug and decide whether to proceed with the investment.

In the next section we take a closer look at traditional economic theories of the firm based on profit maximisation. We then examine in more detail why this objective may not always be an appropriate assumption in health care and investigate theories based on alternative objectives.

4.3 PROFIT MAXIMISATION MODELS

As suggested, traditional theories of the firm are based on the assumption that firms aim to maximise profits. Within this, there are different models depending on the market structure that is assumed. The following market characteristics are particularly important in defining market structure:

- the number of competitors;
- the freedom with which competitors can enter the market;
- whether the different firms in the market sell homogenous, differentiated or unique health care products.

Using these, we can distinguish between four categories of market structure. Table 4.2 shows the key features of these and their applicability in health care. Three of them – perfect competition, monopoly and monopolistic competition – are specific models of market behaviour; the fourth – oligopoly – is actually a compendium term for many different models.

Before describing these models, we will discuss the mathematics of profit maximisation, since that is common to all of the models.

Table 4.2 Alternative market structures

Market structure	Number of firms in the market	Entry into market	Type of product	Control of provider over price	Examples
Perfect competition	Many	Unrestricted	Undifferentiated	None	Internet pharmacies
Monopolistic competition	Many	Unrestricted	Differentiated	Some	Medicines in the medium and long run
Oligopoly	Few	Restricted	Either undifferentiated or differentiated	Some	Hospital services; GP services; private health insurance
Monopoly	One	Restricted/ completely blocked	Unique	Considerable	Medicines in the short run; public health insurance

4.3.1 How Firms Maximise Profits

The level of profit that firms make depends on the difference between the revenue that they receive from sales of their product and the cost of producing it. Revenue is dependent on price and the quantity sold at that price via the demand function analysed in Chapter 2; cost is dependent on the quantity of output via the cost function of Chapter 3. From this information about demand and supply conditions, it is possible to determine the prices and quantities that will maximise the firm's profits and how much profit will be made at that level. To illustrate the key concepts, we will use the example of a profit-maximising fertility clinic which provides services in the form of assisted reproduction techniques (ARTs). It has a large enough share of the local market for ARTs to be aware that it faces a downward-sloping demand curve.

The total profit earned by the clinic (π) is its *total revenue* (*TR*) minus its total costs of production (*TC*):

$$\pi = TR - TC \tag{4.2}$$

The total revenue earned by the clinic is its total earnings from the provision of a specific quantity of ARTs provided, Q:

$$TR = p_Q \times Q \tag{4.3}$$

where p_Q is the price at which ARTs are sold. For example, if the clinic sells 500 ARTs per month at a price of £1700 per ART, $TR = £850\,000$. *Average revenue* (*AR*) is the amount the clinic earns per ART, calculated as

$$AR = \frac{TR}{Q} \tag{4.4}$$

Because we assume that the clinic sells each ART at the same price, *AR* is obviously equal to price. For example, if total revenue is £850 000 and the clinic provides 500 units of ART per month then its average revenue is £1700. However, the same is not true of *marginal revenue* (*MR*), which is the additional revenue derived from providing an additional ART:

$$MR = \frac{\Delta TR}{\Delta Q} \tag{4.5}$$

The reason that this is not necessarily equal to price is that there is a downward-sloping demand curve, and therefore the price is likely to change if the amount sold changes. For example, the clinic could employ an additional nurse and provide an additional 100 ARTs per month, giving a total of 600. However, to sell the additional 100 ARTs the price must be reduced to £1600 each. The total revenue of the clinic is now

£1600 × 600 = £960 000, an increase of £110 000, so MR is £110 000/100 = £1100. This is less than AR, because the increase in revenue due to increased numbers of ARTs sold is offset by a lower AR for every ART sold. In the extreme, MR can even become negative if the revenue increase is outweighed by the loss due to the fall in AR.

How does revenue vary with the number of ARTs provided by the clinic? We can define an AR curve relating AR to quantity. AR is equal to price, so the AR curve is the same as the demand curve, which is the curve relating price to quantity. The MR curve will also be downward sloping, but steeper than the AR curve, reflecting the fact that MR is less than AR at every quantity provided.

We can also define a TR curve which, with downward-sloping AR and MR curves, first rises and then falls. The turning point occurs at the point at which MR becomes negative. The second, third and fourth columns of Table 4.3 gives some illustrative figures for revenue, and the curves derived from these are shown in Figure 4.1.

The next stage is to combine this information with that on cost, which is also related to output: it is assumed in this that all output produced is sold. The fifth, sixth and seventh columns of Table 4.3 show total, average and marginal costs at different levels of output. The key data are plotted in Figure 4.2. In the top graph, we can see that π, which is found by subtracting TC from TR, is maximised at the output where the distance between the TR and TC curves is greatest. In the data this occurs at around 600 ARTs per month. Notice that at this point the slopes of the TR and TC curves, which are, respectively, MR and MC, are equal. This is shown in the bottom graph. Mathematically, it must be the case that the profit-maximising level of output, Q_π, occurs where $MC = MR$.

Table 4.3 Revenue, costs and profits for a profit-maximising fertility clinic providing assisted reproduction techniques (ARTs) with some market power in setting prices

ARTs per month	AR	TR	MR	TC	AC	MC	TR–TC	MR–MC
0		0		100 000			−100 000	
100	2100	210 000	2100	250 000	2500	1500	−40 000	600
200	2000	400 000	1900	360 000	1800	1100	40 000	800
300	1900	570 000	1700	440 000	1466	800	130 000	900
400	1800	720 000	1500	510 000	1275	700	210 000	800
500	1700	850 000	1300	590 000	1180	800	260 000	500
600	1600	960 000	1100	690 000	1150	1000	270 000	100
700	1500	1 050 000	900	810 000	1157	1200	240 000	−300
800	1400	1 120 000	700	950 000	1187	1400	170 000	−700
900	1300	1 170 000	500	1 110 000	1233	1600	60 000	−1100
1000	1200	1 200 000	300	1 290 000	1290	1800	−90 000	−1500

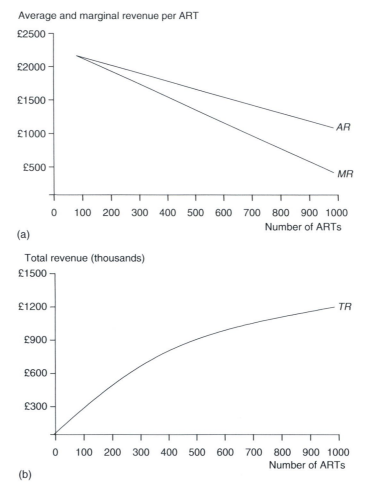

Figure 4.1 Revenue curves for a fertility clinic with some market power in setting prices.

The size of profit at this level of output can be demonstrated using the *AR* and *AC* curves, as in Figure 4.3. The profit per unit of output is the difference between *AR* and *AC* at the specified level of output. This is multiplied by the level of output to give total profits, shown as the shaded area.

The owners of the fertility clinic must earn a minimum amount of profit to prevent them from closing down their business and doing something else instead. This minimum profit can be thought of as a cost because, like other costs, it has to be recovered if the

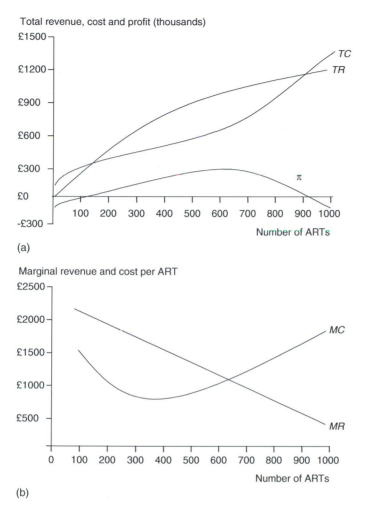

⭕ **Figure 4.2 Revenue, cost and profit curves for a fertility clinic with some market power in setting prices.**

clinic is to continue to operate. It is an opportunity cost because it represents the profit that the owners could have earned in the next-best business alternative; if they can earn more than this running the fertility clinic, they will stay in business. This profit is referred to as normal profit and, because it is counted as a cost it is included in the cost curves. Another type of profit is called supernormal profit. This is profit earned over and above normal profit. Since normal profit is included in the costs, the profit shown by the shaded area in Figure 4.3 is supernormal profit.

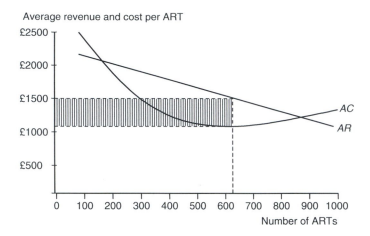

Figure 4.3 Using average revenue and average cost curves to show total profit.

4.3.2 Perfect Competition

Of all of the market models based on profit maximisation, the perfect competition model is the most important, because of its strong conclusions, and also the most controversial, for the same reason. It is based on the following assumptions:

- a large number of sellers in the market;
- freedom of entry into and exit from the market;
- product homogeneity;
- perfect knowledge.

The first three assumptions imply that an individual firm in the market has no control over the price it charges for its goods. This is known as being a *price taker*.

In explaining these ideas and their consequences, we will discuss internet pharmacies as an example of a perfectly competitive market. In recent years there has been a massive increase in the number of companies selling products over the internet, including pharmaceuticals. Many of these companies sell their products directly to consumers, which is known as 'B2C' (business-to-consumers) e-commerce. For consumers, buying medicines from internet pharmacies can have many benefits, including access to drugs for the disabled or homebound, the convenience of being able to shop at any time of the day or night, privacy and anonymity for those who do not want to discuss their medical condition in a public place, and lower prices. However, internet pharmacies also create potential problems. Essentially, three types of internet pharmacy exist: pharmacies that only fill prescriptions written by a patient's doctor; pharmacies that charge for a 'cyber-consultation' and whose cyber-doctor then writes a prescription; and pharmacies that dispense prescription drugs without a physician's prescription (Rost, 2000). The latter two types of pharmacies can present significant problems, such as the sale of unapproved new drugs, sale of prescription drugs without a valid prescription, or marketing of products with fraudulent health claims, as well as bypassing the legitimate health care professional/patient interaction.

One of the benefits of internet pharmacies is that they are making the market for pharmaceuticals more competitive. We can see this by analysing the assumptions of perfect competition in more detail.

The market has a large number of firms so that each individual firm supplies only a small proportion of the total output provided in the market. The implication is that each firm is unable to affect the market price. There are also many buyers, who are also unable to influence the operation of the market. The growth of e-commerce generally has led to many firms selling pharmaceuticals starting up in business online. Since the reach of the Internet is global, companies need to be aware of competitors in the rest of the world and not just regionally or nationally.

In the perfect competition model, there is a distinction between the *short run* and the *long run*, defined by how easy it is for new firms to enter the market and for existing firms to leave it. In the long run there are no barriers to entry or exit and new firms will be attracted into the industry if incumbent firms earn supernormal profits. In the short run freedom of entry and exit is restricted, but only because of the time it takes to start up or close down a firm. Internet companies have lower start-up costs than conventional rivals, because their premises can be smaller with no need for an expensive public 'shop-front', and marketing costs can be relatively low, especially with the use of internet search engines. Lower start-up costs also mean that internet firms have less to lose if the business fails. Therefore, the costs of entry to and exit from the market are lower.

A perfectly competitive industry is defined as a group of firms producing a homogenous – the same – product. The implication of product homogeneity is that buyers are unable to differentiate between the products sold by different firms in the market. While concerns exist surrounding the quality of products bought from internet pharmacies, the products supplied may be just the same as those purchased from other types of pharmacy.

All buyers and sellers in the market have complete knowledge of the conditions in the market. This means that firms are fully aware of market prices, the costs of production, and opportunities for making profits in other markets. Buyers are fully aware of the price, quality and availability of the products in the market. If you buy a product online it is possible to conduct an exhaustive search of suppliers and compare prices for the same product very quickly. This makes price competition more likely.

What Happens in a Perfectly Competitive Market?

The short-run equilibrium in the internet pharmacy market is shown in Figure 4.4. It occurs at price p^* and output Q^*, given by the intersection of the market demand and supply curves. An individual internet pharmacy, as a price taker, must sell its output at price p^*, which is set by the market. As a result, AR is equal to MR and the AR and MR curves are horizontal. At this price the profit-maximising level of pharmaceutical sales, Q_1, is determined by the intersection of the MR and short-run MC curves. The size of the profits earned at this level, which depends on the AR and short-run AC curves, is shown by the shaded area.

In the long run, if businesses in the sector are earning supernormal profits then market supply will increase as new internet pharmacies begin trading and existing businesses increase the scale of their production. The overall effect will be an increase in market supply, as shown in Figure 4.5. At price p_1 firms earn supernormal profit. Therefore total supply in the market increases as the sector supply curve shifts to the right, leading to a fall in the equilibrium market price. Supply will continue to increase, and the price will continue to fall until firms no longer make a profit above the normal level. This is shown in Figure 4.5 at supply curve S_L and price p_L. On this basis, the long-run equilibrium output of the firm is Q_L. Note that no profits above normal are earned at this level of output, since $AR = LAC$.

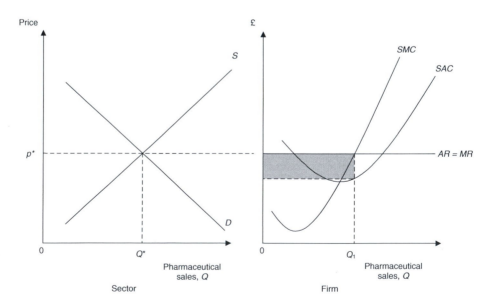

Figure 4.4 Short-run equilibrium in the internet pharmacy sector under perfect competition.

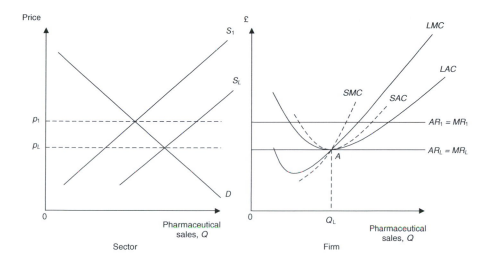

○ **Figure 4.5 Long-run equilibrium in the internet pharmacy sector under perfect competition.**

The condition for the long-run equilibrium of the internet pharmacy market is that LMC is equal to price and LAC:

$$LMC = LAC = p \qquad (4.6)$$

The pharmacy adjusts its size so that it produces the level of output at which LAC is minimised. The long-run equilibrium condition is

$$SAC = SMC = LAC = LMC = p = AR = MR \qquad (4.7)$$

This equilibrium occurs at the bottom of the internet pharmacy's long-run average cost curve at point A. This means that given the current state of technology the firm will in the long run produce its output at the minimum feasible cost. Note also that consumers pay the minimum possible price for their medications, which just covers the marginal cost of production.

4.3.3 Monopoly

A monopoly is a market structure in which there is a single seller of a product. There are no close substitutes for the good sold by the firm, and there are significant barriers to entry. In order for a monopoly to exist there must be barriers to entry for new firms. The main causes of these are as follows.

- The size of the market. This may not be sufficient to support more than one firm. If a monopoly experiences substantial economies of scale, which may only be reaped at large scale levels of production, the industry may be able to support only a single firm. In this case the market creates what is called a natural monopoly, and it is usual for the government to undertake the production of the good or service in order to avoid exploitation of the consumers.

- Lower costs for an established firm. Over and above the barriers caused by economies of scale, an established monopoly may have lower costs of production. This is because the existing firm is likely to have developed specialised production and marketing skills, to be aware of the most efficient production techniques, to have knowledge of the cheapest and most reliable suppliers of raw materials, and to have access to cheaper finance.

- Ownership of raw materials or exclusive knowledge of production techniques.

- Patent rights for a product or production process.

- Government licensing limiting the number of firms operating in a geographical area.

- Limit-pricing policy. This occurs when the existing firm adopts a pricing policy aimed at preventing new firms from entering the industry. This can be combined with other strategies to create barriers to new competition, including intense advertising and continuous product differentiation, all of which render entry for new firms unattractive.

- Brand loyalty. This might arise if the firm produces a unique product that consumers associate with the brand.

In health care, an example of a monopoly is a patented drug. The justification for laws permitting such a monopoly is that developing new medicines is a lengthy and expensive process. It has been estimated in the UK by the Association of British Pharmaceutical Industry that the development process can typically take 10–12 years to go from drug discovery to full-scale manufacture, at a cost of £350 million to the company (ABPI, 2006). For these reasons, as soon as a promising new compound is found, the pharmaceutical company applies for a patent. This gives the company intellectual property rights over the compound for a period of 20 years. Effectively, the company is granted monopoly power in producing the compound, and other companies are legally prevented from producing it. This acts as a reward for the expenditure incurred in bringing the medicine to market, and to encourage future research and development.

What Happens in a Monopoly Market?

We will use the example of a patent for a new type of drug that means there is a single pharmaceutical company in the market. As a result, the demand curve for the company is the demand curve for the whole market. Because the monopolist sells a unique

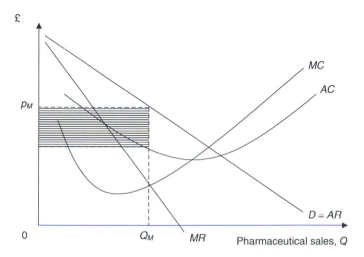

● **Figure 4.6 Monopoly equilibrium for a pharmaceutical company with a medicine under patent in the short run.**

product, it can raise its price and consumers have no alternative product to buy. They must either buy the product at the higher price or not buy it at all. Thus the firm is a *price maker*, and has the downward-sloping AR and MR curves analysed in Section 4.3.1. Combining the cost and revenue curves produces the profit-maximising equilibrium shown in Figure 4.6.

The level of sales assuming profit maximisation is Q_M, which is the point at which $MC = MR$. The price of the medicine at this output is p_M and the level of profits earned by the monopolistic company at this price and output is given by the shaded area.

Since there are barriers to entry in the form of patent laws, the supernormal profit earned by the monopolist will not be eroded in the long run as with perfect competition, though they may be competed away once the patent expires. The only difference between short-run and long-run equilibrium under monopoly is that the long-run equilibrium occurs at the intersection of the MR and long-run marginal cost (LMC) curves. Thus, in contrast with long-run equilibrium under perfect competition, the firm does not operate at the minimum average cost, and price is greater than marginal cost.

4.3.4 Monopolistic Competition

Perfect competition and monopoly are the extremes of possible models based on profit maximisation. While we have identified some examples, few health care markets can in reality be classified as being perfectly competitive or as pure monopolies. This is because most providers of health care do compete with other providers and also have some degree of market power: competition is imperfect. Monopolistic competition is one type of imperfect competition. This model retains the idea from perfect competition that, at least in the long run, there may be many firms in the market, but relaxes the assumption that all products are identical, giving it some monopoly power. It is based on the following assumptions.

- There are many firms competing in the market.
- There are no barriers to entry and exit.
- Each firm sells a differentiated product from its competitors.

The effect of product differentiation is that the firm has some discretion in the determination of price. The firm is not a price taker because its product is sufficiently different from its rivals to allow it to raise its price without losing all its customers. Each firm, however, faces competition from close substitutes in the market, and so this discretion in setting the price is limited. Product differentiation gives rise to a demand curve for the firm that is downward sloping with a corresponding downward-sloping *MR* curve.

What Happens in a Monopolistically Competitive Market?

The market for medicines has some features that conform to monopolistic competition. Figure 4.7 shows the product life cycle for a typical medicine. The general trend is that

Figure 4.7 Product life-cycle for a medicine with and without a class effect. Adapted from the Association of British Pharmaceutical Industry (www.abpi.org).

once it is produced it takes some time for the medicine to build up sales and achieve market share. For example, in its early years the pharmaceutical company needs to persuade doctors to prescribe and use the medicine. Once the medicine has become established it then enters a period of maturity when most profits are made. Finally, as the medicine loses patent protection, generic products enter the market at a lower cost. Sales of the original medicine start to fall because there are close substitutes available.

The bold line shows the life-cycle for a product with no competitor until the patent for the molecule expires. The dotted line shows the product life-cycle assuming there is a similar but differentiated competitor that is available before the patent expires. An example would be a medicine that is based on a different molecule but that falls within the same therapeutic class, such as the statins which we mentioned earlier. While each statin is different, and hence each is awarded a separate patent, all of these drugs fall in the same class and are used similarly by doctors. In this case the market meets the definition of monopolistic competition.

In the period before the medicine's patent expires, but while there are competitors, the profit-maximising equilibrium of the pharmaceutical company is as shown in Figure 4.8. The profit maximising level of output is Q_{MC}, which is sold at price p_{MC}. The diagram is similar to the equilibrium for a monopolist except the demand curve is more price elastic due to the competition from close substitutes in the same therapeutic class. The amount of supernormal profit earned by the firm is given by the shaded area. This

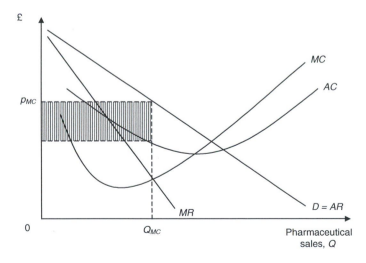

Figure 4.8 Monopolistic competition equilibrium for a pharmaceutical company with a medicine under patent with similar products.

depends on the degree of market power held by the firm, and hence on the slope and position of the demand curve.

When the patent expires in the long run new firms will enter the market and start to provide generic copies of the medicine. This will have two effects:

- The demand curve for the company will shift to the left as the demand for its product contracts.

- The demand curve will also become more price elastic as the number of competitor products increases.

The demand curve will continue to shift leftwards and become flatter as long as super-normal profits are being earned. The long-run equilibrium is reached when the firm earns no profit. At this point there is no incentive for new firms to enter. This is shown in Figure 4.9. The demand curve shifts until it is tangential to the LAC curve. The equilibrium output, given by the intersection of the LMC and MR_L curves, is Q_{MC} and the corresponding price is p_{PC}. At Q_{MC}, AR_L and LAC are equal which means that the firm only earns normal profit.

In reality, under monopolistic competition profits may persist in the long run. This is because firms may use non-price competition to maintain an advantage over their rivals.

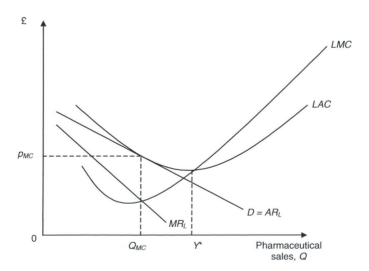

⬤ Figure 4.9 Monopolistic competition equilibrium for a pharmaceutical company with a medicine after patent expiry.

This has two components: product development and product promotion. Product development is concerned with developing a product that will be in high demand and that will have a price-inelastic demand curve owing to a lack of close substitutes. The aim of product promotion, such as advertising, is to shift the demand curve for the product to the right and to make it more price inelastic. The former is achieved by using product promotion to inform potential consumers of the product's existence and availability. The latter is achieved by using product promotion to enhance brand loyalty, thus causing barriers to entry.

In the market for medicines, when a medicine loses patent protection the pharmaceutical company will usually implement marketing strategies to boost sales, including improving the product and re-launching the 'new improved' version. One powerful way the company can try to reduce the loss of sales is to establish a very strong brand identity. Consumers will then stick with the product they know because they do not regard the alternatives as effective substitutes. An effective way of branding is to make the product look unique. This could be achieved by making the tablet or capsule a special shape. Also it can be coloured or produced with special graphics printed on it. A distinctive use of unusual shapes and colours make it more difficult for competitors to produce a medicine that the consumer might confuse with the original. Names, logos and packaging are all protected by registering them as trademarks. This makes direct copying illegal.

4.3.5 Oligopoly

Oligopoly is another type of imperfect competition in which, compared with monopolistic competition, there are fewer firms but more than one, and entry for new firms is restricted. Firms may sell either the same or differentiated products, and they have some control over price. This is the dominant market structure in many health care markets, for example for hospital services and for GP services, where there are more likely to be a few rather than many providers competing with one another, and where the providers have some market power. There are numerous models of oligopoly and we therefore give only a brief overview. The main features of an oligopolistic market are:

- There are barriers to entry for new firms. The main causes of these are the same as for a monopoly.
- Firms are mutually dependent. Each firm will be affected by the decisions made by its rivals. This interdependence arises because there are relatively few firms in the industry producing products that are close substitutes. Firms recognise that the other firms in the industry will be affected by their pricing and output decisions and will react to them. Accordingly, they will attempt to predict the reactions and incorporate these predictions into the decision-making process.

These two characteristics lead to one of two behaviours by oligopolistic firms. Either firms will collude in order to limit competition among themselves or they will compete with each other in order to gain, for example, a larger share of the profits earned by the industry for themselves. The first is called a collusive oligopoly and the second a non-collusive oligopoly.

Collusive oligopoly is more likely to arise when:

- There are only a small number of firms, who are well known to each other.
- There is no government intervention to prevent collusion.
- There is a dominant firm that the other firms will follow.
- Entry into the market by other firms is severely restricted, which makes it unlikely that new firms will enter the market and disrupt the collusion process.
- Firms are prepared to share information about their costs and production methods with each other.

Collusion between firms may be formal or informal (tacit). A formal collusive agreement is called a cartel. A cartel attempts to act like a monopoly, behaving as if it is a single firm. Informal or tacit collusion will usually take the form of price leadership, where firms follow the price set either by a dominant firm in the market (dominant firm price leadership), or by a firm considered to be a reliable gauge of market conditions (barometric firm price leadership).

In the case of a non-collusive oligopoly there is no agreement, formal or informal, between firms. With no collusion, price competition between firms is more likely to occur. Because each firm will be affected by its rivals' decisions – that is because the firms are interdependent – non-collusive oligopolists are required to devise strategies that take into account the impact of their actions on the behaviour of their rivals. Therefore, the behaviour of a firm will depend on how it believes its rivals will react to its policies.

Box 4.4 shows an example of how oligopoly operates in the hospital sector in the United States.

4.3.6 Game Theory

A key feature of oligopolistic markets is that the actions of one firm are dependent on and react to the decisions of other firms. This interdependence is a key feature of oligopoly. Game theory – mathematical models of decision-making that explicitly take into account interdependence – is therefore particularly useful in explaining firms' behaviour in this context. Game theory provides insights into a large number of economic phenomena, but we will here look at it only as an analysis of how firms behave

Box 4.4 Oligopoly in the health care industry: hospitals versus insurance companies

Oligopoly Watch (2003) report a case of oligopoly in the US health care market arising from tensions between insurance companies and hospitals. In Boston in the USA there was an oligopolistic market for health insurance, with three insurance companies controlling around 75% of the market. This gave the insurance companies considerable power over the local hospitals when they tried to obtain discounts in the fees they paid to the hospitals for the services they provided. In response, the hospitals combined to form an oligopoly to increase their market power:

> The most significant [development] was the December 1993 merger of two of the most prestigious [hospitals], Massachusetts General Hospital and Brigham & Women's – a combination that created Partners HealthCare System Inc. 'In order to increase your leverage in a competitive environment, you need to increase your size,' says Richard Averbuch, a spokesman for the Massachusetts Hospital Association. In 1993, metropolitan Boston had 34 separate hospital networks. Today it has 12 – and life for patients is already changing.

> In the fall of 2000, nearly 200 000 of the 900 000 members of one big HMO, Tufts Health Plan, got letters announcing that they would no longer be able to use hospitals or physicians affiliated with Partners. The reason: Tufts wouldn't accept the fee increases Partners wanted. The uproar was enormous. Without Partners, says James Roosevelt Jr., Tufts general counsel, so many HMO members and their employers 'would drop us that we wouldn't have a health network anymore.' Even people who never used Partners' doctors wanted the option of going to the top teaching hospitals in town in case of a serious illness. 'They would switch their health plan even though that wasn't where they normally went for their medical care.' Tufts went back to Partners, and agreed to a fee increase of 30% over three years.'

[*Wall Street Journal* 25/02/2002]

in markets. Specifically, it is used to examine a firm's optimal pricing and output strategy, which depends on its views about how its rivals will behave in a non-collusive oligopoly. In game theory, oligopolistic or other firms are treated as players in a game where for each action by one player another player may choose among several alternative reactions, either at the same time or in a subsequent time period. The actions of rivals are uncertain, yet it may be possible under certain circumstances to choose a strategy that will maximise the firm's expected gain after making due allowance for the effects of rivals' probable actions.

		Hospital A's pricing alternatives	
		Price = £1000	Price = £900
Hospital B's pricing alternatives	Price = £1000	Hospital A's profit = £10 million Hospital B's profit = £9 million	Hospital A's profit = £11 million Hospital B's profit = £5 million
	Price = £900	Hospital A's profit = £8 million Hospital B's profit = £7 million	Hospital A's profit = £9 million Hospital B's profit = £8 million

Figure 4.10 Profits under different scenarios in a non-collusive oligopoly.

To illustrate how game theory might be used to devise an optimal pricing strategy in order to maximise profits, assume a local hospital market with two hospitals, A and B. The health care services provided by the hospitals are close substitutes, so that if their prices differ the hospital with the lower price will supply the larger share of the market. Suppose the hospitals charge one of two prices for each unit of health care they provide: £900 or £1000. Each hospital has a different cost structure, and the total number of patients treated in the market is affected by the combined action of both hospitals. This means that the profit gains of one hospital will not necessarily be equal to the reduction in profit of the other hospital.

Figure 4.10 shows a *payoff matrix* for the two hospitals. Both decide what price to charge for their services, taking into account their rival's possible strategy. Let us assume that each hospital will choose its pricing strategy expecting its rival to take the worst possible action from the hospital's point of view. In this case if hospital A sets its price at £1000 its minimum profit is £8 million, and if sets it at £900 the minimum profit is £9 million. Among these two minima the hospital will rationally choose the largest, which results from the lower price. This is known as a *maximin* strategy, because it maximises the minimum outcome.

For hospital B, if it chooses a price of £1000 the minimum profit it earns is £5 million. If it chooses a price of £900 its minimum profit is £7 million. The maximin strategy for hospital B is therefore also to charge the lower price. If both hospitals have a maximin strategy, then the outcome will be that both will charge the lower price.

Maximin is not the only possible strategy, however. The hospitals could, for example, adopt an optimistic approach that assumes its rival will act in the best possible way from the point of view of the hospital and again choose the pricing policy that will maximise its profits. This is called a *maximax* strategy. Under this strategy, hospital A will again charge £900 since its profits will be maximised at £11 million if hospital B acts favourably by setting a price of £1000. Hospital A will in fact always adopt a low price strategy, since this will maximise its profits whatever price hospital B charges. This is called a *dominant strategy*. However, hospital B does not have a dominant strategy. Under maximax, it will charge a price of £1000, hoping that hospital A will also charge £1000, and thereby maximise its profits at £9 million.

In the next period, the hospitals will review their decisions. In the maximax case, hospital A has a dominant strategy, so it will conclude that it should maintain its price. Hospital B, however, will observe that if hospital A maintains its low price, hospital B will make greater profits if it also charges a low price. If it does change its policy, hospital B's profit will rise to £8 million and hospital A's profits will fall to £9 million. This produces the same pricing policies for the two hospitals as for the maximin case and therefore the same profit outcomes.

Given that both hospitals charge the low price, neither hospital has any incentive unilaterally to change its strategy, if it believes that the other hospital will not change its strategy. Hospital A's profits would fall from £9 million to £8 million if it increased its prices and B did not; hospital B's profits would similarly fall from £8 million to £5 million if it increased its prices and hospital A did not. Unless there is some change in market conditions, the hospitals will continue with their pricing policies and the outcomes will remain the same in subsequent periods. This is known as a *Nash equilibrium* and is a key concept in game theory.

Note that in this case the equilibrium position puts both hospitals in a worse situation compared to a strategy where they both charge a high price, since they both earn a lower level of profit. Nevertheless, it is a stable position, and unless they collude it will persist. A special case of this, where both players have a dominant strategy that leads to an outcome that is worse for both of them than some other pair of strategies, is called a *prisoner's dilemma*. This is named after an example invented by the mathematician A. W. Tucker, of two prisoners interrogated separately about a crime. They both have an incentive to confess, because whatever their accomplice does, they will receive a lower sentence for giving evidence for the prosecution than if they had not confessed. However, if neither prisoner confesses they will both receive a lower sentence than if they both confess.

Many other scenarios can be analysed using game theory, and the outcome need not necessarily be profit maximisation. It could be some other measure consistent with objectives other than profit maximisation such as number of patients treated, or number of staff employed. One advantage of the theory is that each player does not need to know the actual response its rivals will make to a particular strategy it adopts. However, it does need to know what the outcomes will be for each possible response to its actions.

4.4 GOALS OTHER THAN PROFIT MAXIMISATION

Firms may not seek to maximise their profits. One possibility is that a firm depends for its existence on making profits, but does not aim to maximise them. Another is that the firm actually does not intend to make any profits at all, but to break even. Both of these occur in health care, but the second is particularly widespread.

One reason why for-profit health care firms may not aim to maximise profits is that the owners of the firm may not have complete managerial control. The owners of many health care provider units such as hospitals are not usually the managers who make pricing and output decisions on a day-to-day basis. The owners may want to maximise profit, but this view will not necessarily be shared by the manager. Williamson (1963) argued that the separation of ownership and management in firms means that managers have some freedom in setting and achieving the goals within firms. As a consequence, managers will set goals which maximise their own utility. Factors that are likely to affect a manager's utility function include their salary, power, prestige, job security and working conditions.

Therefore, while profit maximisation might be important, it is unlikely to be the only goal for managers. More realistically, firms are likely to be profit satisficers rather than profit maximisers, aiming for a target level of profit rather than the maximum level. This occurs when managers aim to ensure that sufficient profits are earned to satisfy the owners, conditional on the other factors in the managerial utility function.

As mentioned earlier the separation of ownership and management in the health care industry is further complicated by the presence of a third group of influential decision-makers who have autonomy over patient care decisions: health care professionals. They are likely to set goals that maximise their patients' utility functions, assuming perfect agency, or their own utility function, assuming imperfect agency. Either way, it is unlikely that profit maximisation will be the most important goal. Some but not all of the arguments of the managerial utility function are also likely to feature in the utility functions of health care professionals, with an important addition – patient utility. Hence, the likelihood of profit maximisation as a goal of the health care firm will diminish as the power of health care professionals becomes greater.

Many health care providers, particularly those that are publicly owned, are unlikely to be profit maximisers. This can stem from imperfect knowledge on the part of consumers, as discussed in Chapter 2, which results in an agency relationship between patients and health care professionals. Under these circumstances health care providers are instead more likely to favour goals such as utility maximisation, where utility is a function of the quality and quantity of health care services provided.

Even with the public provision of health care and health care professionals as key decision makers it is likely that some health care programmes will be perceived as being under-provided from the viewpoint of some sections of the population. These sections – special interest groups – might comprise patients, family and friends of patients, health care professionals or others who perceive that certain types of health care are under-provided both privately by the market and publicly by the government. These groups may themselves become involved in the provision of health care, and for reasons that are unrelated to profit. An example is the National Childbirth Trust in the UK, which is a registered charity launched in 1957 with the aim of providing information about pregnancy, childbirth and early parenthood to mothers and fathers. This is achieved via a number of routes including antenatal classes, breastfeeding counselling and mother-and-baby groups.

Taken together, the above factors suggest that goals other than profit maximisation are likely to be pursued by many firms in the health care sector. The consequences of this for hospital care in the USA are explored in Box 4.5.

We now examine various alternatives to profit maximisation models.

Box 4.5 The impact of hospital ownership in the United States

Hospitals in the USA are of three basic ownership types: public; private not-for-profit; and private for-profit. Public hospitals are owned by the government at the federal, state, or local level to serve the military, rural residents, the poor, and/or the uninsured. Private not-for-profit hospitals are owned by a voluntary board of trustees to provide hospital care to paying patients and charitable services to the poor. Private for-profit hospitals are owned by private investors to make profits by serving patients in return for a fee. The key features of the three hospital types are shown in Table 4.4.

Most hospitals are in the private not-for-profit category. These include independent-owned community hospitals, church-owned hospitals, and industry-owned hospitals. Publicly owned hospitals form the second largest category, which consists primarily of government-owned county and city hospitals. In the smallest category are the private for-profit hospitals owned by corporations or partnerships and operated for a profit. While there was a general decline in the number of hospitals and beds in not-for-profit hospitals between 1990 and 1997, in the for-profit sector, the number of hospitals increased by 6%, and the number of beds increased by 14%.

The impact of hospital ownership type on a range of key outcomes is generally ambiguous, with different studies yielding conflicting results. Baker *et al.* (2000) provide a comprehensive review of the literature, analysing the impact of hospital ownership on hospital performance and outcomes. Their analysis is based on a review of 69 studies published between 1985 and 1999. The main findings are:

1. The degree of competition faced by the hospital is the major factor that influences the availability of services and pricing behaviour.

2. Administrative costs are increasing in all three hospital types.

3. For-profit hospitals are more profitable than private not-for-profit and public hospitals. Most of the research on profitability, revenue, and cost differences among hospitals is based on data gathered before 1990. Generally, these studies report that, although costs are similar, for-profit hospitals charge more for their services and are more profitable than private not-for-profit and public hospitals.

4. The association between hospital ownership and patient outcomes is unclear. The evidence is mixed and inconclusive regarding the impact of hospital ownership on access to care, morbidity, mortality, and adverse events.

5. Hospital ownership status has an impact on the type and degree of community benefits: public and private not-for-profit hospitals provide better access to care, a wider range of amount and type of health services, and greater involvement in professional education.

4.4.1 Growth Maximisation

Marris (1963) suggested an alternative to the traditional theory of the firm, based on growth maximisation, that may apply in some sectors of the health care industry. Under this model the firm aims to maximise the rate of growth taking into account various

Table 4.4 Hospital ownership types in the United States

Characteristic	Ownership type		
	Public	Private	
		Not-for-profit	For-profit
Owners	The public	Stakeholders	Shareholders
Key decision makers	Government officials	Volunteer Board of Trustees	Paid corporate officers
Goals	Multiple (for example equity, efficiency), often conflicting, frequently change with elections	Ambiguous	Profit maximisation
Sources of finance	Government, fees	Patient fees and charges, donations	Patient fees and charges
Market	Determined by government	Mission-driven, determined by clients	Determined by people's buying power
Number of hospitals			
1990	1767	3191	749
1997	1530	3000	797
% change	−14	−6	+6
Number of beds (000s)			
1990	1055	657	101
1997	699	591	115
% change	−34	−10	+14

Adapted from Baker *et al.* (2000).

indicators of size such as the demand for the products of the firm, output, revenue and market share.

The justification for this goal is that while there may be a separation of ownership and management in firms, both with different goals, growth maximisation is correlated with profit maximisation – the goal of the owners of the firm – and other factors such as salaries, prestige and job security, which are likely to feature in the managerial utility function. Thus growth maximisation can result in the joint maximisation of both the owners' and managers' utility.

Growth in the size of the firm may be achieved either by internal expansion or by merger and acquisition. A merger is the result of a mutual agreement by two firms to come together. An acquisition arises when a firm succeeds in a takeover bid for another

Table 4.5 Mergers and takeovers related to Pfizer and GlaxoSmithKline

Company 1	Company 2	Date	New company name
Pfizer			
Parke-Davis	Warner-Lambert	Early 1970s	Parke-Davis, Warner-Lambert
Pharmacia	Upjohn	1995	Pharmacia and Upjohn
Pfizer	Warner-Lambert	2000	Pfizer
Pharmacia and Upjohn	Monsanto	2000	Pharmacia Corp.
Pfizer	Pharmacia Corp.	2003	Pfizer
Pfizer	Pharmacia	2003	Pfizer
GlaxoSmithKline			
Beecham Group	SmithKline Beckman Corporation	1989	Smithkline Beecham
Glaxo	Wellcome	1995	Glaxo Wellcome
Glaxo Wellcome	Smithkline Beecham	2000	GlaxoSmithKline

Source: Royal Pharmaceutical Society of Great Britain (2004).

firm. Mergers and takeovers in the pharmaceutical industry are common. Two of the largest pharmaceutical companies are Pfizer and GlaxoSmithKline. Table 4.5 illustrates how these companies have grown in recent years as a result of mergers and takeovers.

4.4.2 Behavioural Theories of the Firm

Cyert and March (1963) developed a generalised behavioural theory of the firm which recognised that firms are generally not simple organisational units with a single goal and a single decision-making unit, but instead are complex organisational units with multiple goals and multiple decision-making units of different groups that are involved in the activities of the firm. These groups include managers, owners, workers and customers. Each group has its own demands on the firm, which may conflict with the demands of other groups. For example, managers want high salaries, power and prestige; owners want high profits; workers want high wages and good working conditions; customers want low prices and good-quality goods and services.

In this model the top management ultimately sets the goals of the firm through continuous bargaining with the different groups. The goals take the form of aspirations, or wishes, rather than strict maximising constraints.

Using this information the firm in a behavioural theory of the firm does not aim to maximise a single dimension of output, but instead seeks to attain a satisfactory performance in all relevant output dimensions in order to satisfy the wishes of the different groups. Hence the firm is a satisficing organisation rather than a maximising one, aiming to achieve satisfactory power, prestige and salaries for managers, a satisfactory level of profits for the owners, satisfactory wages and working conditions for workers, and satisfactory low prices and quality for consumers.

An example of this type of model in the hospital sector is given by Harris (1977). He argues that a hospital comprises two separate firms or divisions – the medical staff and the administration. Medical staff comprise the 'demand division', and are responsible for patient care decisions and ordering services from the administration – the 'supply division' – who are referred to as ancillary departments. These comprise laboratory, radiology, pharmacy and intensive care services, operating rooms, and the blood bank, plus other general services such as laundry and admissions services. The firms interact with each other in a complex way, and have their own managers, objectives, pricing strategies and constraints. The goals for the medical staff are related to patient outcomes, in their role as agents for patients, and their individual earnings. The administration is likely to be more concerned with maximising profit, maximising the utilisation of services and avoiding spare capacity.

4.4.3 Utility Maximisation

Newhouse (1970) developed a model of utility maximisation, which was applied to the hospital sector. In the Newhouse model the hospital aims to maximise both the quantity and quality of services provided subject to a financial constraint. Quality and quantity are each measured in a single dimension and together comprise the output of the hospital. The quantity of services Q could be measured in several ways, such as:

• the number of patients treated;
• the number of patient-days of care provided.

Quality k could be measured in number of dimensions including:

• the expertise of the clinical staff;
• the status and prestige of the institution and its staff;
• the quality of care, as viewed by patients;
• the quality of care as measured using routinely collected statistics, for example readmission rates, length of stay, incidence of hospital-acquired infection;
• the non-health care characteristics of provision, for example the quality of the food and the décor.

The assumptions underpinning the Newhouse model are as follows.

1. The demand for the hospital's services are a function of, *inter alia*, the quality of the care provided: $D = AR = f_1(k)$, where higher values of k denote higher quality. Other things held constant, k has a positive impact on demand.

2. The average costs of production are also determined, *inter alia*, by the quality of services provided: $AC = f_2(k)$. Other things held constant, k has a positive impact on AC.

3. The financial constraint faced by the hospital is that it breaks even. This occurs at the level of output Q at which $AR(k) = AC(k)$. If there is more than one point where this holds, the hospital will choose the one with the highest output.

4. The utility of the hospital U is a function of the quality and quantity of services provided: $U = f_3(k,Q)$.

The outcome of the model is shown in Figure 4.11. Given quality level k_1 with corresponding cost and revenue curves $AC(k_1)$ and $D(k_1) = AR(k_1)$, the equilibrium (break even) level of output for the firm is Q_1. Depending on the relative movement of the cost and revenue curves as k changes the new equilibrium quantity might be higher or lower than Q_1. Figure 4.11 shows a situation in which, following an increase in quality from k_1 to k_2, the relative impact on the cost and revenue curves is such that Q_2 lies to the right of Q_1. Eventually, however, it is likely that increases in quality produce an increase in demand that is more than offset by the increase in costs. This is shown in the figure by an increase in quality from k_2 to k_3, which results in a new equilibrium output Q_3, which lies to the left of Q_2.

As k runs over its feasible range of values this will produce a locus of equilibrium quality–quantity combinations. This yields the quality–quantity frontier as shown by FF in Figure 4.12, which at lower levels of quality, below k_B, shows a positive relation-

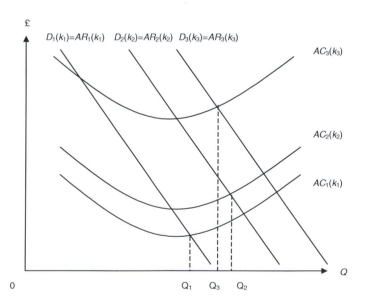

Figure 4.11 Quantity–quality trade-off in the Newhouse model.

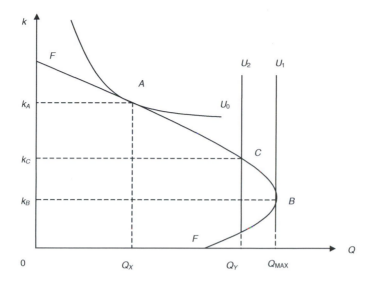

Figure 4.12 Quantity–quality frontier derived from the Newhouse model.

ship between k and Q. Eventually, at higher levels of k, above k_B, the frontier bends back, demonstrating a quality–quantity trade-off.

The decision maker will choose a combination of quality and quantity on the frontier that maximises their utility. This will occur where the frontier is tangential to the highest attainable indifference curve. Assuming that $U = f(k,Q)$ and that there is a diminishing marginal rate of substitution between k and Q, then the indifference curves will have the usual shape, as shown for example by U_0. In this case the equilibrium quality and quantity combination is k_A and Q_X, which occurs at point A.

If the goal of the decision maker is quantity maximisation, subject to a break-even financial constraint, then $U = f(Q)$ and the decision maker's indifference curves will be vertical. The equilibrium of the firm is given by point B in Figure 4.12, which is on the highest attainable indifference curve U_1, with level of output Q_{MAX} at quality k_B.

An alternative case, also discussed by Newhouse, is where quality, rather than being a component of the decision maker's utility function, instead acts as a constraint. Thus, the maximisation problem facing the firm is to maximise output subject to a given level of quality and breaking even. Suppose the minimum acceptable quality is k_C. In this case the equilibrium position is given by the intersection of the highest attainable indifference curve U_2 and FF, yielding an equilibrium quantity Q_Y.

4.4.4 Maximising Net Income per Physician

In the final model in this section we consider Pauly and Redisch's (1973) model of the hospital as a physicians' cooperative. In this model physicians have control over the operation of the hospital and act as net-income-maximising agents in which role they seek to maximise the sum of money incomes of all staff physicians. The model assumes that the group of attending staff physicians have control of the hospital and are able to appropriate the profits earned. Net income per physician is given by:

$$\frac{\pi}{M} = \frac{p_Q Q - p_x x}{M} = \frac{TR - TC}{M} \qquad (4.8)$$

where π is the total profit earned by the hospital, which is appropriated by the physician staff M. p_Q is the price of the output Q and p_x is the price of the non-physician inputs x. Figure 4.13 depicts the equilibrium of the hospital under these conditions. The physician supply curve S_0 is upward sloping. The net income per physician curve passes through the origin – net income per physician is zero with no physicians employed – and is inverted U-shaped. This is due to the relative shape of the cost and revenue curves assuming the hospital is a price taker, and is based on the shape of the π curve in Figure 4.2.

Under a 'closed staff' situation in which the existing physicians determine the number of physicians employed, the optimal physician staff size is M^*, where the net income per physician is $(\pi/M)_{MAX}$. Alternatively under an 'open staff' system, where any physician who chooses to do so can become a member of staff, the equilibrium number of physicians employed is M_1 with net income per physician given by $(\pi/M)_S$. This arises from the intersection of the net income per physician curve and S_0.

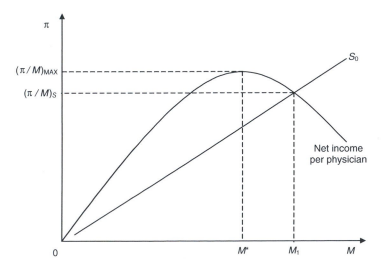

Figure 4.13 Maximising net income per physician.

SUMMARY

1. A firm is an economic unit that produces and sells goods, such as medical equipment, or services, such as dental care or health insurance. An industry is a collection of firms that sell similar products, such as the pharmaceutical, insurance or hospital industries. An industry is the supply side of the market. To analyse the supply of health care we therefore need to develop a theory of the firm, which can be used to explain how health care firms behave.

2. A useful framework with which to analyse supply of health care is the structure–conduct–performance paradigm. Supply is strongly influenced by the market structure within which the health care firm operates. For example, a hospital operating in a highly competitive environment – the structure – may conduct its activities differently from a hospital with few or no competitors. The more competitive the environment the more aggressive the hospital may have to be to attract patients and revenue in terms of the price of services provided and the quality of care. This conduct will in turn influence the performance of the hospital, which may be measured in a variety of dimensions such as the number of patients treated, revenue earned, or profitability.

3. Economists traditionally assume that firms aim to maximise their profits. The profit-maximising level of output occurs where the marginal revenue received from sales of the product equals the marginal cost of producing it. There are different models of profit maximisation depending on the market structure that is assumed.

4. Market structure is commonly defined by the number of competitors in the market, the freedom with which competitors can enter the market, and whether the different firms in the market sell homogenous, differentiated or unique health care products. Common market structures are perfect competition, monopoly, monopolistic competition and oligopoly.

5. In perfect competition there are a large number of sellers in the market, there is freedom of entry and exit, firms sell undifferentiated products and there is perfect knowledge. Firms have no control over price: they are price takers. The implication of these assumptions is that in the long run firms will earn zero profits. An example of perfect competition in the health care industry is given by internet pharmacies.

6. A monopoly is a market structure in which there is a single seller of a product. There are no close substitutes for the good sold by the firm, and there are significant barriers to entry. An example of monopoly in the health care industry is given by the market for medicines: pharmaceutical

companies, having found a new compound, are granted a patent that gives them monopoly power to produce the compound. This acts as a reward for the expenditure incurred in bringing the medicine to market, and to encourage future research and development.

7. With monopolistic competition there are many firms competing in the market, there are no barriers to entry and exit and each firm sells a differentiated product from its competitors. An example of monopolistic competition in the health care industry is given by the market for medicines when a product's patent may not have expired but there may be competitors producing a product in the same class of drugs; hence the firm will have some market power. In the long run after the patent has expired new firms will enter the market and start to provide generic copies of the medicine.

8. Oligopoly occurs where there are only a few firms in an industry, but more than one, and entry for new firms is restricted. An important characteristic of oligopolies is that firms are mutually dependent. Oligopolistic firms may collude in order to limit competition among themselves, and this collusion may be formal (in which case the oligopoly is called a cartel) or informal. In the case of a non-collusive oligopoly there is no agreement, formal or informal, between firms. With no collusion, price competition between firms is more likely to occur. Owing to the interdependence of oligopolistic firms, non-collusive oligopolists are required to devise strategies that take into account the impact of their actions on the behaviour of their rivals. An example of oligopoly in the health care industry is hospitals acting collusively in order to increase their revenue.

9. Game theory is an approach that can be used to examine the optimal strategy of the firm, depending on its views about how its rivals will behave, in a non-collusive oligopoly.

10. While the goal of profit maximisation may be applied to some sectors of the health care industry (for example, the pharmaceutical industry), goals other than profit maximisation also rise. This is due to the divorce of ownership and managerial control, autonomy of health care professionals, and special interest groups.

11. Common alternatives to profit maximisation in the health care industry include: growth maximisation; behavioural theories, which recognise that health care firms are complex organisational units with multiple goals and multiple decision-making units; utility maximisation, where utility is a function of the quality and quantity of care provided; and maximising net income per physician.

Chapter 5

Markets, Market Failure and the Role of Government in Health Care

5.1 INTRODUCTION

In Chapter 4 we examined the way in which the characteristics of a market – such as the number of firms and barriers to entry – influence the way in which firms behave with respect to pricing decisions, output and profits. This chapter extends our consideration of markets by asking the questions: Are private health care markets competitive? Do health care markets produce allocations of resources that are efficient? What might go wrong – and what should the government do about it?

We begin with a simple proof of one of the most fundamental conclusions of economics: where markets are 'perfectly' competitive, this will lead to efficiency in the allocation of resources. We then consider whether the assumptions underpinning the perfectly competitive model apply to health care markets in the real world, and the characteristics of health care that often lead to market failure. We conclude with an examination of the rationale for government involvement in the production and consumption of health care to address these market failures.

5.2 USING PERFECTLY COMPETITIVE MARKETS TO ALLOCATE RESOURCES

5.2.1 Equilibrium in Competitive Markets

In Chapter 1 we introduced a simple model of the demand for and supply of health care in private markets. The key characteristic of perfectly competitive markets is that they tend towards equilibrium. Mismatches between demand and supply are resolved by market forces – shortages of goods and services will drive prices up; unsold goods will result in prices falling. Prices result from interactions between buyers and sellers, and will adjust to clear the market.

We noted in Chapter 1 that health care is an economic good: it is scarce relative to our wants for it. The problem of scarcity means that we are faced with difficult questions concerning what health care to produce, how to produce it, and who should receive it. If health care were bought and sold in competitive markets, those questions would be resolved as follows.

- First, through the price system, the market decides which types of health care and how much of each type should be produced, by finding the price at which the quantity demanded equals the quantity supplied. The equilibrium quantity corresponding to this price defines how much of each health care programme should be provided.

- Secondly, health care will be supplied by health care providers willing to supply health care at the equilibrium price. In an effort to maximise profits, health care will be produced in a manner which is technically efficient.

- Thirdly, health care will be purchased by those consumers who are willing and able to pay the equilibrium price. Access to health care is based on ability to pay and not other factors such as need.

5.2.2 The Efficiency of Competitive Markets

One of the most important results of economic theory is the *First Fundamental Theorem of Welfare Economics*. This states that a perfectly competitive market will generate an allocation of resources that is efficient for society. This idea is the basis for many economists' arguments in favour of free markets and minimal government interference.

We must first define what we mean by social efficiency, since this is a much broader concept than those of technical and productive efficiency that we have used so far. Economists have a very specific definition of social efficiency, which rests on the concepts of Pareto improvements and Pareto optimality. These will be explained in more detail in Chapter 8. Briefly, if it were possible to make changes to the health care system, for example in terms of the health care programmes provided, and these changes benefited some people without making anyone else worse off, then this is described as a *Pareto improvement*. When all Pareto improvements have been made – when it is not possible to make anyone better off without making someone else *worse* off – then the health care system is said to be Pareto efficient, Pareto optimal or socially efficient.

Under certain assumptions, perfectly competitive health care markets, in the precise sense described in Chapter 4, can be shown to be Pareto efficient. In a competitive market, a rational health care decision maker, for example a consumer or a health care provider, will choose to undertake an activity, for example to purchase or provide health care, so long as the gain from doing so exceeds the extra cost incurred. That is, an activity is worth doing as long as the private marginal benefit to the decision maker (PMB) exceeds the private marginal cost (PMC), or $PMB > PMC$. If the gain is less than the extra cost ($PMB < PMC$), then the decision maker should undertake less of the activity. If the gain equals the extra costs ($PMB = PMC$), then they have achieved private efficiency; the decision maker is acting efficiently in his or her own private interest.

By analogy, Pareto efficiency will be achieved when the gains to society rather than individual decision makers (the social marginal benefit, SMB) are equal to the marginal cost to society (SMC). In a perfectly competitive health care market, *private* efficiency is achieved, in the sense that individuals choose quantities of health care that maximise their utility, and firms produce quantities of health care that maximise their profits, and price adjusts to ensure equilibrium. So long as there are no 'spillover effects' – costs or benefits to society over and above those experienced by individual consumers and producers in the market transaction, discussed in Section 5.3.1 – then the private marginal benefits will exactly equal the marginal *social* benefits ($PMB = SMB$) and the private marginal costs equal the marginal *social* costs ($PMC = SMC$). In these circumstances, the market equilibrium will be socially optimal, that is, Pareto efficient.

We will explain the efficiency of competitive health care markets using the example of the internet pharmacy market, first discussed in Chapter 4 as an example of perfect competition. This proof proceeds in four stages.

First, the privately efficient level of consumption of internet pharmaceuticals is achieved when $MU \, (= PMB) = p^C \, (= PMC)$. Under perfect competition, the marginal benefit to a consumer from consuming pharmaceuticals is their marginal utility (MU) from consumption. MU falls as consumption increases; that is, there is diminishing marginal utility of consumption. The marginal cost of consumption is the price the consumer

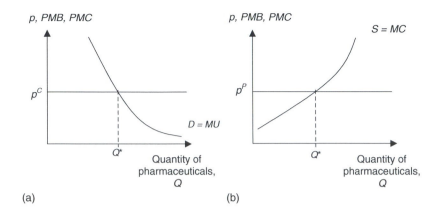

◯ **Figure 5.1 Private efficiency of the internet pharmacy market.**

has to pay, p^C, which is set by the market. A rational consumer will continue to consume pharmaceuticals up to the point where $MU = p^C$, or where the private marginal benefit from consumption equals the private marginal cost. This is shown by Q^* in Figure 5.1(a). Note that the MU curve tells us how much of the good is consumed at each price; it is therefore also the demand curve (that is, $D = MU$).

Secondly, the privately efficient level of production of internet pharmaceuticals is achieved when p^P (= PMB) = MC (= PMC). The marginal benefit to the internet pharmacy from providing pharmaceuticals is its marginal revenue, which under perfect competition is equal to the price p^P. The internet pharmacy is a price taker and so price is set by the market. Under profit maximisation, the pharmacy will supply pharmaceuticals up to the point where p^P (= MR) = MC, or where the private marginal benefit from production equals the private marginal cost. This is shown by Q^* in Figure 5.1(b). Note that the MC curve tells us how much of the good is supplied at each price; it is therefore also the supply curve (that is, $S = MC$).

Thirdly, private efficiency is achieved when $MU = p = MC$. Under perfect competition, this is achieved because the same price is faced by both the consumers and producers in the internet pharmacy market. In other words, $p^C = p^P$ and the privately efficient levels of consumption and production are achieved simultaneously.

Fourthly, Pareto efficiency is achieved when $SMB = MU = P = MC = SMC$. With no externalities, private marginal benefits will equal the marginal social benefits ($PMB = SMB$) and private marginal costs will equal the marginal social costs ($PMC = SMC$). Therefore, the equilibrium prices and quantities yielded by a competitive market will also be Pareto efficient.

5.3 MARKET FAILURE IN HEALTH CARE

In the real world most health care markets rarely if ever achieve Pareto efficiency. For example, the First Fundamental Theorem relies crucially on markets being perfectly competitive – and *any* breakdown in the underlying assumptions, such as freedom of market entry and perfect information, will lead to distortions in prices, quantities and social inefficiency. The term 'market failure' is used to cover all circumstances in which Pareto efficiency is not achieved by the market. The main causes of market failure in health care are discussed below.

5.3.1 Externalities

Externalities, or spillover effects, are costs and benefit incurred in the consumption or production of goods and services that are not borne by the individual consumer or producer. The spillover effects may be positive or negative. Whenever other members of society are affected beneficially by a spillover effect, there are said to be external benefits. Whenever other members of society are affected adversely there are external costs.

Health care markets will not lead to Pareto efficiency if there are externalities. To see this, note that the full marginal cost to society from the production or consumption of health care (SMC) is equal to the private marginal cost (PMC) plus the marginal external cost (MEC), and the marginal benefit to society (SMB) is equal to the private marginal benefit (PMB) plus the marginal external benefit (MEB). Hence, consumption and production decisions made in the market, which are based on private marginal costs and benefits, will not equal social marginal costs and benefits if the marginal external cost or the marginal external benefit is non-zero.

There are four types of externality:

- **External costs of production ($MEC > 0$; $SMC > PMC$)**
  These might arise if, for example, a firm producing pharmaceuticals dumps its waste in a river, or pollutes the air. In this case the pollution caused by the firm will impose a positive external cost on society.

- **External benefits of production ($MEC < 0$; $SMC < PMC$)**
  Imagine a pharmaceutical firm undertaking research to identify a new compound to bring to market. If a promising compound is discovered this will eventually lead to the publication of scientific papers on the pharmacological properties of the compound. Patent laws prevent other firms from copying the product, but the research undertaken by the firm may identify useful avenues of research for other firms. In

this case there may be external benefits of production arising from the research and development process.

- **External costs of consumption (*MEB* < 0; *SMB* < *PMB*)**
  The consumption of cigarettes and alcohol may lead to external costs of consumption. In addition to their effects on individual health, their consumption may also have negative effects on the rest of society in terms of passive smoking and antisocial behaviour.

- **External benefits of consumption (*MEB* > 0; *SMB* > *PMB*)**
  Public health interventions such as vaccines may have external benefits of consumption. This is because they can have a direct health benefit on others by reducing their chances of ill health.

Whenever there are external benefits there will be too little consumed or produced in the market. Whenever there are external costs there will be too much consumed or produced in the market.

5.3.2 Caring Externalities

The sorts of externalities described above are sometimes referred to as 'selfish externalities'. An *altruistic* external benefit of consumption – sometimes referred to as the 'caring externality' – may arise from knowing that an individual is receiving the health care they need, even if this does not impact directly on the health of others.

This is shown in Figure 5.2. An individual, when determining what level of health care to consume, will choose the level at which the private marginal benefit from consump-

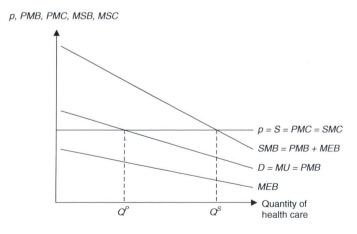

Figure 5.2 Pareto inefficiency with caring externalities.

tion equals the private marginal cost, given by Q^P. However, there are external benefits of consumption, in other words there is a positive marginal external benefit, to others from the consumption of health care by the individual, shown by the line MEB ($MEB > 0$). Hence, the marginal benefits to society from consumption are given by the line SMB, which lies above PMB, and the socially efficient level of consumption that occurs where $SMB = SMC$ is Q^S, which is greater than Q^P.

The existence of caring externalities in Sweden is discussed in Box 5.1.

Box 5.1 Caring externalities in Sweden

Jacobsson *et al.* (2005) investigated the existence of caring externalities and examined whether the magnitude of the marginal external benefit of caring externalities is related to the severity of the illness being treated. They posit a utility function given by

$$U_i = U(C_i, H_1, H_2, \ldots, H_n)$$

where U_i is the utility of individual i, C is the consumption of goods and services, H is health (which is itself a function of health care received) and there are $i = 1, 2, \ldots, n$ individuals in society. The caring externality arises when the utility of individual i is an increasing function of the health care received by other individuals in society.

To investigate the magnitude of the marginal external benefit of the caring externality, the authors conducted a survey of 180 individuals in Sweden. Respondents were first asked how much they would be willing to pay in Swedish Kronor (SEK) for a cure from each of six ill-health states ranging from slight illness to completely disabled (the ill health categories were slight (= 1), moderate, considerable, severe, very severe, completely disabled (= 7)). This was called the 'internal preference group'. They were then asked how much they would be willing to pay for an improvement in the ill-health state of someone else, even if it meant the respondent must relinquish some of their own health care consumption for the benefit of the other person. This was called the 'caring externality group'. To analyse the magnitude of internal preferences and caring externalities in relation to the degree of severity of the health states, a ratio was constructed in which the sum of the willingness to pay for the two mildest health states was divided by the sum of the willingness to pay for the two most severe health states.

Caring externalities were found in all health states, with 52% of respondents willing to pay to cure another individual in the mildest ill-health state. The mean value of the willingness to pay for the improvement in health of another individual was smaller than that for the respondent in all ill-health states. Across all respondents the mild/severe ratio for the internal preference group was 0.30, while for the caring externality group it was 0.17. The authors suggest that this indicates 'a higher evaluation related to level of severity for caring externalities than for internal preferences'.

This study gives an indication of the size of the marginal external benefit associated with caring externalities. The authors conclude: 'Our results indicate that more attention and resources should be directed to severe health states, as compared to mild health states, than advocated by internal preferences in order to obtain more efficient resource allocation in the health care sector.'

5.3.3 Market Power

Whenever there is a monopoly or imperfect competition, the market will fail to allocate goods and services in a Pareto efficient manner: the monopoly will provide less health care than is Pareto efficient. This is shown in Figure 5.3 in the case of a patented drug. As discussed in Chapter 4, a monopolist producing a patented drug is a price maker and has a downward sloping $D = AR$ curve, and therefore the MR curve is below the AR curve. A profit-maximising monopolist will produce at the level of output where

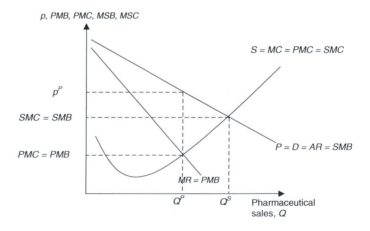

Figure 5.3 Pareto inefficiency with market power.

$MR = MC$, at output level Q^P in the figure. The Pareto efficient output is at the higher level Q^S, which occurs where $MSB = MSC$.

5.3.4 Public Goods

Public goods are goods which may be jointly consumed by everyone. Specifically, public goods have two characteristics. The first is non-rivalry. This means that the consumption of a good or service by one individual will not prevent the consumption of the same good or service by others. The implication is that non-rival goods tend to have large marginal external benefits, which makes them socially very desirable but privately unprofitable to provide. Commonly used examples of non-rival goods include street lighting and pavements.

The second characteristic is non-excludability. This means that it is not possible to provide a good or service to one individual without letting others also consume it; that is, it is not possible to exclude others from consumption. Non-excludability means that individuals can obtain the benefits from consuming a non-excludable good without paying for it. Because there is no incentive for individuals to pay for non-excludable goods, this leads to a *free-rider problem*, in which individuals are unwilling to pay for goods and services if other individuals will pay for them. The implication is that if everyone free-rides then the good or service will not be provided at all, which might lead to a loss to society. Examples of non-excludable goods include lighthouses and national defence.

When goods have these two features they will not be provided in a private market. This is because there is no incentive for private individuals to pay for them. Generally, public goods are provided by the government, who then compels individuals to finance their provision via some form of taxation. Note the distinction between public goods, which are non-rival and non-excludable goods or services, and publicly provided goods, which are goods or services that are provided by the government.

Pareto efficiency requires that the level of provision of a public good occurs where $SMB = SMC$. Since public goods are jointly consumed, the marginal social benefit is obtained by summing the private marginal benefits across all individuals. This is shown in Figure 5.4. Two individuals, Dave (D) and Nancy (N), receive private marginal benefits from consumption given by PMB^D and PMB^N, respectively. The marginal social benefit is the vertical sum of the private marginal benefits at each level of consumption, SMB. With a marginal social cost given by SMC the socially efficient level of provision is Q^S. At this level of provision, Dave would be prepared to pay price p^D and Nancy would be prepared to pay p^N, which equates the private marginal cost with the private marginal benefits at the socially efficient level for each individual. Because both Dave and Nancy will free-ride, the good will be provided by the government and they will both be compelled to pay the price via taxation.

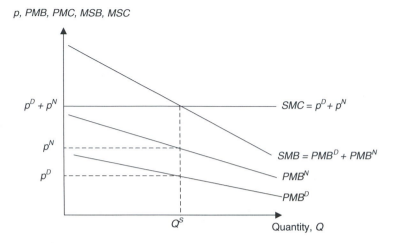

○ **Figure 5.4 Pareto inefficiency with public goods.**

Most health care products and services are *not* public goods because they are both rival and excludable. The receipt of health care by one person will usually prevent another person from consuming that same health care – for example, one person's admission to a hospital bed prevents another from using it. Further, those who do not pay for health care could usually be excluded from consuming it. However, there are some health care programmes that do have public good properties. An example is public health measures aimed at preventing the spread of bird flu – see Box 5.2.

5.3.5 Information Imperfections

Market failure also arises in health care due to imperfect information. These arise in health care due to uncertainty and to imperfect knowledge.

Certainty in health care markets implies that buyers know exactly what health care they wish to consume, when they want to consume it, and how they can obtain it. Certainty is required for Pareto efficiency because consumers need to know the quantity of health care they would like to demand and providers need to know the quantity of health care to provide. If consumers have certainty, they are able to budget their finances in order to be able to afford their consumption. With uncertainty, a market is unable to function properly because consumers and producers do not know how much of a good to demand and supply. They are therefore unable to equate the private marginal benefits of consumption with the private marginal costs.

There is certainty in the market for many of goods and services. For instance, in the market for chocolate bars, individuals know which items they would like to purchase.

Box 5.2 Public goods in health care: preventing a bird flu pandemic

Like humans, birds are susceptible to flu. There are currently 15 known types of bird flu, and the type currently causing concern is strain H5N1, which can be fatal in humans. Bird flu spreads via migratory birds, which can then pass it on to domestic birds, and then on to humans. It was thought only to infect birds until the first human cases were confirmed in Hong Kong in 1997. Humans catch the disease by being in close contact with live infected birds: the birds excrete the virus in their faeces, which then dry and become pulverised, and are then inhaled.

By February 2007, the World Health Organization (WHO) confirmed 272 cases of H5N1 in humans worldwide, which have resulted in 166 deaths. If the virus mutates and gains the ability to pass between humans, experts predict there may be between 2 million and 50 million deaths worldwide.

A variety of public health measures have been taken to try to stop the spread of bird flu. The WHO has devised a rapid-response plan to detect and contain a global flu pandemic (WHO, 2005). Millions of farmyard birds have been culled, and millions more have been vaccinated and confined indoors where they are less likely to be contaminated by migratory birds. Regions where the disease has been found have been quarantined and some countries have banned imports of live birds and poultry products.

These measures have public good aspects. With the imposition of controls, the protection provided is non-rival in the sense that if one individual is protected then others are also protected. It is also non-excludable in that it is not possible to exclude people in a region from being protected, and individuals who do not pay for the protection privately cannot be excluded from receiving it.

Also, it is possible for individuals to predict when they would like to buy chocolate bars and how they can obtain them. The assumption of certainty may also hold for certain aspects of health care. For example, pregnancies may be planned and it is possible to predict the timing of a birth and the cost of health care services required. Therefore, consumers of maternity services will know how much health care to demand, and providers know how much health care to supply. However, the consumption of the majority of health care services cannot be planned in this way. This is because illness and deteriorations in health are often sudden and unexpected. Therefore, there is uncertainty in the market and the demand for health care cannot be predicted in advance.

While the uncertainty surrounding the demand for health care certainly implies that markets may not allocate health care resources in a Pareto efficient manner, the problem of uncertainty can be addressed with the introduction of health insurance. The subject of health insurance and the various effects that insurance has on the demand and supply for health care services are discussed in Chapter 6.

Unless consumers and producers are well informed, they may take actions that are not in their best interests; they will be unable to equate private marginal benefits of consumption and production with the private marginal costs, and therefore private efficiency (and so Pareto efficiency) is unlikely to be achieved.

The assumption of perfect knowledge on the part of consumers means that they are aware of their health status and of all the options open to them to maintain or improve their health. Although this may be the case for some illnesses, it is clearly not the case for the majority. Therefore, the market for health care is characterised by imperfect knowledge. Unfortunately, perfect knowledge is especially important in the market for health care since making the wrong decision may have much more serious consequences than the decision whether or not to, say, consume a chocolate bar.

The fact that there is imperfect knowledge in health care does not necessarily undermine the usefulness of health care markets, because individuals are able to seek the help of suitably qualified and knowledgeable health care professionals whose job is to provide expert advice on health and health care: health care providers are available to provide the information that individuals need to formulate health care consumption decisions. Hence health care providers find themselves placed in the position of offering expert advice to consumers about health care. However, the same providers also supply health care and receive revenue from the services they provide. Therefore, the supplier of health care is in a position to influence the demand for health care, and supply and demand are no longer independent. Consumers of health care may be unable to act free of self-interested advice from health care providers, and the market may fail to provide an efficient level of health care. Issues surrounding the existence and consequences of this problem – physician-induced demand – were discussed in greater detail in Chapter 2.

5.4 GOVERNMENT INTERVENTION IN HEALTH CARE

Governments intervene in the market for health care for two main reasons: because health care markets fail to achieve Pareto efficiency and are inequitable. From a societal perspective it might be viewed that health care should be provided according to need and not ability to pay. The government might therefore become involved directly in the provision of health care in order to ensure greater access for certain population groups, for example low income groups and children, who might otherwise not receive the health care they need. We focus more fully on the issue of equity in health care in Chapter 7, but issues of equity are also relevant to the following discussion.

In the attempt to address these two issues there are several policy instruments that governments might use in the market for health care.

5.4.1 Direct Government Involvement in the Finance and Provision of Health Care

The government might be involved directly in the financing of health care programmes, making the public pay for them via taxation. The government might also provide some forms of health care directly. For example, hospitals might be publicly owned. The government might also be involved in the finance of health care, via the provision of public health insurance, which may be universal or applied to certain population groups. In this case, health care might typically be provided for free or at very low cost at the point of receipt and the public would be required to pay for health care via some form of taxation.

There are various examples from around the world that illustrate these types of involvement. In some European countries hospital care is both financed and provided within a single government-based system; for example in the National Health Service in the UK both the finance and provision of health care are mainly controlled by the government. Primary care in many countries is provided by self-employed general practitioners (private provision) who receive much of their funding from the government (public funding). In the USA, private insurance companies might contract with hospitals of various ownership types. These include publicly owned hospitals, and privately owned not-for-profit and for-profit hospitals. In this case, while the finance of health care is mainly private, health care provision may be public or private. We consider in more detail the role of the government in the finance and provision of health care in Chapter 6.

5.4.2 Taxes and Subsidies

When there are market imperfections Pareto efficiency will not be achieved: marginal social benefit will not equate with marginal social cost. This means that a different level of output would be more socially desirable.

Government can introduce taxes or subsidies to correct these imperfections. Taxes are introduced on activities where the current level of provision in the market is greater

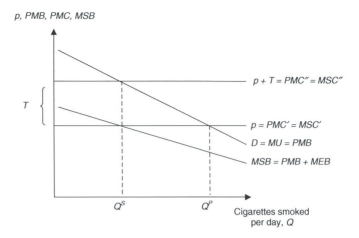

○ **Figure 5.5 Imposing a tax to offset the external costs of consumption associated with cigarette smoking.**

than the Pareto efficient level. Subsidies are introduced when the current level of provision is lower than the socially efficient level.

In the case of externalities, the government could impose a tax equal to the marginal external cost, or grant a subsidy equal to the marginal external benefit. One obvious area in which taxes might be used is to correct for external costs of consumption. For example, cigarette smokers pollute the air for other people but may take no account of this when deciding how much to smoke. Via passive smoking, this can give rise to a consumption externality. The Pareto efficient level of cigarette consumption might be achieved via the introduction of a tax. This is illustrated in Figure 5.5. The Pareto efficient level of cigarette consumption is Q^S, which is given by the intersection of the *SMB* and *SMC'* curves. The privately efficient level of consumption is higher at Q^P. If a tax were levied on each unit of consumption of value equal to T, then the price (and private marginal cost and marginal social cost) would rise to $p + T$ as shown in the figure. The privately efficient level of consumption is now also Q^S.

5.4.3 Regulation

Governments influence the allocation of resources in the health market by establishing rules and regulations. At one extreme the government might prohibit certain activities entirely because of the adverse consequences they have on health: for example, the production and consumption of certain types of recreational drugs. At the other extreme the government might compel individuals to undertake certain activities, judging it is in their best interests to do so: for example, making the wearing of seat belts in cars or the wearing of cycle helmets mandatory. In addition, the government might regulate the market, determining the conditions under which goods and services are produced or consumed. Regulation in health care can take many different forms, including price-setting, quantity-setting and quality controls.

The pharmaceutical market is one of the most heavily regulated markets. Governments intervene in the pharmaceutical market for a number of reasons (Maynard, 1993). First, they intervene in order that only safe, efficacious and cost-effective drugs are marketed. As a consequence of this the process of getting a new drug to market becomes longer and more expensive. Secondly, they reward innovation with patent protection. The goal of patent legislation is to reward the producers of innovative drugs by giving them monopoly power for a period in which they can earn a reasonable reward. In a free market there will be an underinvestment in research and development on pharmaceuticals owing to the free-rider problem. Safety and efficacy legislation erodes the life of patent protection. Thirdly, they impose utilisation policies. A number of policies can be introduced with a view to constraining pharmaceutical expenditure costs, particularly physician prescribing behaviour. These are summarised in Box 5.3. Fourthly, governments intervene in the pharmaceutical market to enhance competition. In Chapter 4 we looked at mergers and acquisitions in the pharmaceutical industry. Governments intervene in the market for medicines to prevent anti-competitive behaviour through these actions. Finally, the government may intervene to regulate prices and profits in the pharmaceutical industry. They may do this because of monopoly power, patient insensitivity to costs in a publicly funded health care system where health care is effectively free at the point of receipt, and physician insensitivity to costs and price changes. Box 5.4 discusses the regulation of profits in the pharmaceutical industry in the UK.

5.4.4 Provision of Information

When market failure in health care arises due to imperfect knowledge, the government may help to correct the problem via the provision of information. An example is the provision of information for the general public on the benefits of certain types of health care. Box 5.5 considers an example of the provision of information by the government to reassure the population about the safety of the MMR vaccine.

5.4.5 Theory of Second Best

If Pareto efficiency is achieved in the health care market, then we say that the first-best allocation of health care resources has been achieved. Unfortunately, in reality health

Box 5.3 Policies to control utilisation in the market for pharmaceuticals

Bloor and Maynard (1993) discuss various policies to control utilisation in the pharmaceutical market.

DEMAND-SIDE POLICIES

1. *User (prescription) charges.* These can be used to raise revenue, to reduce prescribing of unnecessary medicines and to reduce the number of visits to physicians.

SUPPLY-SIDE POLICIES

2. *Generic prescribing.* Prescribing generic alternatives to brand-name drugs becomes possible when a drug goes out of patent. This also encourages price competition. When drugs go out of patent there may be considerable savings to be made by prescribing cheaper generics that are usually produced by companies not involved in research and development. Generic drugs may be different in quality from brand-name drugs and can have different formulations. Brand-name drugs may actually increase in price with the introduction of generics in an attempt to indicate superior quality.

3. *Hospital formularies.* These are preferred prescribing lists used in hospitals with the intention of providing guidelines for effective and cost-effective prescribing (without necessarily dictating which drug to use).

4. *Limited lists.* These are related to hospital formularies. They limit the range of drugs prescribable via the health care system. For example, particular drugs in certain therapeutic areas may not be prescribable (that is they are banned or made available over-the-counter only).

5. *Data on prescribing habits and cost.* The dissemination of data on physician prescribing habits is an attempt to influence prescribing behaviour of doctors by providing information about individual and mean prescribing patterns to increase awareness of costs.

6. *Indicative prescribing budgets.* Indicative prescribing amounts have been set for prescribers based on factors including existing prescribing costs, numbers and ages of patients and local social and epidemiological factors.

Box 5.4 Regulating profits in the pharmaceutical industry in the UK

In Box 4.1 we examined the revenues and profits earned by pharmaceutical companies in the USA. Bloom and van Reenen (1998) discuss various ways in which the government could intervene to regulate prices and profits in the pharmaceutical industry.

RPI–X REGULATION

This is a form of price regulation where in each period drug prices are raised by the rate of inflation (the increase in retail price index [*RPI*]) minus a certain percentage (*X*) to take account of expected increases in efficiency. For example, if the rate of inflation were 5% and if the regulator expected the pharmaceutical company to reduce its costs by 3%, then price rises would be limited at 2%. *RPI-X* regulation provides pharmaceutical companies with incentives to cut production costs, since any cost savings feed directly into profits. With this form of regulation there may be difficulties in setting a value for *X*, and since this method only deals with changes in prices there are difficulties in using it to deal with new products. *RPI-X* regulation also gives no incentive to limit the quantity of medicines supplied by pharmaceutical companies.

RATE OF RETURN REGULATION

This is a form of profit regulation in which prices are limited to levels that give 'acceptable' profits. Typically, this type of regulation is of the form $TR^* = TVC + rK$ where TR^* is the maximum permitted total revenue, TVC is the total variable cost of production, r is the normal rate of return on capital, and K is the value capital. For example, if a pharmaceutical company's TVC were £5 million, K were £25 million and r were judged by the regulatory body to be 6%, then the firm would be permitted to charge a price that would yield a TR^* of £5 m + 0.06 × £25 m = £6.5 million. One disadvantage of rate of return regulation is that it may encourage inefficiency because the regulated company has no incentive to decrease costs.

THERAPEUTIC BENEFIT PRICING

Under this system doctors adjudicate prices on the basis of their therapeutic benefit (for example, higher prices for the most beneficial drugs). This method encourages firms to develop socially beneficial drugs, leading to a positive relationship between profits and social value. Problems arise in determining the price consistent with a specific therapeutic benefit.

INTERNATIONAL REFERENCE PRICING

This involves constructing a weighted average of prices in other countries. It is reliant on the pricing methods used in other countries.

THERAPEUTIC REFERENCE PRICING

This method involves grouping therapeutically similar drugs together and reimbursing only for the cost of the cheapest in the group. This will have the effect of driving prices downwards towards those of the lowest in the group. This method of regulation does not address pricing of monopoly drugs still on patent.

Since 1978, UK NHS expenditures on branded pharmaceuticals have been regulated by the Pharmaceutical Price Regulation Scheme (PPRS), which is based on rate of return regulation. Each year, pharmaceutical companies trading with the NHS are required to make financial returns to the Department of Health, which assesses the company's profitability in relation to targets that are set to ensure that profits and prices are 'reasonable'.

Box 5.5 The MMR vaccine

The MMR vaccine provides immunisation against measles, mumps and rubella. It is commonly given to children at around 1 year of age; a booster dose is usually administered at 3 to 5 years of age. The MMR vaccine is widely used around the world, having been administered in over 90 countries since its introduction in the 1970s (NHS Immunisation Information, 2004).

Controversy has arisen surrounding the safety of the MMR vaccine because some scientists and parents argue that it increases the risk of autism and other disorders such as Crohn disease. In February 1998, the authors of a paper published in the journal *The Lancet* suggested a link between the MMR vaccine and autism (Wakefield *et al.*, 1998). As a result, uptake of the MMR vaccine fell sharply, leading to fears of a measles epidemic.

Further controversy was generated about the research when it emerged that there was an undisclosed conflict of interest in the submission of the original *Lancet* paper. This meant that the paper would probably not have been published. The result was a partial retraction of the paper by some of its authors.

Owing to the controversy and uncertainty surrounding the safety of the MMR vaccine and the potential effect on uptake, the Department of Health and others have stressed and continue to stress that extensive research in numerous studies shows no link between MMR and autism. The Department of Health continues to try to reassure parents about the safety of the MMR vaccine, stating categorically that there is no link between MMR and autism. In a Department of Health press release on 12 January 2001 the Chief Medical Officer, Professor Liam Donaldson, said: 'Scare stories clearly worry parents but giving children separate vaccines unnecessarily exposes them to the risk of life-threatening infection. MMR remains the safest way to protect our children.'

care markets will invariably deviate from the first-best rules owing to market failure – the first-best allocation of resources is not achieved.

Market failure implies a role for government intervention in health care. The general idea is that by intervening appropriately in parts of the health care sector where the first-best allocation of resources is not achieved – for example through the use of taxes, subsidies, regulations and direct provision and finance – the government may be able to improve social welfare.

Given that the first-best allocation is not achieved in the health care market, this has lead economists to ask whether we achieve the second-best allocation of resources – that is the best one that is feasible given the existence of market failures – by following the first-best rules whenever possible. The answer to this question is no. This is known as the *theory of second best*: if we accept that Pareto efficiency is not achieved in all parts of the health care market, then attempting to achieve Pareto efficiency by addressing market failures wherever possible is often not desirable. The theory of second best implies that the pursuit of perfect competition is not necessarily a desirable goal in health care if the first-best allocation of resources is not achievable.

To illustrate this point, suppose that a pharmaceutical company enjoys a monopoly in the provision of a particular medicine. Also suppose that in the production of the medicine the pharmaceutical company imposes an external cost of production on society in the form of pollution. Given that the pharmaceutical company imposes a negative production externality on society, should the government intervene to reduce its monopoly power, that is, attempt to achieve the first-best rules of perfect competition whenever possible? In this case the answer is no: reducing the monopoly power enjoyed by the company and making the market more competitive will increase the output of the pharmaceutical company, and lower its prices, which creates an even bigger negative production externality – there will be even more pollution. Overall society may be worse off than if the government had not reduced the monopoly power. To reach the first-best allocation would require further intervention, such as a pollution tax, to take account of the externality problem.

5.5 GOVERNMENT FAILURE

There are various reasons why government intervention may be desirable in the market for health care. However, this is not to say that government intervention is unambiguously a good thing. For government intervention to be desirable it must be able to improve efficiency and equity. Government intervention may not be desirable if it fails to do this. This might happen because the government has imperfect knowledge about the marginal social benefit and marginal social cost of consumption and production of health care. In this case it is unlikely the government will be able to intervene to achieve Pareto efficiency.

In addition to imperfect knowledge, there may be relative inefficiencies in the public provision of goods compared to private provision. These may arise from the level of bureaucracy and administration in government; because there is a lack of market incentives (for example, the absence of significant competition, the lack of a threat of bankruptcy and difficulties in measuring performance in the public sector); because there is a multiplicity of conflicting objectives in government arising from the interaction of different departments; and because of continual changes in government policy resulting from the political business cycle.

If the problems created by government intervention are greater than the problems overcome by the intervention that arise from market failure, then there is *government failure* and a strong case for only limited government intervention.

A common criticism made against the public sector is that it is overly bureaucratic and inefficient. The implication is that government intervention in health care leads to a waste of scarce health care resources. An alternative view is that administration costs are lower when health care finance and provision fall under the auspices of government authorities rather than the private market with many firms, each with their own red tape and bureaucracy. Box 6.7 compares health care administration costs in the USA (predominantly private market-based) and Canadian (predominantly government-based) health care systems, and finds that these are much lower in the government-based system.

Next, in Chapter 6, we analyse in more detail one specific cause of market failure in health care, namely uncertainty. We focus on the solutions to this problem in terms of health insurance and then consider alternative methods of health care financing.

SUMMARY

1. If health care were bought and sold in a perfectly competitive market, this would determine what types of health care to produce, how to produce them and who receives them. The price system determines which types of health care and how much of each type are produced, by finding the price at which the quantity demanded equals the quantity supplied. The equilibrium quantity corresponding to this price defines how much of each health care programme should be provided. Health care will be supplied by health care providers willing to supply health care at the equilibrium price. In an effort to maximise profits, health care will be produced in a manner that is technically efficient. Health care will be purchased by those consumers who are willing and able to pay the equilibrium price. Access to health care would be based on ability to pay and not other factors such as need.

2. Pareto, or social, efficiency occurs when it is not possible to make someone better off without making someone else worse off. The First Fundamental Theorem of Welfare Economics states that the allocation of resources in a perfectly competitive market will be Pareto efficient.

3. In the real world, health care markets rarely if ever achieve Pareto efficiency. The term market failure is used to cover all circumstances in which Pareto efficiency is not achieved by the market. Four causes of market failure that arise in health care are externalities, market power, public goods and information imperfections.

4. Externalities are spillover effects (positive or negative) incurred in the consumption or production of goods and services in the market. Health care markets will not lead to Pareto efficiency if there are externalities. This is because private marginal costs and/or private marginal benefits deviate from the social marginal costs and/or social marginal benefits. An example of an externality in health care is the caring externality, which is an altruistic external benefit of consumption.

5. Whenever there is a monopoly or some form of imperfect competition, the market will fail to allocate goods and services in a Pareto efficient manner. For instance, a monopoly will provide less health care than is Pareto efficient.

6. Public goods are non-rival, non-excludable goods that are jointly consumed by everyone. Public goods will not be provided in a perfectly competitive market because there is no incentive for private individuals to pay for them; they will free-ride.

7. Information imperfections arise in health care because of uncertainty and imperfect knowledge. Uncertainty can be addressed via the introduction of health insurance. Imperfect knowledge can lead to physician-induced demand.

8. Governments intervene in the market for health care because markets fail to achieve Pareto efficiency and because markets can be inequitable. There are several policy instruments that governments might use to intervene in the market for health care: direct involvement in the finance and provision of health care; taxes and subsidies; regulation; and the provision of information.

9. The theory of second best states that if we accept that Pareto efficiency is not achieved in all parts of the health care market then attempting to achieve Pareto efficiency by addressing market failures wherever possible may not be desirable.

10. Government intervention in the market for health care is not unambiguously a good thing in the presence of market failure. There may be government failures which mean that intervention does not improve Pareto efficiency and equity. In addition, there may be inefficiencies in the public provision of goods compared to private provision.

Chapter 6

Health Insurance and Health Care Financing

6.1 UNCERTAINTY IN HEALTH CARE

As we have already noted, uncertainty is an important cause of market failure in health care. In this chapter we shall consider the implications of uncertainty, and other issues, for decisions about the way in which health care is funded.

It may be possible to predict future health states associated with chronic conditions, and to predict the magnitude of ill health at the aggregate level, thereby allowing an individual assessment of the probability of future ill health. Generally, however, an individual's future health state is uncertain. While it may be possible to predict future demand for health care that is unrelated to the onset of ill health, such as prevention or cosmetic surgery, the demand for many types of health care is uncertain.

More specifically, health care is typically consumed under conditions of uncertainty with respect to the timing of health care expenditure (that is, when people become ill) and the amount of expenditure on health care that is required (that is, what treatment is required and how much it will cost to become well again). They are at risk from unexpected ill health and of incurring possibly large unplanned expenditures for treatment. Health care expenditures may be 'catastrophic' if they require individuals to spend a significant proportion of their income at the same time that illness may be reducing their ability to earn. As a result, they may be unable to afford the health care that they need.

The usual solution to such problems is insurance. This consists of an insurance contract between an insurance provider and individuals who consider themselves to be at risk of ill health. When an individual buys health insurance he or she enters into an agreement with the insurer to pay an agreed price, called an insurance premium, in exchange for a payout to be made to the insured should they become ill.

Insurance works in the following way. Suppose that a group of 100 people each have a 1% chance in a year of becoming ill, which would require treatment costing £1000. It is likely therefore that in a year one person out of the group will become ill, so the group's total expenditure would be £1000. If each pays £10 into a fund, they will accumulate £1000, which is exactly enough to meet their total expenditure. So, by *pooling risks* each of them converts an uncertain possible loss of £1000 to a certain loss of £10.

The model of health care markets we have used up to this point can be characterised as in Figure 6.1. There are two parties in the market for health care: households, who demand health care and pay for it out of their own pocket; and health care providers, who supply health care in return for payments made by households. With the introduction of health insurance as a means of addressing uncertainty, a third party – an insurance company – is introduced, as shown in Figure 6.2.

In the first part of this chapter we look at these issues in more detail and investigate the demand for and supply of health insurance. We develop a model of health insurance and examine the main features of the market for health insurance. In the second part of the chapter we develop that model and use it to explore the various ways in which health care is financed in the real world. We begin by looking

Figure 6.1 Two-party health care market model.

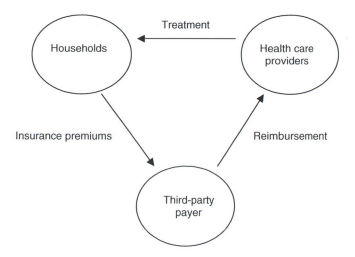

Figure 6.2 Third-party health care market model.

Box 6.1 Mind the gap: 45 million uninsured Americans

Data released by the US Census Bureau (2005) showed that the number of Americans without health insurance cover (either public or private) was 45.8 million in 2004, or 15.7% of the total population. This represents an increase of 800 000 people over the number uninsured in the year 2003, of nearly 6 million compared with the year 2000, and of nearly 15 million since 1987. The proportion with no health insurance was not distributed uniformly across the population. For example, individuals with low income were more likely to be uninsured (24.3% of people with an annual income below $25 000 were uninsured, while for people with annual income over $75 000 the percentage was 8.4%). African American (19.7%) and Hispanic (32.7%) ethnic groups were much more likely to be uninsured than white non-Hispanic groups (11.3%). Because these individuals are required to pay for their health care directly, that is out of their own pocket, they are at risk from potentially catastrophic health expenditure.

Figure 2.8a shows that the USA spends more money per person on health care than any other country. The difference between the magnitude of US health care expenditure and the number of Americans who are uninsured has been famously described as 'a paradox of excess and deprivation' (Enthoven and Kronick, 1989).

at attitudes towards risk and investigating why individuals will pay to reduce uncertainty via insurance.

6.2 ATTITUDES TO RISK

The role of health insurance in addressing uncertainty in the demand for health care depends on attitudes to risk. We distinguish between risk and uncertainty in the following way: uncertainty exists when any one of a number of states of the world may occur and we do not know which one will arise. Risk exists when the probability of each possible state of the world occurring can be estimated.

To define attitudes to risk we first need to understand the concept of a fair gamble. Suppose an individual is offered a 50% chance of winning £10 and a 50% chance of losing £10. On average the individual would expect to make no money because the expected value of the gamble is zero: $(+10 \times \frac{1}{2}) + (-10 \times \frac{1}{2}) = 0$. A gamble like this, which has an expected value of zero, is called a fair gamble. A fair gamble is one which, on average, will make exactly zero profit.

Now suppose that the individual is offered a 25% chance of winning £20 and a 75% chance of losing £10. This is an unfavourable gamble. The expected value is negative and the individual will lose £2.50 on average. If the chances of winning and losing are reversed, this is a favourable gamble because on average the gamble will be profitable; the expected value is positive and the individual will gain £2.50 on average.

We can use these ideas to classify attitudes to risk. A risk-averse individual will refuse a fair gamble. This does not mean that they will never undertake risky behaviour, only that the gamble needs to be sufficiently favourable to overcome their dislike of risk. The more risk-averse the individual, the more favourable the gamble must be. A risk-neutral individual is indifferent between accepting and not accepting a fair gamble. A risk-neutral individual will only accept a favourable gamble and will refuse an unfavourable gamble. A risk-loving individual will accept a fair gamble, and may even accept an unfavourable gamble. The more risk-loving an individual, the more unfavourable the gamble must be before the individual will not bet.

Risk attitudes arise from two sources. One is that risk aversion may be due to a specific disutility from taking chances, and risk loving to utility from gambling. However, as the next section demonstrates, there is another explanation; that a fair gamble in money terms may not be a fair gamble in utility terms.

6.3 DIMINISHING MARGINAL UTILITY OF INCOME

Given the uncertainty facing consumers of health care, and their attitudes to risk, we examine the demand for health insurance using the notion of diminishing marginal utility of income. We first introduced the concept of diminishing marginal utility in Chapter 2 to explain the shape of indifference curves. In Figure 6.3, $U(Y)$ shows the total utility attained by the individual at each level of income. The slope of the $U(Y)$ curve gives the marginal utility of income. As income Y rises, the $U(Y)$ curve becomes flatter and the marginal utility of income diminishes.

Suppose that an individual has an initial level of income Y_0 with utility $U(Y_0)$ and is offered a gamble with possible outcomes Y_1 and Y_2 and associated utilities $U(Y_1)$ and $U(Y_2)$, respectively. The probabilities of each outcome are p_1 and p_2, respectively. The individual's expected income $E(Y)$ and expected utility $E(U)$ are

$$E(Y) = \overline{Y} = p_1Y_1 + p_2Y_2 \tag{6.1}$$

$$E(U) = \overline{U} = p_1U(Y_1) + p_2U(Y_2) \tag{6.2}$$

Let us also suppose that $p_1 = p_2 = {}^1/_2$, which means that $\overline{Y}$ is halfway between Y_1 and Y_2 and $\overline{U}$ is halfway between $U(Y_1)$ and $U(Y_2)$. The fact that $Y_0 = \overline{Y}$ implies that the

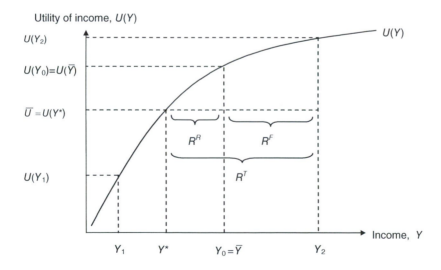

Figure 6.3 Diminishing marginal utility of income.

gamble is a fair one. The expected utility from the gamble $\bar{U}$ is less than the utility associated with the initial level of income $U(Y_0)$. Therefore, the individual will choose not to take the fair gamble; they will choose the certainty of Y_0. This implies that the individual is risk averse, and that risk-averse individuals have diminishing marginal utility of income.

6.4 THE DEMAND FOR HEALTH INSURANCE

6.4.1 Total Premium

We can also use Figure 6.3 to investigate the demand for health insurance: how much individuals are willing and able to pay for it. Suppose an individual has an initial level of income given by Y_2, with utility $U(Y_2)$. If they become ill and require health care they incur a treatment cost equal to $Y_2 - Y_1$, and their income falls to Y_1, with utility $U(Y_1)$. Suppose the probability that the individual becomes ill is p_1; then the probability that they do not become ill is p_2 (since $p_1 + p_2 = 1$). The individual's expected income and expected utility if they are uninsured are $\bar{Y}$ and $\bar{U}$, respectively.

The maximum amount of money the individual is prepared to pay for health insurance, R^T, is $Y_2 - Y^*$. The reason for this is that the individual will pay for insurance as long as the utility it yields is at least as high as the utility they would achieve if they did not buy insurance. Starting at the initial level of income Y_2 with utility $U(Y_2)$, the largest insurance premium an individual would pay would be one that reduced their utility to $\bar{U}$, which is their expected utility without insurance (and which has a corresponding income of Y^*). If they had to pay more than $Y_2 - Y^*$, then their utility would fall below $\bar{U}$ and they would not buy insurance.

The total premium R^T can be disaggregated into two components: a fair premium R^F and a risk premium R^R.

6.4.2 Fair Premium

If the individual is uninsured their expected income is $\bar{Y}$. Their expected loss is therefore $Y_2 - \bar{Y}$. This is the amount of income that they would expect to lose on average if they were uninsured and is called the fair premium, R^F. This is equal to the probability of becoming ill (p_1) multiplied by the lost income if they become ill ($Y_2 - Y_1$):

$$R^F = Y_2 - \bar{Y} = Y_2 - p_1 Y_1 - p_2 Y_2 = (1 - p_2)Y_2 - p_1 Y_1 = p_1 Y_2 - p_1 Y_1 = p_1(Y_2 - Y_1) \qquad (6.3)$$

6.4.3 Risk Premium

If someone pays a fair premium for health insurance, then it is exactly equal to the amount that they would lose, on average, if they were uninsured. In reality, people are generally willing to pay more than this because they are risk averse.

Risk averse individuals are willing to pay, on top of the fair premium, a risk premium R^R. The magnitude of the risk premium depends on their degree of risk aversion, which determines the value of the certainty introduced by health insurance over the uncertainty of being uninsured. To see this, note that the expected utility $\bar{U}$ might be obtained either as the expected utility from an uncertain income depending on whether or not they become ill with outcomes Y_1 and Y_2 (with an expected income $\bar{Y}$) or the utility from a certain income Y^*. Therefore, the individual is indifferent between an uncertainty with expected income $\bar{Y}$ and a certain income Y^*. The value in monetary terms of the certainty to the individual is therefore $\bar{Y} - Y^*$. This is the risk premium R^R.

The model is summarised in Table 6.1. The maximum premium the individual is prepared to pay R^T is equal to the fair premium R^F plus the risk premium R^R. Note that with insurance income is the same whether they become ill or not (Y^*), thereby removing any uncertainty.

6.5 RISK POOLING

We have shown that health insurance removes uncertainty facing individuals with respect to the timing and magnitude of health care expenditure. After the purchase of insurance the uncertainty is passed from the insured to the insurer. Why do insurers take on the risks that their customers are prepared to pay to avoid? The answer is that

Table 6.1 Demand for health insurance

		Not ill	Ill
(i)	Income if uninsured	Y_2	Y_1
(ii)	Probability	p_2	p_1
(iii)	Expected income if uninsured	$\bar{Y}$	$\bar{Y}$
(iv)	Payout if insured	0	$Y_2 - Y_1$
(v)	Fair premium, R^F	$Y_2 - \bar{Y} = p_1(Y_2 - Y_1)$	$Y_2 - \bar{Y} = p_1(Y_2 - Y_1)$
(vi)	Risk premium, R^R	$\bar{Y} - Y^*$	$\bar{Y} - Y^*$
(vii)	Total premium, R^T [(v) + (vi)]	$Y_2 - Y^*$	$Y_2 - Y^*$
(viii)	Income if insured [(i) + (iv) − (vii)]	Y^*	Y^*

Box 6.2 A worked example of the demand for health insurance

Suppose a 55-year-old male with hypertension is considering whether to buy health insurance to cover himself from the risk of incurring treatment costs for coronary heart disease (CHD) over the next year. He has a probability of 5% of developing CHD, and an initial level of income of £20 000. If he does develop CHD, then the treatment required will cost £5000. If he is uninsured, his income will fall to £15 000. Without insurance, the expected loss is £5000 × 0.05 = £250. This is the fair premium. Given his level of risk aversion it is the case that $U(18\ 500) = 0.95 \times U(20\ 000) + 0.05 \times U(15\ 000)$, and therefore the maximum premium he is prepared to pay for insurance is £1500. The risk premium is £1250. If he had to pay more than £1500, his utility would fall below $U(18\ 500)$ and he would be worse off buying insurance than if he were uninsured. This is shown in the figure below.

the insurance provider is able to pool its risks. It can do this using the law of large numbers, which we first came across in Chapter 3 in the context of increasing returns to scale. This basically says that predictions based on larger samples have smaller confidence intervals. Put another way, the larger the number of events of a particular type the more precise their predictions of the average outcome will be. Using the law of large numbers, individuals may face uncertainty but insurance providers, who insure a large number of individuals, may face approximate certainty. Using the example of CHD risk, our 55-year-old male with hypertension does not know whether or not he will get CHD in the next year, but the CHD rate in the population for 55-year-old males with hypertension is known. It is the relative certainty of the average outcome resulting from the law of large numbers that allows insurance providers to provide insurance profitably.

6.6 THE SUPPLY OF HEALTH INSURANCE

We have investigated the size of the premium that people will pay for health insurance and the reason why insurance providers are able to take on the risks of those whom they insure. In this section we consider the price at which insurance providers will supply health insurance. We saw previously that the expected loss for an uninsured person is given by $p_1(Y_2 - Y_1)$. This is the average payout that the insurance provider would expect to make to each individual it insures. The total premium charged by the insurance provider θ is defined as

$$\theta = p_1(Y_2 - Y_1) + F \qquad (6.4)$$

where F is called the loading factor. This covers the insurance provider's administration costs and the profit it needs to earn for each insured individual to remain in the market. This is the price at which health insurance will supplied in a competitive insurance market.

6.7 THE MARKET FOR HEALTH INSURANCE

In this section we bring together the earlier arguments and analyse the market for health insurance. A private health insurance market will exist as long as it is possible to supply health insurance at a price that people are prepared to pay. On the demand side, people will be prepared to pay an amount R^T equal to the fair premium (their expected loss) plus a risk premium that depends on their degree of risk aversion. Insurers will be prepared to supply health insurance at a price equal to

Box 6.3 Worked example of the supply of health insurance

Using the example in Box 6.2, the insurance provider knows that the man has a probability of 5% of developing CHD, and that if he does develop CHD the treatment required will cost £5000. It therefore calculates that the expected loss – the average payout it expects to make to him is £5000 × 0.05 = £250.

The average costs to administer the insurance contract held with each insured person are £25 per year and the additional administration and other costs of dealing with a claim are £600. Suppose the probability that someone will make a claim is equal to the probability of illness (that is, there are no bogus claims). The expected costs of dealing with a claim are £600 × 0.05 = £30. To remain in the market the insurance provider needs to earn a certain level of profit which it will achieve if it charges a mark-up of £150 on every person that it insures. Combining all these elements the loading factor the insurance provider charges is £25 + £30 + £150 = £205, and the price at which insurance is supplied is £250 + £205 = £455.

the expected loss plus a loading factor, F. Hence, a market for health insurance exists only if

$$R^R \geq F \Leftrightarrow \bar{Y} - Y^* \geq F \tag{6.5}$$

This indicates that for a health insurance market to exist an individual's degree of risk aversion, represented by $\bar{Y} - Y^*$, must be sufficient to cover the insurance provider's administration costs and profit.

6.8 HEALTH INSURANCE MARKET FAILURES

Unfortunately, even if equation (6.5) holds, a number of problems arise with the introduction of health insurance markets in practice which may limit their success in adequately dealing with uncertainty in health care.

6.8.1 Adverse Selection

Adverse selection arises when exactly the wrong people, from the point of view of the insurance provider, choose to buy insurance: those with a relatively high probability of illness. To illustrate the basic idea, suppose that an insurance provider has estimated that the average person requires £500 of treatment each year. The insurance provider therefore sets the insurance premium at £950, including a loading factor of £450. Individuals whose probability of illness is lower than average will probably choose not to buy insurance at this price, unless they are sufficiently risk averse that they are prepared to pay a risk premium of at least £450. Those who are most likely to buy health insurance are high-risk people who are most likely to become ill. Suppose they require on average treatment that costs £2000 each year. Clearly the insurance provider will make a loss if it insures only these people. One obvious solution is to raise the insurance premium, for example to £2450. This has two implications: the average person is deprived of insurance (they will refuse to pay this amount) and premiums continually increase until insurance is not attractive to anyone except those with the highest risks of illness. This has been referred to as the 'adverse selection death spiral' (see for example Buchmueller and DiNardo, 2002).

Adverse selection arises because of the asymmetry of information between individuals who wish to buy insurance, who often have a good idea of their own risk status, and the insurance provider, who does not know the risk a specific individual has of becoming ill but does know the *average* risk in the population. Insurance providers base their assessment of the risk of an individual becoming ill on the broad experience of the whole population, which includes high-risk and low-risk people. This is known as *community rating*, where insurance premiums are calculated on the basis of average probability in the population. Any individual who feels that their probability of illness is greater than the community rate will have an added incentive to insure, and those with a lower than average probability may choose not to insure unless they are sufficiently risk averse.

Suppose the numbers of high-risk, medium-risk and low-risk individuals in the population are N^H, N^M and N^L, respectively. The probability of illness in each group is p^H, p^M and p^L, respectively, where $p^L < p^M < p^H$, and the insurance premiums that individuals in each group are prepared to pay are θ^H, θ^M and θ^L, respectively, where $\theta^i = p^i(Y_2 - Y_1) + F$ for $i = L, M, H$ and $\theta^L < \theta^M < \theta^H$. The insurance company knows N^H, N^M and N^L, but does not know to which group any single individual belongs who wishes to buy insurance. They decide to set a community rate θ^{C1} payable by everyone and equal to the average of the amounts each group is prepared to pay weighted by the proportion of the population in each group:

$$\theta^{C1} = \left[\frac{p^L N^L + p^M N^M + p^H N^H}{N^L + N^M + N^H} \right](Y_2 - Y_1) + F \tag{6.6}$$

Suppose $\theta^L < \theta^{C1} < \theta^M < \theta^H$. This community rate will be unacceptable to the low-risk group because it is more than they are prepared to pay. They will therefore drop out of the health insurance market and will be uninsured.

If the insurance provider supplies health insurance at price θ^{C1} it realises that the low-risk group will drop out and that it will make a loss if only the high- and medium-risk groups remain in the market. It will therefore set a revised community rate θ^{C2} based now on the weighted average premium the remaining two groups will pay:

$$\theta^{C2} = \left[\frac{p^M N^M + p^H N^H}{N^M + N^H} \right](Y_2 - Y_1) + F \tag{6.7}$$

Since $\theta^M < \theta^{C2} < \theta^H$, the new community rate is more than the medium-risk group is prepared to pay; they too will drop out. It is not feasible for the insurance provider to charge θ^{C2} to the high-risk group, so it will finally set a rate given by

$$\theta^{C3} = p^H(Y_2 - Y_1) + F \tag{6.8}$$

In this case $\theta^{C3} = \theta^H$, and only those with the highest risk of illness will buy health insurance. If p^H is close to 1, then insurance is no longer feasible and the insurance market will collapse. A real-world example of this phenomenon is given in Box 6.4.

There are two broad approaches that might be adopted to prevent adverse selection. The first is experience rating, where the insurance provider sets a different insurance premium for different risk groups; for example, the high-risk, medium-risk and low-risk groups are set separate premiums of θ^H, θ^M and θ^L, respectively. Those who apply for health insurance might be asked to undergo a medical examination and to disclose any relevant facts concerning their risk status. There are two problems with this approach. First, the cost of acquiring the appropriate information may be prohibitive. This cost will be passed on to insured individuals in their insurance premiums via the loading factor and may mean that health insurance is no longer affordable or attractive. Secondly, it might encourage insurance providers to 'cherry pick' individuals, only choosing to provide insurance to the low risk. This may mean that high-risk individuals are unable to obtain health insurance at all.

An alternative solution is to make health insurance compulsory. The problem of adverse selection arises because low-risk individuals drop out of the market. By making health insurance compulsory this is prohibited and adverse selection will not arise. This approach is typically used with publicly provided health insurance discussed later in the chapter. It may be inequitable to low-risk individuals, who effectively subsidise the health insurance payments of those with higher risks.

6.8.2 Moral Hazard

Health insurance changes the economic incentives facing both the consumers and the providers of health care. One manifestation of these changes is the existence of moral hazard, which is takes the form of excess use of services. Moral hazard arises when it

Box 6.4 Adverse selection in health insurance in practice

Cutler and Zeckhauser (1997) give an example of adverse selection in the health insurance market in the university sector in the USA in the 1990s. Traditionally, employees of Harvard University were offered various types of private health insurance plan, with the employee paying a small proportion of the premium (the average was around $500 per annum) and the university paying the major share (around $6000 per annum).

From 1992 a new plan was also offered, run by Blue Cross/Blue Shield of Massachusetts. After an initial run-in period, employees were charged more or less the same for the new plan cost as they were for the other plans, and it succeeded in enrolling 20% of Harvard University employees. Then in the mid-1990s the university faced a budget deficit. In an effort to cut costs it encouraged the health insurance providers to charge lower premiums, saying that it would implement an equal contribution rule. This rule meant that the additional costs of more expensive plans would be paid by the employees and so by cutting its premiums an insurance provider would attract employees. The long-standing insurance providers were able to cut their premiums, while the new entrant was not. The upshot was that employee charges in the new plan increased considerably to an average of around $1000 and, as expected, there was a reduction in enrolment in 1995 from 20% to 15%. The employees who switched provider were healthier and younger than those who remained with the new plan, and as a result Blue Cross/Blue Shield made a loss from the plan in 1995. It therefore had to raise premiums in 1996. This rise led to an increase again in employee charges for the remaining enrolees to an average of more than $2000 and unsurprisingly enrolment fell again, this time to 9%. Those who left were again shown to be younger and healthier than those who stayed, and as a result the provider made a loss again in 1996. In 1997 it was clear that for the plan to break even charges would have to be increased substantially yet again, which was untenable both for the university and for Blue Cross/Blue Shield. The new plan was disbanded. As noted by Cutler and Zeckhauser: 'The adverse selection "death spiral" twisted swiftly.'

is possible to alter the probability of the insured event, p_1 (that is, the probability of illness), or the size of the insured loss, $Y_2 - Y_1$ (that is, the payout required by the insurance provider). Moral hazard can be avoided as long as insured individuals cannot influence p_1 and $Y_2 - Y_1$. If they can, p_1 and $Y_2 - Y_1$ are said to be endogenous; if they are free from influence then p_1 and $Y_2 - Y_1$ are exogenous.

With endogenous p_1, individuals can influence the probability of the insured event. In many cases in health care this will probably not arise: it seems unlikely that, given the intrinsic unpleasantness of being ill and of receiving treatment, anyone would choose to put themselves at greater risk of illness just because any treatment they required would be paid for by their health insurance provider. However, one example where this might arise in health care is planned pregnancy, which can be influenced by individual action. As a result, the probability of making a claim is not exogenous and it is usual for pregnancy to be excluded from private health insurance plans. Complications of pregnancy are often covered, however, because they are exogenous.

In the case of endogenous $Y_2 - Y_1$, individuals can influence the size of the payout that the insurance provider is obliged to meke. This problem might be caused by either the consumers or the providers of health care. Consumers have an incentive to bring about additional benefits to themselves at the expense of the insurance provider. This is perfectly rational economic behaviour: individuals increase consumption in response to a lower price. As shown in Figure 6.4, the extent of the problem depends on the price elasticity of demand. Suppose the equilibrium price under perfect competition is p^*. With health insurance the price facing the insured individual is zero, shown by p^0. If demand is perfectly inelastic, as in Figure 6.4(a), then with insurance the units of health care consumed are the same as at the perfectly competitive equilibrium. If demand is price elastic, as in Figure 6.4(b), then the introduction of health insurance causes the demand for health care to rise ($Q^* < Q^0$).

This problem might also be caused by health care providers, resulting in producer moral hazard. In this case the excess payout by the insurance provider is instigated by health

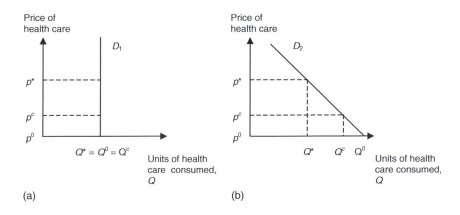

Figure 6.4 Moral hazard and price elasticity.

care providers who demand more health care for their patients in their role as agent. We examined this issue – supplier-induced demand – in Chapter 2.

A number of mechanisms can be used to reduce moral hazard. The first is *co-insurance*. Many insurance policies require that when an event occurs the insured shares the insured loss $Y_2 - Y_1$ with the insurer. The co-insurance rate is the percentage of the insured loss that is paid by the insured. The co-payment is the amount that they pay. For example, with a co-insurance rate of 10% on an insured loss of £2500 the insured would be required to make a co-payment of £250 and the insurer would pay the remaining £2250.

The second mechanism is deductibles. A deductible is an amount of money the insured pays when a claim is made irrespective of co-insurance. The insurer will not pay the insured loss unless the deductible is paid by the individual. For example, a deductible of £100 would mean that the insured would pay the first £100 of all insured losses claimed for. This is also sometimes referred to as an *excess*.

The effect of co-insurance and deductibles is to increase the price of health care from zero to some positive value. For example, p^c in Figure 6.4 represents a copayment that the insured is required to pay to their insurer if they make a claim. Assuming health care is price elastic, demand will then fall from Q^0 to Q^c.

The third mechanism is no-claims bonuses. These are payments made by insurers to discourage claims. They usually take the form of reduced insurance premiums in the next period. Suppose an individual currently pays an insurance premium θ^1. If they make no claim on an insured loss in the current period, then in the following period they receive a no-claims bonus equal to $\theta^1 - \theta^2$. The premium they are charged by the insurer will be θ^2, where $\theta^1 > \theta^2$. Suppose the insured requires treatment that costs $Y_2 - Y_1$. If $Y_2 - Y_1 > \theta^1 - \theta^2$, then treatment costs more than the no-claims bonus and it makes sense for the insured to claim a payout to cover the insured loss from the insurer and forgo the no-claims bonus. If, on the other hand, $\theta^1 - \theta^2 > Y_2 - Y_1$, it makes financial sense for the individual not to claim from the insurer, to pay the cost of treatment $Y_2 - Y_1$ out of their own pocket, and obtain the no-claims bonus in the next period. No-claims bonuses typically discourage insurance claims where the payout by the insurer is small.

6.8.3 Non-Price Competition

The introduction of insurance can have a perverse effect on cost-minimising decisions of health care providers: with the introduction of health insurance it is unlikely that providers will supply health care at least cost, nor is there an incentive

Box 6.5 Moral hazard and prescription charges in the UK

Prescription charges were introduced in the UK National Health Service in 1952. They were removed in 1966, but reintroduced in 1968, and they have been in use ever since. From 1 April 2005 the prescription charge was £6.50. The prescription charge is a flat fee, and remains unchanged irrespective of the cost of the drug dispensed. Certain population groups are exempted from paying the charge, including children, the elderly, those in full-time education, pregnant women, those earning low incomes, and individuals with certain medical conditions.

The prescription charge has been heavily criticised by patient groups, professional bodies and the pharmaceutical industry. For example, the Royal Pharmaceutical Society of Great Britain (2005) has argued that its value as a deterrent on drug use is limited for a number of reasons:

1. Owing to exemptions, around 50% of the population are exempt from paying prescription charges, and over 85% of prescriptions are obtained free of charge.

2. About 60% of prescriptions cost less than the charge.

3. Many anomalies exist. For example, patients with some diseases such as hypothyroidism pay no charges even for unrelated medicines, while some groups, such as older people, are entirely exempt, irrespective of their financial circumstances.

4. While an additional benefit from the point of view of the government is that it raises revenue (around £500 million per annum), this accounts for only 6% of the total net ingredient cost of all prescriptions dispensed.

for them to do so. This is because price is no longer important to patients. The effect of health insurance is to reduce the price of health care to the insured from the market price to zero or, if there are co-payments or deductibles, to a price above zero but below market price. Having paid the insurance premium, the insured receives all services covered by the insurance contract for free, at the expense of the insurer.

If they have a free choice of provider, then, since health care is effectively free, patients may select a health care provider not on the basis of price but instead on the basis of non-price factors such as comfort, available facilities and the quality of food. This will cause health care costs to rise as providers compete for patients on these factors.

Since the problem with non-price competition is essentially one of cost escalation, the adverse effects of non-price competition can be addressed with the introduction of policies for cost containment.

6.8.4 Incomplete Coverage

Another problem that arises in health insurance markets is incomplete coverage. Even if adverse selection does not occur, some population groups might find it difficult to buy health insurance. Low-income groups may not be able to afford health insurance, even if it is charged at the fair premium rate and there may be incomplete coverage for high-risk groups.

With respect to the latter, there will be incomplete coverage when the probability of illness tends towards 1 (that is, payout by the insurance provider is a certainty). Recall from equation (6.4) that the total premium charged by the insurance provider, θ, is equal to $p_1(Y_2 - Y_1) + F$. As $p_1 \to 1$, then $p_1(Y_2 - Y_1) \to (Y_2 - Y_1)$ and the premium charged by the insurance provider exceeds the insured loss $[\theta > (Y_2 - Y_1)]$ owing to the loading factor. Using the example in Boxes 6.2 and 6.3, if the probability of CHD for this man was in fact equal to 1 he would have to pay a premium of £5205 to cover treatment costs of £5000. In this case private health insurance will not be offered because there is no demand for it. In health care this problem can arise for people with chronic or congenital illnesses, such as cancer, if they attempt to buy health insurance after the condition has been diagnosed. Typically, private health insurance providers exclude treatment for pre-existing conditions, precisely because the probability of requiring treatment is too high to insure. The likelihood of incomplete coverage is compounded in low-income, high-risk groups, for example, older people.

Incomplete coverage might be remedied using cost-containment policies, which will cause treatment costs to fall. If this reduction is passed by the insurer on to the insured, then premiums may become more affordable. Another solution would be to make health insurance compulsory and calculate individual insurance premiums not on the basis of individual risk but on ability to pay. This would mean that low-income and high-risk groups would be more likely to be able to afford health insurance. Addressing the problem of incomplete coverage in this way provides an important justification for tax-based health systems and those based on social health insurance.

6.9 A HEALTH CARE FINANCING FRAMEWORK

In the last section we outlined various reasons why the health insurance market might fail to provide appropriate protection from catastrophic expenditure. In light of the problems discussed, various different health care financing systems have developed in the real world. The framework that we will use to analyse these systems is shown in Figure 6.5 and comprises four key elements:

- the type of third party payer;
- the method by which health care providers are reimbursed;
- the extent of integration between third-party payers and health care providers;
- the ways in which health care is financed.

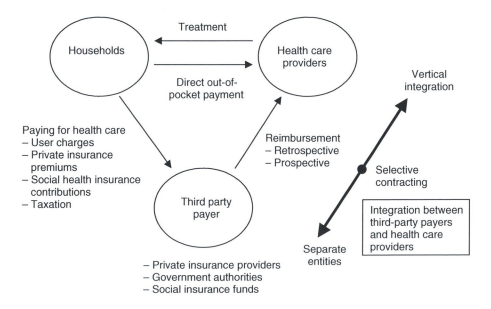

Figure 6.5 Health care financing framework.

6.10 THIRD-PARTY PAYERS

In the basic insurance model used so far, health insurance is supplied by an un-specified insurance provider. In reality, the third-party payer can be one of three broad types: private insurance companies; the government; or social insurance funds.

Private insurance companies operate in the same way as any private firm, with the making of profits as their main goal, although in health care insurance there are many companies that are not-for-profit.

In tax-based systems, the third-party payer is the government (local, regional or national). In effect it acts as both a provider of insurance and a purchaser of health care. The government therefore has considerable market power in setting payments for health care providers for the services it purchases. Any lower payment rates achieved may be passed on to households. Additionally, with a dominant large insurance pro-vider administration costs may be lower than in a system with many individual private health insurance providers, each with different payment systems and their own bureau-cracy (see Box 6.6).

In social health insurance systems, the third-party payer is effectively the social insur-ance fund, which is usually independent of direct government control. There might be numerous individual funds or a single national fund with market powers equivalent to those of government authorities.

6.11 REIMBURSEMENT

The method of reimbursement relates to the way in which health care providers are paid for the services they provide. It is useful to distinguish between reimbursement methods because they can affect the quantity and quality of health care. We focus on methods for reimbursing hospitals.

6.11.1 Retrospective Reimbursement

Retrospective reimbursement at full cost means that hospitals receive payment in full for all health care expenditures incurred in some pre-specified period of time. Reim-bursement is retrospective in the sense that not only are hospitals paid after they have

Box 6.6 Health care administration costs in the USA and Canada

Woolhandler *et al.* (2003) calculated and compared the administrative costs in the USA (where third-party payers are predominantly private insurance providers) and Canadian (predominantly government authorities) health care systems in 1999. They included the following cost components: insurance overheads; employers' costs to manage health care benefits; hospital administration; administrative costs of practitioners; nursing home administration; and administrative costs of home care agencies. Data were obtained from published sources, surveys of physicians, employment data, and detailed cost reports filed by hospitals, nursing homes and home care agencies. The costs for each component were summed and those for Canada were converted to 1999 US dollars using gross domestic product purchasing power parities.

Health care administration accounted for 31.0% of total health care expenditures in the USA compared with 16.7% in Canada. The results showed that in the USA, total health care administration costs in 1999 were US$294.3 billion, or US$1059 per capita. In Canada, they were US$9.4 billion, or US$307 per capita. This represented a difference of US$752 per capita. If this difference were applied to the 1999 US population, the total excess administrative cost would be US$209 billion.

The authors conclude that large saving might be made in the USA if administrative costs could be reduced by implementing a Canadian-style government-based health insurance system. The authors end their paper with the question: 'Is $294.3 billion annually for US health care administration money well spent?'

provided treatment, but also in that the size of the payment is determined after treatment is provided. Total reimbursement ρ is given either by

$$\rho = W \times AC \tag{6.9}$$

or by

$$\rho = W \times (S \times I) \tag{6.10}$$

where W = workload (for example, number of cases treated), AC = average cost of services provided per case, S = number of services provided per case, and I = fee per item of service. Which model is used depends on whether hospitals are reimbursed for actual costs incurred, or on a fee-for-service (FFS) basis.

The main features of retrospective reimbursement are that in the actual costs model hospital income depends on workload and the actual costs incurred. In the FFS model reimbursement depends on workload and the services provided. I may be set by competition or by the third-party payer. Since hospital income depends on the actual costs incurred (actual costs model) or on the volume of services provided (FFS model) there are few incentives to minimise costs. For example, hospitals might encourage excessively long lengths of stay or may over-order diagnostic tests.

6.11.2 Prospective Reimbursement

Prospective reimbursement implies that payments are agreed in advance and are not directly related to the actual costs incurred. This does not mean that the hospital receives the payment in advance, only that the size of the payment is determined in advance. Since payment is not directly related to the actual costs incurred, incentives to reduce costs are greater, but payers may need to monitor the quality of care provided and access to services. If the hospital receives the same income regardless of quality, there is a financial incentive to provide low-quality care for minimum effort and minimum cost.

Prospective reimbursement can take two forms. With global budgeting the size of the budget paid to the hospital is set prospectively across the whole range of treatments provided. It is unrelated to the actual costs incurred and to workload. This provides a financial incentive to constrain total expenditure ($= W{\times}AC$). Global budgeting gives overall expenditure control to the third-party payer, but because the way in which the global budget is distributed throughout the hospital is not specified, the allocation of the global budget within the hospital may not be efficient. The size of the global budget might be set historically with an additional adjustment made each year to account for inflation and changes in case-mix, or it might be set according to a resource allocation formula based on the size of the need-weighted population served by the provider. In the latter case, the incentives of the global budget will depend on the precise components of the formula.

With prospectively set cost per case, the amount paid per case ($S{\times}I$) is determined before treatment is provided. By setting the costs per case prospectively, reimbursement is divorced from the costs incurred (AC) or the services provided per case (S), which generates incentives for cost containment. Total reimbursement can still be increased by increasing workload. So, unlike global budgeting, this method does not provide overall expenditure control to the third-party payer.

An example of prospectively set costs per case is the diagnostic-related groups (DRG) pricing scheme introduced into the Medicare system in the USA in 1984, and subsequently used in a number of other countries (see Boxes 6.7 and 6.8). Under this scheme, DRG payments are based on average costs per case in each diagnostic group derived from a sample of hospitals. Total reimbursement achieved by a hospital is given by

$$\rho = W \times (DRG) \tag{6.11}$$

where DRG is the DRG-based prospective payment.

The precise effect of this type of reimbursement will depend on the actual costs incurred by the hospital. If $DRG < AC$, hospitals will reduce AC until $DRG = AC$; hospitals have

Box 6.7 Global budgeting versus prospectively set costs per case in Italy

In 1995, health care reforms in Italy included the introduction of a DRG pricing scheme in the hospital sector, with the aims of controlling the growth of hospital costs and making hospitals more accountable for their productivity. Previously hospital services had been reimbursed using global budgeting. Louis *et al.* (1999) examined the impact of the scheme on length of stay, health outcomes and quality of care.

Using hospital discharge data for the period 1993 to 1996 for 32 hospitals in the Friuli-Venezia-Giulia region of Italy, they examined changes in hospital admissions, length of stay, mortality, severity of illness and readmission rates. The main findings were that inpatient admissions decreased by 17.3% over the period, and the mean length of stay decreased from 9.1 days to 8.8 days. The fall in inpatient admissions was compensated by an increase in less costly day-case procedures, whose use increased by 700% over the period. For eight of the nine conditions studied (appendicitis, diabetes mellitus, colorectal cancer, cholecystitis, bronchitis/chronic obstructive pulmonary disease, bacterial pneumonia, coronary artery disease, cerebrovascular disease, but not hip fracture) severity of illness worsened over the period. Changes in mortality over the period were found to be small.

The authors concluded that the introduction of the DRG pricing scheme had the predicted effects, showing a trend towards reduced costs (substituting day-cases for inpatient admissions and reduced length of stay) with a negative effect on some health outcomes.

Box 6.8 Healthcare Resource Groups (HRGs) and payment by results in the NHS

'Payment by results' (PbR) is a prospective reimbursement system used to commission NHS-funded health care services from NHS providers. The units of currency in this system are Healthcare Resource Groups (HRGs), which are standardized categories of clinically similar treatments that consume roughly equal amounts of health care resource – similar to, and indeed derived from DRGs.

In essence, there now exists a national 'tariff' of prices for each HRG, which is the basis on which secondary care services are commissioned for patients, and which determines the revenues hospitals receive from each of their activities.

The aim of PbR is to 'provide a transparent, rules-based system for paying trusts. It will reward efficiency, support patient choice and diversity and encourage activity for sustainable waiting time reductions. Payment will be linked to activity and adjusted for casemix.' (www.dh.gov.uk/PolicyAndGuidance/OrganisationPolicy/FinanceAndPlanning/NHSFinancialReforms/fs/en).

HRGs are also the basis for a proposed Programme Budgeting system (see Chapter 12) for the NHS.

an incentive to minimise costs. If, on the other hand, $DRG > AC$, hospitals will increase costs until $DRG = AC$. They will spend more on amenities in order to improve their competitive position in the health care market, which will cause AC to rise.

Predicted effects of the DRG pricing scheme are cost shifting, patient shifting and DRG creep. Cost shifting and patient shifting are ways of circumventing the cost-minimising effects of DRG pricing by shifting patients or some of the services provided to patients out of the DRG pricing scheme and into other parts of the system not covered by DRG pricing. For example, instead of being provided on an inpatient basis, treatment might be provided on an outpatient basis where it is reimbursed retrospectively. DRG creep arises when hospitals deliberately or inadvertently classify cases into DRGs that carry a higher payment, indicating that they are more complicated than they really are. This might arise, for instance, when cases have multiple diagnoses.

6.12 INTEGRATION BETWEEN THIRD-PARTY PAYERS AND HEALTH CARE PROVIDERS

The way in which health care providers are reimbursed for the services they provide is a crucial determinant of health care costs and the quality of services provided. Retrospective reimbursement is likely to lead to an escalation in health care costs, while prospective reimbursement leads to concerns over quality and access. The problem from the point of view of the third-party payer is how best to monitor the activities of health care providers, and how to encourage them to act in a mutually beneficial way. This problem might be reduced if health care providers and third-party payers are linked in some way so that they share common goals.

There are three levels of integration between third-party payers and health care providers. In the first, the third-party payer and the health care provider are separate entities with separate aims and objectives. The goals of health care providers may not be consistent with those of insurance providers. In the second, there is selective contracting, with the third-party payer agreeing to steer individuals insured on their plans to selected providers and, in return, the selected providers charge lower prices to the third-party payer. Typically the third-party payer will undertake utilisation reviews to check the appropriateness of the selected providers' practices with respect to the cost and quality of care. In the third, there is vertical integration in which the insurance provider and the health care provider merge to become different parts of the same organisation. Vertical integration means that a single organisation provides health care in return for payment of an insurance premium. Because the two entities are parts of the same organisation, they have common goals with respect to the cost and quality of care. Integration between third-party payers and health care providers is a key feature of managed care.

Managed care organisations (MCOs) have arisen predominantly in the private health insurance sector in the US health care system as a means of controlling spiralling health care costs arising from the traditional private health insurance model (sometimes referred to as an indemnity plan). As noted in the previous section, a key feature of managed care is the integration between the third-party payer and the health care provider. Typically, health care is provided by an MCO to a defined population at a fixed rate per month. The payments made by individuals are lower than with direct out-of-pocket payment or indemnity plans. In return for paying lower premiums, enrolees are required to receive health care from a limited number of providers with whom the MCO has negotiated lower reimbursement rates. There are three broad types of MCO, reflecting the extent of integration between third-party payers and health care providers.

6.12.1 Preferred Provider Organisations

In return for payment of an insurance premium, preferred provider organisations (PPOs) provide insured individuals with two options when they require treatment. First, they can use the PPO's preferred providers – those with which it contracts selectively in return for lower reimbursement rates. By using the preferred provider individuals face lower user charges, and so the reduced costs of care with the preferred provider are passed on to the individual. Secondly, individuals may choose to use a different provider outside the network of preferred providers but with higher user charges. Patients can choose freely which option they prefer because there is no gatekeeper to authorise the type of care selected; but there is obviously a financial incentive to use the preferred providers.

6.12.2 Health Maintenance Organisations

In its simplest form, the main feature of a health maintenance organisation (HMO) is that the insurance company and the health care provider vertically integrate to become different parts of the same organisation. The HMO provides health care to the individual in return for a fixed fee (insurance premium), thus combining the role of third-party payer and health care provider. Usually HMOs provide comprehensive health care but stipulate that all care is to be provided by an authorised provider integrated with the HMO in some way. HMO members are assigned a primary care physician who has a gatekeeper role and authorises any health care provided; the individual must pay an additional charge for any treatment not authorised.

There are four broad types of HMO, reflecting different relationships between the third-party payer and the health care provider. In the *staff model* the HMO employs physicians directly. In the *group model* the HMO, instead than employing staff, contracts with a group practice of physicians for the provision of care. In the *network model* the HMO contracts with a network of group practices. Finally, in the case of *independent practice associations* physicians in small independent practices contract to service HMO members.

6.12.3 Point-of-Service Plans

Point-of-service (POS) plans are a mixture of PPOs and HMOs. As with PPOs, in return for payment of an insurance premium patients have two options when they require treatment: use the preferred provider network with lower user charges; or use non-networked providers on less favourable terms. Unlike PPOs, however, POS plans employ primary care physician gatekeepers who authorise any health care provided by the preferred provider network. In this way, POS plans are like HMOs.

Box 6.9 HMO performance in the USA

The potential advantages of HMOs over indemnity plans are that they can reduce health care costs by incentivising health care providers to charge lower prices and to encourage patients to choose cheaper providers. They also tend to emphasise potentially cost-saving prevention and health promotion practices that encourage individuals to stay healthy. The potential disadvantages are that they may limit access to care and may result in reduced quality in an effort to reduce costs.

Miller and Luft (2002) undertook a systematic review of the peer-reviewed literature from 1997 to mid-2001 to investigate various dimensions of HMO performance relative to non-HMOs in the USA. They identified 79 studies and HMO performance was judged according to whether the findings were favourable to HMOs relative to non-HMOs and whether the findings were statistically significant. The outcome measures included quality of care, access to care, patient satisfaction, prevention practices, length of hospital stay and use of expensive resources.

The authors reported that HMOs had generally lower length of stay and use of expensive resources, indicating that they were successful in reducing health care costs. They also tended to provide more prevention activities. It was noted that while in some studies HMOs resulted in lower quality and worse access, in total the effects were ambiguous. This was interpreted to mean that quality and access were not uniform and that they varied across providers, plans (HMOs and non-HMOs), and geographical areas. Patient satisfaction was generally lower with HMOs than with non-HMOs.

Summarising their work, Miller and Luft state: '. . . [I]f quality is comparable for HMO and non-HMO plans, then many HMO enrolees who have a choice among plans seem willing to accept lower satisfaction for lower out-of-pocket payments. Based on the findings from the articles reviewed here and in the past, the trade-off overall does not appear to be one of lower quality of care for lower out-of-pocket payments.'

They conclude by saying: 'The consistently mixed quality-of-care results for HMO versus non-HMO plans over the past two decades suggests that for HMOs to meet the vision of their advocates and as a whole outperform PPO and indemnity plan quality of care, nothing less than a systematic revamping of health care information systems, incentives, and clinical processes may be required. It remains to be seen whether such a revamping will occur.'

6.13 OPTIONS FOR HEALTH CARE FINANCING

In this section we discuss options for insurance-based health care financing. The exposition draws heavily on Mossialos *et al.* (2002).

6.13.1 Private Health Insurance

This type of health insurance has all the main features of the basic insurance model developed in the first part of this chapter. Individuals enter into contracts with insurance providers voluntarily, and pay premiums out of their own pocket or are paid by their employers as part of their salary package or both. Private health insurance is usually supplied by providers for profit, though it can also be offered by public bodies or by not-for-profit organisations. The size of the insurance premium is usually based on the risk status of the insured individual. Patients may be required to pay user charges, in the form of co-payments or deductibles, to cover all or part of the costs of their health care.

Private health insurance can be substitutive, when it provides the only form of insurance cover for an individual; complementary, when it provides cover for health care that is excluded or not fully covered by the compulsory insurance system; or supplementary, when its role is to increase subscriber choice of provider and improve access. Private health insurance can be provided via indemnity plans or MCOs.

6.13.2 Social Health Insurance

Social insurance is based on the notion of 'solidarity', whereby workers, employers and government each contribute to the financing of health care by paying into a social insurance fund. Payments by employees can be fixed, or related to the size of their income, but are not related to individual risk. The size of the contribution might be set by the government, by an association of insurance funds or by individual funds. There may be upper and lower income thresholds above and below which contributions are not levied. Many countries finance their social insurance funds by means of a hypothecated pay-roll tax, each firm paying an amount depending on the number of people they employ. The social insurance funds are usually independent of direct government control.

Membership of social health insurance funds may be assigned according to occupation or region of residence, or individuals may be free to choose a fund. Children are covered through their parents' funds, and husbands and wives who do not work are covered by their spouses' funds. Contributions can be made into social health insurance funds for retired and unemployed individuals either by the state, or via pension funds and unemployment funds.

6.13.3 Taxation

Taxation-based systems usually cover the whole population. Finance for health care is mainly taken from taxes, which are collected by the government at the local, regional or national levels. They can be general (tax revenues are pooled together and allocated according to budgetary decisions made by the government) or hypothecated (earmarked specifically to pay for health care); direct (levied on individuals or firms) or indirect (determined by the amount of consumption); compulsory or non-compulsory; and based or not based on ability to pay. This does mean that a person's payments for health care are not related to their risks.

6.13.4 The Key Features of Health Care Systems

The key features of each system are summarised in Table 6.2. The table also includes the mechanisms available in each system for dealing with health insurance market failures (adverse selection, moral hazard, non-price competition, incomplete coverage).

Box 6.10 discusses the public's view about the performance of different health care systems, based on data in Table 6.3.

Box 6.10 The performance of health care systems: The public's view

Most health care systems are financed from a variety of sources, including taxation, social health insurance, private health insurance and out-of-pocket payments. The top panel in Table 6.3 shows the sources of health expenditure in five countries (Australia, Canada, New Zealand, UK, USA). Each has a mix of public and private funding sources. Four countries are predominantly tax-based, with a high proportion of public expenditure and a low proportion of social security expenditure (representing social health insurance). The other country (the USA) is financed mainly from private sources (out-of-pocket expenditure and prepaid private health insurance plans).

The fact that most countries rely on a mix of revenue sources means that it is difficult to evaluate a health care system's performance based on the nature of the health care financing system. Bearing this in mind, Blendon *et al.* (2003) undertook a survey of 750–844 'sicker adults' in each of the five countries. Telephone interviews were conducted with respondents during March–May 2002 and their views were elicited on a variety of issues relating to their satisfaction with the health system in their country and the major problems associated with it.

A large minority of respondents in each country had negative views about their health care system. The proportion reporting they were 'not very satisfied' or 'not at all satisfied' ranged from 31% in the UK to 48% in New Zealand. In no country was the proportion reporting they were 'very satisfied' greater than 25%.

When respondents were asked to list the two biggest problems facing their health care system there were marked differences across countries. Unsurprisingly for a predominantly private health insurance system, the high cost of health care and inadequate coverage of services were major concerns in the USA. These were far less important in the other countries, but inadequate government funding was important. This is also unsurprising in predominantly publicly funded systems. Reflecting these findings, when asked what was the single most important thing the government could do to improve care, respondents in all countries except the USA said increased public spending on health care. The government policy endorsed most frequently by US respondents was to improve coverage of services or people.

While there were differences in responses that are clearly related to the way in which each health care system is financed, the authors of the paper conclude: 'Interestingly, despite clear structural differences among the systems, findings in all five countries reveal consistent dissatisfaction among surveyed populations with general health system quality.' Taken at face value the findings of the survey suggest that the type of health care financing system has little bearing on overall satisfaction, though it does influence the causes of dissatisfaction.

Empirically, most health care systems are a mix of the types discussed above. For policy makers the challenge is to ensure an appropriate financing mix to meet the relevant policy objectives. Potentially important objectives are equity or fairness in the finance and distribution of health care. We turn our attention to these issues in Chapter 7.

Table 6.2 Key features of insurance-based health care financing systems

	Private health insurance	Social health insurance	Taxation
Key features	1. Insurance is voluntary 2. Premiums are paid by the individual and/or their employer 3. Premiums are based on individual risk status 4. Insurance providers may be profit maximisers or have goals other than profit maximisation 5. Insurance provision may be via indemnity plans or MCOs	1. Insurance is compulsory for all or part of the population 2. Premiums are usually paid in the form of a hypothecated payroll tax 3. Payments are related to ability to pay, usually as a proportion of income; they are not related to individual risk 4. Payments are made into a social insurance fund	1. Insurance is compulsory for the whole population 2. Premiums are paid in the form of tax payments made to the government 3. Payments are related to ability to pay; they are not related to individual risk 4. Taxes can be: direct or indirect; general or hypothecated; set locally, regionally or nationally
Countries with predominantly this type of system	USA	France, Germany, Luxemburg, the Netherlands	Denmark, Finland, Ireland, Italy, Norway, Portugal, Spain, Sweden, UK
Dealing with adverse selection	Experience rating	Compulsory insurance	Compulsory insurance
Dealing with moral hazard	1. Co-insurance 2. Deductibles 3. No-claims bonuses 4. Retrospective reimbursement 5. Selective contracting and vertical integration between third-party payers and health care providers	1. Co-insurance 2. Deductibles 3. Retrospective reimbursement 4. Selective contracting and vertical integration between third-party payers and health care providers	1. Co-insurance 2. Deductibles 3. Retrospective reimbursement 4. Selective contracting and vertical integration between third-party payers and health care providers
Dealing with non-price competition	1. Co-insurance 2. Deductibles 3. No-claims bonuses 4. Retrospective reimbursement 5. Selective contracting and vertical integration between third-party payers and health care providers	1. Co-insurance 2. Deductibles 3. Retrospective reimbursement 4. Selective contracting and vertical integration between third-party payers and health care providers	1. Co-insurance 2. Deductibles 3. Retrospective reimbursement 4. Selective contracting and vertical integration between third-party payers and health care providers
Dealing with incomplete coverage	1. Retrospective reimbursement 2. Selective contracting and vertical integration between third-party payers and health care providers	Compulsory insurance in which payments are related to ability to pay	Compulsory insurance in which payments are related to ability to pay

Table 6.3 Health system financing and public satisfaction

	Australia	Canada	New Zealand	UK	USA
National Health Accounts					
Total expenditure on health as % GDP	9.5	9.6	8.5	7.7	14.6
Per capita GDP in international dollars	28 277	30 429	21 943	27 959	36 056
Public expenditure on health as % total expenditure on health	67.9	69.9	77.9	83.4	44.9
Private expenditure on health as % total expenditure on health	32.1	30.1	22.1	16.6	55.1
Social security expenditure on health as % public expenditure on health	0	2.1	0	0	30.8
Out-of-pocket expenditure on health as % private expenditure on health	61.4	50.3	72.6	55.9	25.4
Prepaid plans as % private expenditure on health	22.7	42.1	25.9	18.6	65.7
Satisfaction with health system (%)					
Very satisfied	15	21	14	25	18
Fairly satisfied	48	41	36	41	36
Not very satisfied	21	23	32	21	25
Not at all satisfied	14	13	16	10	19

Sources: National Health Accounts: WHO (2006). Satisfaction with health system: Blendon *et al.* (2003).

SUMMARY

1. At the individual level, ill health is usually unpredictable. This means that the demand for many types of health care is uncertain and that consumers typically operate under conditions of uncertainty. Health care expenditures may be 'catastrophic' if they require individuals to spend a significant proportion of their income on health care as a result of unforeseen or unexpected illness.

2. Problems arising from the existence of uncertainty may be addressed by health insurance which is a contract between an insurance provider and an individual who considers themself to be at risk of ill health. When an individual buys health insurance they enter into an agreement with the insurer to pay an agreed price, called an insurance premium, in exchange for a payout to be made to the insured should they become ill.

3. Individuals choose to buy health insurance because they are risk averse. This means that they will refuse a fair gamble (a gamble which, on average,

will make exactly zero profit). The amount of money an individual is prepared to pay for insurance is equal to the fair premium, which is their expected loss if uninsured, plus a risk premium which reflects their degree of risk aversion.

4. Insurance companies are able to supply health insurance because they can pool risks across a large number of insured individuals. The total premium charged by insurance providers is equal to the fair premium plus a loading factor, which covers the insurance provider's administration costs and the profit it needs to earn to each insured individual to remain in the market.

5. Adverse selection is a source of insurance market failure and arises because of the asymmetry of information between individuals who wish to buy insurance and the insurance provider. Because of this asymmetry the insurance provider may set a community rate for insurance which will be more attractive to high-risk individuals. This will mean that people with low risks will choose not to buy insurance, and premiums can spiral until the insurance market collapses. Adverse selection may be addressed by experience rating and compulsory insurance.

6. Moral hazard is a problem of excess use of health care. It arises when it is possible to alter the probability of illness or the size of the payout required by the insurance provider. Moral hazard may be reduced by co-insurance, deductibles and no-claims bonuses.

7. Non-price competition arises when health care providers compete for patients not on the basis of price but on other factors such as comfort, available facilities and the quality of food. This will cause health care costs to rise.

8. Incomplete health insurance coverage is likely to be a problem for low-income groups and for high-risk groups even if health insurance is charged at the fair premium rate.

9. Four crucial elements of the health care financing framework are: the third party payer; the ways in which health care is paid for by households; the method of reimbursement; and the integration between third-party payers and health care providers.

10. There are three broad types of third-party payer in health care: private insurance providers; the government; and social insurance funds.

11. Methods of paying for health care include user charges, private insurance premiums, social health insurance contributions and taxation.

12. Reimbursement may be retrospective or prospective. Retrospective reimbursement gives weak incentives for cost containment. Prospective

reimbursement can take two forms: global budgeting; and prospectively set costs per case.

13. There are three levels of integration between third-party payers and health care providers: they can be separate entities; there can be selective contracting; or there can be vertical integration.

14. Managed care organisations have arisen predominantly in the private health insurance sector in the US health care system as a means of controlling spiralling health care costs. A key feature of managed care is the integration between the third-party payer and the health care provider. There are three broad types of managed care organisation: preferred provider organisations; health maintenance organisations; and point of service plans.

15. The main options for health care financing are private health insurance, social health insurance and tax-based systems.

Chapter 7

Equity in Health Care

7.1 INTRODUCTION

The way in which health care systems are organised and funded is, as we have shown in Chapters 5 and 6, important for efficiency. It also has important implications for the way that heath care is distributed among individuals. The aim of this chapter is to consider equity – that is, fairness – in relation to the distribution of health care and in the financing of health care.

Equity is an important policy objective in almost every health care system (Box 7.1 illustrates its importance to the NHS in the United Kingdom). However, what is actually meant by equity might well differ across countries. The precise meaning and importance of equity at the health system level will depend upon factors such as cultural beliefs and attitudes.

While there is no uniquely correct way of defining equity, it is informative nonetheless to consider it in a systematic way. A useful distinction, which will be made frequently throughout this chapter, is between horizontal and vertical equity. Horizontal equity refers to the equal treatment of equals – for example, the extent to which those who are equal with respect to health status have equal access to health care. Vertical equity refers to the unequal treatment of unequals – for example, the extent to which those who are unequal with respect to income differ with respect to how much they have to contribute towards the costs of health care. We will also develop a taxonomy of other

Box 7.1 The equity foundations of the NHS in the United Kingdom

Whitehead (1994) discusses the reasons why the NHS was established. She argues that the introduction of the NHS in 1948 grew out of a realisation by the government of the time that the pre-NHS system was 'inequitable, inefficient, and near to financial collapse'. In the 1930s, only 43% of the population were covered by the national insurance scheme; they were mainly men in manual and low-paid occupations and they were covered only for GP services. Around 21 million people were not covered by any health insurance, and faced potentially catastrophic expenditure should they become ill. Additionally, there was an uneven distribution of services, with deprived areas in particular being poorly served in terms of the quantity and quality of available health services. According to Whitehead:

> Against this background a wide consensus formed in the 1940s about the need to build a more equitable service and what the principles and values of such a service should be. The concept of equity in the NHS articulated by Aneurin Bevan, the minister of health responsible for introducing the NHS, was multifaceted, incorporating the following principles:

> **A service for everyone:** Everyone was to be included in the scheme as of right, without having to undergo a means test or any other test of eligibility.

> **Sharing financial costs and free at the point of use:** In the words of Bevan: 'It has been the firm conclusion of all parties that money ought not to be permitted to stand in the way of obtaining an efficient health service.' The method of funding chosen, through general taxation, was linked to the ability to pay.

> **Comprehensive in range:** There was a clear commitment to extend coverage – to preventive, treatment, and rehabilitation services, covering mental as well as physical health, chronic as well as acute care.

> **Geographical equality:** With the intention of creating 'a national service, responsive to local needs', came a commitment to improve the geographical spread of services.

> **The same high standard of care for everyone:** The Royal Commission [Merrison, 1979] emphasised that this principle must be based on levelling up, not levelling down: 'The aim must be to raise standards in areas where there are deficiencies but not at the expense of places where services are already good.'

> **Selection on the basis of need for health care, not financial position in situations of scarcity:** People had the right to expect that no one would be able to gain access to a service ahead of others, by money or social influence.

The encouragement of a non-exploitative ethos: To be achieved by maintaining high ethical standards and by minimising incentives for making profits from patients.

(Whitehead, 1994)

It is clear that considerations of equity played a pivotal role in the establishment of the NHS. This also explains why equity continues to be an important objective for the NHS today.

equity concepts. In addition we will describe how equity might be measured, with respect to both finance and distribution.

As noted in Chapter 1, the analysis of equity has both positive and normative aspects. Positive analysis is commonly undertaken to describe or measure the distribution of health and of health care use, and of the way in which payments for health care are shared between individuals in society. We will show in this chapter how economists undertake analyses of this kind. As we shall also see, economists usually analyse equity with respect to some measure of equality, such as whether people with the same ability to pay for health care make equal payments, or whether people with equal needs for health care have equal utilisation. Normative analyses are needed to make judgements about which equalities define equity, and which inequalities define inequity. For example, are inequalities in payments for health care, or in health care use or in health, across income groups, inequitable?

We begin by looking at equity in the finance of health care, that is, whether or not the way in which health care is paid for is fair. For example, do certain individuals in society, such as the poor, pay more for health care than they ought to? In the second part of the chapter we focus on distribution, which considers various equity principles and how they affect the distribution of health and health care. For example, do some individuals in society receive more health care that they ought to?

7.2 EQUITY IN THE FINANCE OF HEALTH CARE

The literature on equity in the finance of health care has focused largely on the extent to which health care is financed according to ability to pay, and in particular on whether individuals with different levels of income make appropriately different payments – that is, whether there is vertical equity. Much less attention has been paid to horizontal equity, which considers the extent to which individuals with the same income make the same payments.

7.2.1 Vertical Equity

The extent to which payments for health care vary by income can be measured by the progressivity of the health care financing system. The principle of progressivity in this context can be seen with reference to the hypothetical example in Table 7.1. Column 1 shows income deciles in a hypothetical population. The first decile shows the income and amount spent financing health care for the poorest 10% of the population. The second income decile shows the amounts for the second poorest 10% of the population, and so on. Column 2 shows the mean annual income across all individuals in each income decile. This shows that the poorest 10% of individuals earn a mean annual income of £2000, while the richest 10% of individuals earn a mean annual income of £100 000. Columns 3 to 5 show three hypothetical scenarios examining the amount of money (and in brackets the proportion of their income) that individuals in each decile spend on health care.

In a *progressive* financing system, the proportion of income that is used to pay for health care rises as income rises. This is shown in column 3. In a *regressive* financing system (column 4), the proportion of income that is used to pay for health care falls as income rises. In a *proportional* financing system the proportion of income paid does not vary with the level of income (column 5). Note that it is the *proportion* of income that is spent on health care that is relevant for determining the progressivity of the health care financing system, not the actual amount of income that is spent. Column 4, for example, demonstrates a regressive system even though rich people spend more money on health care than poor people. Economics can describe a system in terms of

Table 7.1 Amount and proportion of income spent financing health care, by income decile

1	2	3	4	5
Income decile	Mean annual income (£)	Annual amount spent paying for health care (%)		
		Progressive	Regressive	Proportional
1	2 000	160 (8)	340 (17)	240 (12)
2	5 000	450 (9)	800 (16)	600 (12)
3	9 000	900 (10)	1 350 (15)	1 080 (12)
4	14 000	1 540 (11)	1 960 (14)	1 680 (12)
5	20 000	2 400 (12)	2 600 (13)	2 400 (12)
6	27 000	3 510 (13)	3 240 (12)	3 240 (12)
7	35 000	4 900 (14)	3 850 (11)	4 200 (12)
8	45 000	6 750 (15)	4 500 (10)	5 400 (12)
9	65 000	10 400 (16)	5 850 (9)	7 800 (12)
10	100 000	17 000 (17)	8 000 (8)	12 000 (12)

vertical equity, but statements about the fairness of these types of financing system rely on value judgements about fairness.

7.2.2 Kakwani's Progressivity Index

One way in which the progressivity of health care financing can be measured is Kakwani's progressivity index (Kakwani, 1977), which measures the extent to which health care finance departs from proportionality. The basic ideas can be illustrated with reference to Figure 7.1, which shows concentration curves for income and for payments for health care.

The curve CY is the (prepayment) income concentration curve, which is sometimes referred to as the *Lorenz curve* for income. It plots the cumulative proportion of the population, ranked according to income, against the cumulative proportion of income. The shape of CY measures the degree of inequality in the distribution of income. If income were equally distributed throughout the population – if everyone earned the same income – then CY would coincide with the 45° line, which delineates equality. If all income were earned by a single individual then CY would be ⌐-shaped. By definition of the *x*-axis, CY must lie on or below the 45° line. In Figure 7.1, CY indicates that the poorest 50% of the population earn 30% of total income.

CP is the payment concentration curve. This plots the cumulative proportion of the population ranked according to prepayment income, against the cumulative proportion of health care payments. The shape of CP measures inequality in the distribution of

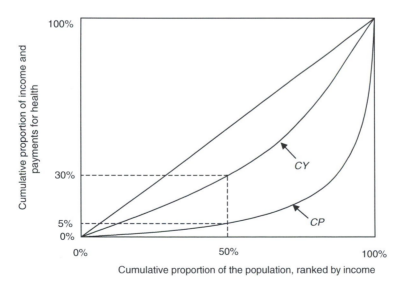

Figure 7.1 Concentration curves for income and for payments on health care.

payments for health care. If payments were equally distributed throughout the population – if everyone paid the same for health care – then CP would coincide with the 45° line. If all health care were paid for by the richest individual in the population, then CP would be ⌐-shaped. Conversely, if all health care were paid for by the poorest individual, then CP would be Γ-shaped. Hence, CP may lie on, above or below the 45° line. In Figure 7.1, the CP curve indicates that the poorest 50% of the population contribute 5% of the total payments for health care.

If payments as a proportion of income are constant across the income distribution, so that the source of health care finance is proportional, then CY and CP coincide. If payments as a proportion of income rise with income – that is, payments are progressive – CP lies below CY. If payments as a proportion of income fall with income – that is, they are regressive – CP lies above CY. As shown in Figure 7.1, CP lies below CY, which indicates that the financing system is progressive: the poorest 50% of the population earn 30% of income but contribute only 5% of payments for health care. Therefore, the richest 50% of the population earn 70% of total income and contribute 95% of all payments for health care. Payments for health care must therefore account for a larger proportion of income of the richest 50% of the population than they do of the poorest 50% and the health care financing system is progressive.

The concentration index for income, IY, is twice the area between CY and the 45° degree line. IY is sometimes referred to as the *Gini coefficient* for income. IY may take values in the range 0 to +1. If all income is earned by a single individual then $IY = +1$. If income is equally distributed so that CY coincides with the 45 degree line then $IY = 0$.

The concentration index for payments, IP, is twice the area between CP and the 45° line. IP may take values in the range −1 to +1. If all health care is paid for by the richest individual in the population then $IP = +1$. If all health care is paid for by the poorest individual then $IP = -1$, and if payments are equally distributed throughout the population then CP will coincide with the 45° line and $IP = 0$.

Kakwani's progressivity index K is defined as

$$K = IP - IY \qquad (7.1)$$

This is twice the area between CY and CP. If the financing system is progressive then CP lies below CY, and $IP > IY$, and $K > 0$. If the financing system is regressive then $K < 0$. If it is proportional then $K = 0$. Values of K range from −2 (all payments for health care are paid by the poorest person, and all income is earned by a single person) to +1 (all payments for health care are paid by the richest person, and income is equally distributed).

The overall index for a financing system consisting of more than one source of finance is the weighted average of the indices for the individual sources, where the weights are the proportions of each source of total health expenditure. This means that the progressivity of the health care financing system depends on the proportion of total health expenditure raised from each source of finance and the progressivity of each source. Another feature of K is that it is possible for a source of finance to be progressive (or regressive) at one income level but then regressive (or progressive) at another income level. The implication is that CY and CP will cross. Calculating K as the difference between IP and IY implies that the effects at different income levels will offset one another.

7.2.3 The Relationship between Progressivity and Health Care Financing Systems

The progressivity of health care finance will be affected by the type of financing system. Chapter 6 described three broad types of health care financing: private health insurance; social health insurance; and tax-based systems. Combining these with direct out-of-pocket payments for health care results in four main financing methods.

Figure 7.2 shows the mix of health care financing methods in 13 countries, illustrating the percentage of total health expenditure that is tax-based or financed by social health insurance. There are three main clusters. In the bottom right corner are countries whose

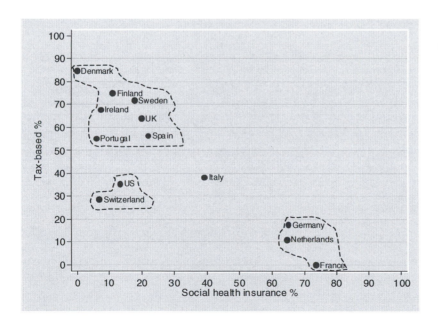

Figure 7.2 Percentage of total health expenditure that is tax-based or financed by social health insurance in 13 countries. Based on data from Wagstaff *et al.* (1999).

health care system is financed predominantly via social health insurance (France, Germany and The Netherlands). In the top left corner are countries with a predominantly tax-based system (Denmark, Finland, Ireland, Portugal, Spain, Sweden and the UK). Switzerland and the USA lie in the bottom left corner and are predominantly privately financed, mainly by private health insurance. The health care system in Italy is financed by an equal mix of taxation and social health insurance.

Box 7.2 discusses the progressivity of health care finance measured in these countries. Evidence suggests that health care systems that are based mainly on social health insurance tend to be regressive; those that are tax-based tend towards progressivity; and those that are based predominantly on private health insurance are highly regressive.

7.2.4 Horizontal Equity

Horizontal inequity in the finance of health care arises when individuals with the same ability to pay for health care, for example with the same income, pay different amounts for it.

The reasons for horizontal inequity depend on the type of health care financing system. In a tax-based system horizontal inequity will arise with direct taxation if local taxes vary across regions. It arises with indirect taxation if individuals in the same income group consume different amounts of taxable goods. With social health insurance there is horizontal inequity if households with similar incomes are members of different social health insurance schemes with different payment schedules. This might arise because they are in different occupation groups – social health insurance schemes tend to be occupation-specific. In the case of private health insurance, because it is not compulsory, individuals with the same income may make unequal payments if they choose to buy different levels of insurance cover. Also, individuals with the same income will pay different private insurance premiums if they have different risk status. With direct out-of-pocket payments, horizontal inequity can arise because of individual variation in the incidence of ill health and preferences for use of health care services across individuals with the same income.

Various measures of horizontal inequity in finance have been developed. One of the more commonly used was proposed by Aronson *et al.* (1994). In their approach, horizontal inequity is measured by the variation in health care payments, or in their case taxes, among groups of individuals or households with the same prepayment income. If there is no variation within each group, there is horizontal equity. If there is variation, there is horizontal inequity. Typically, the variation in payments for health care is measured using the concentration index for payments CP shown in Figure 7.1 for each prepayment income group. An overall index of horizontal inequity is constructed by taking a weighted sum of these concentration indices across all the groups.

Box 7.2 Progressivity of health care finance

Wagstaff *et al.* (1999) investigated the progressivity of health care finance in 13 countries. Data on prepayment income, direct out-of-pocket payments on health care and payments for private health insurance were collected primarily from household surveys in each country. Data on social health insurance payments and tax-based payments were either obtained from the same surveys or computed using data on the incidence of social health insurance payments and direct and indirect taxes from tax files combined with the household survey data on income.

Progressivity indices for total payments for health care in 12 of the countries, combining tax-based payments, social health insurance payments, private health insurance and direct out-of-pocket payments are shown below.

Country	K
France	0.0012
Germany	−0.0452
Netherlands	−0.0703
Denmark	−0.0047
Finland	0.0181
Portugal	−0.0445
Spain	0.0004
Sweden	−0.0158
UK	0.0518
Switzerland	−0.1402
USA	−0.1303
Italy	0.0413

Source: Wagstaff *et al.* (1999).

Combined with Figure 7.2, the progressivity indices show that in those countries whose health care system is financed predominantly via social health insurance (France, Germany and The Netherlands) health care finance is either proportional (K is close to zero) or regressive. In Germany and The Netherlands the system is more regressive than in France owing to the exclusion of high-income groups from the social health insurance system. In countries with a predominantly tax-based system (Denmark, Finland, Spain, Sweden and the UK) the health care financing system is either proportional or progressive. The main exception is Portugal, where total payments are regressive. This is due to the large proportion of direct out-of-pocket payments in Portugal. In Switzerland and the USA, where there is a greater reliance on private health insurance, the financing system overall is highly regressive. In Italy, where the health care system is financed by an equal mix of taxation and social health insurance, total payments are progressive.

Little empirical work has been undertaken to investigate horizontal inequity in health care finance using measures such as these. This is because they are 'cumbersome' to compute, since they involve calculating many concentration indices for payments – one for each income group (Wagstaff and van Doorslaer, 1997). In one of the few studies to attempt an analysis of horizontal inequity in health care finance, van Doorslaer *et al.* (1999) analyse health care financing mixes in 12 OECD countries and decompose overall inequality in health care payments into a vertical inequity component, a horizontal inequity component and a re-ranking component, which accounts for the extent to which a financing system causes individuals to move up or down the income distribution. The findings show that vertical inequity is much more important in explaining inequality in health care payments than horizontal inequity and re-ranking, but that their relative importance varies by the type of finance. For example, tax-based payments and social health insurance payments tend to have less horizontal inequity than private health insurance payments and direct out-of-pocket payments.

7.3 EQUITY IN DISTRIBUTION

In addition to equity in finance, there usually exists within most health care systems a concern that health care is distributed in an equitable way. In this section we consider this in more detail. The first question we ask is what is the 'distribuendum' – that is, the thing that we want to distribute fairly? Three plausible candidates are health care, health and utility.

7.3.1 Equity in the Distribution of Health Care, of Health or of Utility?

Health economists are interested in the health care sector of the economy, for example, in the optimal way of organising health care systems and of producing specific health care goods and services. This interest in health care leads understandably to a view that it is equity in the distribution of *health care* that should be the focus of equity in distribution.

However, and in keeping with Grossman's (1972) model, health care services are demanded largely because of their effect on *health*. This explains why, for instance, health economists are interested not just in the supply of health care discussed in Chapter 4, but also in its impact on the health of patients (see Chapter 10, which looks specifically at measuring and valuing health care output). This suggests that it is health – not health care – that should be the focus of equity in distribution. Proponents of this view include Williams and Cookson (2000), who argue that equity in health is a more fundamental objective than equity in health care, and that focusing on health care ignores all other possible ways for improving health.

Pursuing the line of reasoning that health care is a means to an end and not an end in itself, it is the case that many health care services have as their output things other than improvements in health. For example, a health education programme that increases awareness of the symptoms of meningitis aims, among other things, to provide information to reassure people about their health, though it may not influence their health directly; in-vitro fertilisation enables infertile couples the opportunity to experience parenthood; tattoo removal provides the opportunity to avoid social stigmatism, Viagra™ provides the opportunity to enjoy increased sexual pleasure, and dental veneers provide the opportunity to improve one's appearance. In these cases, the goal is to improve utility rather than to improve health. If we take the view that the appropriate distribuendum is determined by the goal of health care, then equity in distribution might plausibly be couched in terms of utility.

Whether the focus should be on health or utility depends on whether we believe that resource allocation should depend only on the utility obtained by individuals – a stance known as welfarism – or whether it should also depend on factors other than utility, such as health, which is associated with extra-welfarism. In Chapter 8 we compare and contrast welfarism and extra-welfarism in more detail.

7.3.2 Some Concepts of Equity

Having discussed what it is that we want to distribute fairly, another relevant question is what is the appropriate concept of equity to use in order to achieve this? As we mentioned at the start of the chapter, there are many concepts of equity that could be pursued; these are limited only by our capacity to think about the different ways in which resources could be allocated. It is unsurprising therefore that so many concepts of equity are discussed in the literature. In this section we will focus on the concepts that are commonly mooted by health economists. These are utilitarianism, equal health, equal expenditure, equal access, equal use, maximin and the fair innings.

It is worth bearing in mind that some of these may constrain the distribuendum. For example, Williams and Cookson (2000), who advocate equity in the distribution of health, show that 'the principle of equal access to health care places ethical constraints on the health possibility set: it rules out all attainable health outcomes that require unequal access to health care'. An example in the case of physiotherapy services is that equity in the distribution of health might be achieved only by limiting access to those with the most severe musculoskeletal problems, which is at odds with the principle of equal access.

Utilitarianism is the view that the most desirable states of the world are those that maximise society's welfare. With strict utilitarianism, society's welfare is the equal-weighted sum of the utilities of every member of society. Weighted utilitarianism allows differential weights to be applied to the utilities of different individuals or groups of individuals. Utilitarianism has a long history in philosophy dating back to Jeremy Bentham and John Stuart Mill in the eighteenth and nineteenth centuries. The principle is consistent with our discussion of demand in Chapter 2, where we assumed, at least at the outset, that the consumers of a good are utility maximisers. Restated, a policy of strict utilitarianism would aim to distribute health care in such a manner that the greatest good was achieved for the greatest number of individuals. One implication is that it might increase inequality, which is at variance with many other equity concepts that aim for equality in some dimension. For example, suppose a policy maker has the option of introducing a public health campaign that would increase physical activity levels in the general population. Research suggests that the campaign would reduce slightly the prevalence of obesity and hence provide a small positive effect on health for a large proportion of the population. To fund the programme, the policy maker would have to stop funding an expensive ultra-orphan drug that treats paroxysmal nocturnal haemoglobinuria (PNH), which is a potentially life-threatening condition that affects around one or two people per million each year. After applying a principle of strict utilitarianism, the policy maker chooses to fund the public education campaign – the sum of the small improvements in health over a large number of people is greater than the sum of the substantial loss of health experienced by the small number with PNH. While society's welfare has increased, there is an increase in inequality because the health of the majority improves at the expense of those with PNH. Thus, while strict utilitarianism treats everybody equally in terms of how they contribute to social welfare, it may exacerbate inequality in outcomes. These inequalities may be vitiated by placing more weight on certain individuals in society, for example those with PNH. In this case the policy maker may be less likely to choose the public health campaign and there is less inequality. A more formal description of utilitarianism, in which we construct social welfare functions (SWFs) for both strict and weighted utilitarianism, is provided in Chapter 8.

The concept of *equal health*, where health is measured for example in terms of quality-adjusted life years (see Chapters 9 and 10) or some other measure of mortality and morbidity, is closely related to the principle of *reducing inequalities* in health, and might be applied within age and sex groups. One feature of this concept is that achieving equal health may involve imposing restrictions on how people live their lives. For instance, smoking cigarettes is unlikely to be consistent with equal health. Another feature is that the influence of health care on health is limited. Other factors such as diet, lifestyle, education, economic activity and housing are equally or perhaps more important determinants of health. Hence, it becomes difficult to answer the question of how best to allocate scarce health care resources to achieve equal health, which is often the concern of health economists.

In the case of *equal expenditure* each person receives the same share of health care spending. As it stands this ignores the distribution of need across society (see

Chapter 1 for a more detailed discussion of how economists define this) but it could be amended to equal expenditure for equal need. This is similar to *equal use* for equal need because it ignores preferences for health and for health care and, in the case of risky health care programmes, it ignores attitudes to risk. To illustrate, suppose two people have the same need for a crown to be fitted on one of their teeth. One person dislikes going to the dentist but the other does not. With equal use for equal need the aim would be for both individuals to visit the dentist and get a crown fitted. An alternative is to focus on *equal access* for equal need, in which individuals with equal needs have the same *opportunity* to access health care. With this concept, individuals in equal need may legitimately have unequal use owing to different preferences or attitudes to risk; the person who does not like going to the dentist might legitimately not do so.

Equal access for equal need is frequently cited as an appropriate equity principle (see for example Mooney, 1983, and Mooney *et al.*, 1991), though it is difficult to formulate a usable definition of equal access. One option is that the two individuals needing crowns described above have equal access if the costs incurred by them in receiving treatment are valued equally – that is, if they face the same access costs. These costs include travel costs and time costs as well as monetary costs arising directly for health care. These will depend on geographical factors (travel distances, travel times, availability of transport), waiting times for treatment, and information known by patients. Equal access should also account for differences in income or some other measure of ability to pay, since this is also a determinant of access (Olson and Rodgers, 1991). Note that this means that access is both a supply-side and a demand-side phenomenon. The upshot is that while one person might legitimately visit the dentist and the other might not, with the principle of equal access it would be unacceptable if it were for reasons other than preferences or risk aversion – for example, if one individual was better informed than another about dental services on offer, was more proficient at accessing dental care, or incurred lower costs. Because access is difficult to measure, most empirical studies tend to focus on equal use for equal need (see Section 7.3.3).

The concept of *maximin* was introduced in the context of game theory in Chapter 4. Simply put, the maximin principle is that when making choices, the preferred option is the one whose worst outcome is least bad. This idea was developed into a concept of equity based on distributive justice by Rawls (1971). He identified equitable behaviour as that which would be chosen by individuals if they were placed under a 'veil of ignorance'. Under this veil, every person is ignorant of the position they will have in society. They will not know, for instance, whether they will be rich or poor, or healthy or unhealthy. Rawls argued that, placed in this situation, individuals would adopt a maximin principle: a risk-minimising strategy that maximises the position of the least well off. This principle is also sometimes referred to as the *difference principle*. Applied simply to health care, it would mean that health care is distributed to maximise the health of the most ill individuals in society. The Rawlsian social welfare function is discussed in more detail in Chapter 8. An opposing view to that of Rawls was put forward by Nozick (1974), who argued that any distribution of goods and services such as health care is acceptable as long as it comes about in a free exchange between consenting adults and is made from a 'just' starting position. With this *libertarian* view the distribution is acceptable even if large inequalities emerge from the process. This is in direct contrast to Rawls' *egalitarian* view that inequalities in distribution must benefit the least well off.

The final concept we consider in this section is the *fair innings* approach, introduced by Harris (1985) and advocated more recently by Williams (1997). This is based on the idea that everyone is entitled to some common quantity of lifetime health measured, for example, in terms of quality-adjusted life years. Anyone failing to achieve this has been 'cheated', while anyone getting more than this is 'living on borrowed time' (Williams, 1997). To operationalise the principle, Williams proposes that health care services for individuals facing less than a fair innings should be valued more highly than for individuals expecting a fair innings or more. He demonstrates how weights might be computed for different population groups to accomplish this. Williams shows that the fair innings principle is particularly relevant to the issue of differential treatment of the young and the old, though it also applies to other population groups, distinguished for example by socioeconomic status. He concludes: 'The analysis suggests that this notion of intergenerational equity requires greater discrimination against the elderly than would be dictated simply by efficiency objectives' (Williams, 1997).

7.3.3 Measuring Equity in Distribution

While there are many theoretical concepts of equity in distribution, the measurement of equity requires an empirically testable definition. To this end the literature on equity measurement focuses mainly on two concepts. The first is horizontal inequity, and in particular whether individuals with the same need for health care have the same use of health care services. As we shall see, far less attention has been paid to vertical equity, which in this context is usually interpreted to mean whether individuals with different levels of ill health have appropriately different levels of use. The second concept that is often the focus of empirical analysis is equal health, and in particular, the extent to which inequalities in health vary systematically with socioeconomic status.

In order to investigate horizontal and vertical equity in health care use, positive analysis is required to identify the factors that determine the use of health care services. Normative analysis is then required to distinguish which of these factors *ought* to affect use and which ones ought not to. Factors which ought to affect use are referred to as *need variables* and those which ought not to are *non-need variables*. Using this distinction it is possible to generate more practical definitions of horizontal and vertical inequity and relate them to inequality. There is inequality when individuals have different levels of health care use. There is horizontal inequity when use is affected by non-need variables. This means that individuals with the same need consume different amounts of care. There is vertical equity when individuals with different needs consume appropriately different amounts of health care.

7.3.4 Horizontal Inequity

Most empirical studies of factors affecting the use of health services find that it is determined by morbidity, age, gender, income and other measures of socioeconomic status, ethnicity and supply. They typically use regression analysis to measure the impact of these factors on use, and examine the effect of each factor after controlling for the other factors. Making normative judgements about whether these factors are need or non-need variables allows us to test for – that is, to identify – horizontal inequity. Most studies tend to classify socioeconomic status and ethnicity as non-need variables.

In the case of income, if we believe that use ought not to vary by income and it does, this indicates horizontal inequity with respect to income. If income is positively correlated with use – that is, the rich have more use than the poor – there is pro-rich horizontal inequity. Conversely, if the poor have greater use there is pro-poor horizontal inequity. Analogous arguments apply for other measures of socioeconomic status, for example education, economic activity and social class.

With ethnicity, suppose we make a simple distinction between white and non-white ethnic groups. If whites have more use than non-whites after controlling for need then there is pro-white horizontal inequity. Conversely, if non-whites have more use than whites there is pro-non-white horizontal inequity. This ignores cultural differences in attitudes to use. Some evidence on this is provided in Box 7.3, which examines evidence of inequity in the use of health care by income and ethnic groups in the NHS in England.

The discussion so far has focused on how to identify horizontal inequity. The extent of horizontal inequity can be quantified using concentration indices for health care and for need. The basic ideas are illustrated using Figure 7.3.

The curve CC is the health care concentration curve. This plots the cumulative proportion of the population, ranked according to income, against the cumulative proportion of health care received. The shape of CC measures the degree of inequality in the distribution of health care across income groups. If everyone received the same health care then CC would coincide with the 45° line. If all health care were provided to the richest individual in the population then CC would be ⌐-shaped. Conversely, if it were all provided to the poorest person then CC would be Γ-shaped. CC is closely related

Box 7.3 Inequity and inequality in the use of health care in England

Morris *et al.* (2005) undertook a regression-based analysis of the determinants of health care use in England. The analysis was based on data from three years (1998–2000) of the Health Survey for England, which contained comprehensive individual level data on the determinants of four types of NHS use: GP consultations; outpatient visits; day case treatment; and inpatient stays. Factors affecting use were morbidity, age, gender, income, education, economic activity, social class, ethnicity and supply. The authors found that morbidity, measured using a number of measures including self-assessed general health, limiting long-standing illness, and types of illness, had the expected positive effects on all forms of use.

The results below show the estimated effects of income and ethnicity on selected measures of use.

	GP visits	Outpatient visits	Inpatient stays
Income	Insig.	+ve	Insig.
Ethnic group			
Black Caribbean	Insig.	Insig.	Insig.
Black African	Insig.	Insig.	Insig.
Black Other	Insig.	Insig.	Insig.
Indian	+ve	Insig.	Insig.
Pakistani	Insig.	−ve	Insig.
Bangladeshi	Insig.	−ve	Insig.
Chinese	Insig.	−ve	−ve
Other	Insig.	−ve	Insig.

Source: Morris *et al.* (2005).

Controlling for morbidity and the other factors, income has a positive effect on outpatient visits – that is, the rich were more likely to have an outpatient visit than the poor – but does not have a significant effect on GP consultations or on inpatient stays. The effects of ethnicity are illustrated with reference to the white ethnic group. Relative to whites, those in the Indian group are more likely to visit a GP. Those in the Pakistani, Bangladeshi, Chinese and Other groups were less likely to have an outpatient visit than whites, and those in the Chinese group were less likely to have an inpatient stay.

Overall, the analysis provides some evidence of inequality in the use of health care services with respect to income and ethnicity. In particular, the results indicate that some non-white groups have lower than expected use of certain types of hospital services. The interpretation is complicated by potentially unobserved cultural differences, which may legitimately affect the use of health services. However, if cultural preferences were socially created, including within the health care system, then this reduces their legitimacy. The authors also argue that these factors might be expected to have a smaller impact on hospital services than GP visits because doctors exert more influence over hospital utilisation than over GP utilisation. If so, these results are evidence for pro-white horizontal inequity in the case of hospital services.

to the concentration index for health care, IC, which is twice the size of the area between CC and the 45° line. IC may take values in the range −1 to +1. If all health care is received by the richest individual in the population, then $IC = +1$. If all health care is received by the poorest individual then $IC = −1$. If health care is equally distributed throughout the population then $IC = 0$.

CN is the need concentration curve. It plots the cumulative proportion of the population ranked according to income against the cumulative proportion of need in the

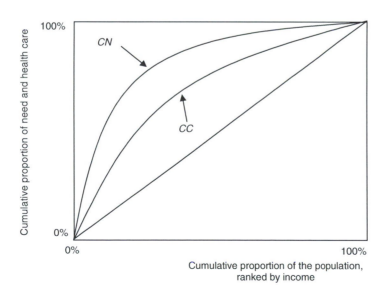

Figure 7.3 Concentration curves for need and for health care.

population. It measures inequality in the distribution of need for health care and is defined analogously to the health care concentration curve. CN may lie on, above or below the 45° line. The concentration index for need, IN, is related to CN. It may take values in the range −1 to +1. If only the richest individual in the population has need for health care, then CN is ⌐-shaped and $IN = +1$. If only the poorest individual has need then CN is Γ-shaped and $IN = -1$.

The measure of horizontal inequity – the horizontal inequity index, HI – is defined as

$$HI = IC - IN \qquad (7.2)$$

This is twice the area between CC and CN. If there is pro-poor horizontal inequity then CC lies above CN, and $IC < IN$, and $HI < 0$. If there is pro-rich horizontal inequity then $HI > 0$. If there is horizontal equity then $HI = 0$. Values of HI range from −2 (all health care is provided to the poorest person, and all the need is concentrated in the richest person) to +2 (all health care is provided to the richest person, and all need is concentrated in the poorest person). The curves in Figure 7.3 show pro-rich horizontal inequity.

The HI index measures horizontal inequity 'on balance' (Wagstaff and Van Doorslaer, 2000) in the sense that if for some types of need there is pro-rich horizontal inequity but for others there is pro-poor horizontal inequity then CC and CN cross. The two effects will offset one another in the index.

Box 7.4 discusses HI indices for primary and secondary health care in various countries in Europe and the USA.

7.3.5 Vertical Equity

Vertical equity considers the extent to which individuals with different needs for health care have appropriately different levels of use. Testing for vertical inequity requires strong judgements about the way health care use ought to vary across individuals with different levels of need. This implies normative statements about the relative merits of the effect of health care on individuals with different levels of need, and positive statements about the effects of this. As a consequence, most empirical studies of equity in the distribution of health care have tended to focus on horizontal inequity using the methods outlined in the previous section.

As noted by Abasolo *et al.* (2001), a necessary but not sufficient test for vertical equity is whether higher levels of need – usually represented by more severe morbidity – are associated with higher levels of use. For this test, information on appropriate use at different morbidity levels is not required; all that is needed is that those with greater

Box 7.4 Horizontal inequity in health care use in Europe and in the USA

Van Doorslaer *et al.* (2000) measured horizontal inequity in health care use for various countries in Europe and the USA. They computed *HI* indices for GP contacts, outpatient medical specialist visits, all physician contacts, inpatient days and aggregate imputed expenditure. Data on health care use, income, and need were obtained for each country from individual level surveys. Need was defined as the health care use that an individual was expected to receive given their age, gender, self-assessed general health, whether or not the individual suffered from one or more chronic conditions, and the type of chronic conditions suffered. Results for all physician contacts (GP contacts and outpatient medical specialist visits combined) and inpatient days are shown below.

Country	All physician contacts	Inpatient days
Denmark	0.045	−0.076
Finland	0.039	−0.061
East Germany	0.034	−0.033
West Germany	−0.010	−0.033
Netherlands	0.047	−0.064
Sweden	0.034	−0.036
Switzerland	−0.004	0.047
UK	0.011	−0.058
USA	0.044	−0.008

Source: Van Doorslaer *et al.* (2000).

In most countries there is evidence of pro-rich horizontal inequity in terms of physician contacts. Conversely, in terms of inpatient care days, there is pro-poor horizontal inequity across all the countries studied except for Switzerland.

The pro-rich inequity in physician contacts does not seem to be associated with country-specific health care system characteristics. The authors conclude: '[T]here is little or no evidence of significant inequity in the distribution of health care overall, though in half of the countries, significant pro-rich inequity emerges for physician contacts. This seems to be due mainly to a higher use of medical specialist services by higher-income groups and a higher use of GP care among lower-income groups. These findings appear to be fairly general and emerge in countries with very diverse characteristics regarding access and provider incentives' (Van Doorslaer *et al.*, 2000).

morbidity receive more health care. Further decisions about vertical inequity are not possible without information or normative judgements concerning the appropriate level of use at different levels of need.

In one of the few studies to attempt to test for and measure vertical inequity, Sutton (2002) analysed the relationship between health status and use of GP services at different levels of health status among health survey respondents in Scotland. He found a generally negative correlation, that is, those with higher health status had lower use, but the relationship was unexpectedly positive at low levels of health status. Taking the normative view that the appropriate negative linear relationship between health status and health care use at the higher levels of health status should apply across the whole range of health status, this provided a method of testing for vertical inequity and measuring its extent. The results indicate pro-healthy vertical inequity: more healthy individuals had higher than expected use given their level of need. Subsequent analyses found that 'divergence between the current allocation of health care and the target allocation of health care therefore falls disproportionately on the poor, although the estimate of vertical inequity is not significant' (Sutton, 2002). Sutton concludes: 'The results of this study are consistent with the widespread concern that the high primary care needs of some individuals are "squeezed" by the less important demands of others' (Sutton, 2002).

7.3.6 Inequalities in Health

As discussed in Section 7.3.1, it has been argued that concerns about the distribution of health care arise from more deep-seated concerns about the distribution of health. Therefore, in a discussion about measuring equity in distribution it is useful to examine the measurement of equity in the distribution of health, which focuses on health inequalities.

There is a huge literature on analysing inequalities in health, much of it emanating from the public health field. This tends to focus on testing whether ill health measured in lots of different ways varies by population groups, such as by socioeconomic status and by ethnicity. We focus here on the type of analyses that tend to be undertaken by economists. Some of the work by economists measures pure inequalities in health. This looks at inequalities in health across individuals irrespective of their socioeconomic status or other factors.

There is also a body of work by economists that focuses on measuring the extent of socioeconomic inequalities in health by quantifying the inequality in ill health between the rich and the poor. This might typically be measured using the concentration curve approach described above. In this context the approach uses the ill health concentration curve (see Figure 7.4).

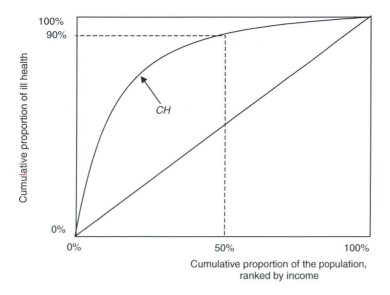

Figure 7.4 Ill health concentration curve.

The ill health concentration curve *CH* plots the cumulative proportion of the population, ranked according to income, against the cumulative proportion of ill health in the population, measured in some way such as by the presence of disease or life expectancy. The concentration index for ill health, *IH*, is twice the size of the area between *CH* and the 45° line. *IH* may take values in the range −1 to +1, depending on whether ill health is concentrated in the richest individual in the population (*CH* is ⌐-shaped and *IH* = +1) or in the poorest individual (*CH* is Γ-shaped and *IH* = −1). If everyone has the same health then *CH* will coincide with the 45° line and *IH* = 0. In Figure 7.4 the poorest 50% of the population incur 90% of ill health – there is a pro-poor distribution of ill health.

Box 7.5 presents an example of an analysis estimating concentration indices for ill health in nine countries.

Once inequity in health care has been identified, policy makers may choose to intervene to bring about a more equitable allocation of health care services. Given the likelihood of market and government failures in health care, as discussed in Chapter 5, a more explicit method for determining what health care services should be provided may be required. In light of the discussion in this chapter, such a method would ideally allow

Box 7.5 Ill health concentration indices in nine countries

Van Doorslaer *et al.* (1997) computed ill health concentration indices in nine countries using individual level survey data for adults from 1982 to 1992 on health and income. Income was measured as disposable household income per equivalent adult. Health was measured by self-assessed general health measured on a three-, four- or five-point scale in each survey.

Values of the ill health concentration indices for the nine countries are reported below.

Country	*IH*
Finland	−0.0566
East Germany	−0.0436
West Germany	−0.0571
The Netherlands	−0.0660
Spain	−0.0732
Sweden	−0.0347
Switzerland	−0.0696
UK	−0.1148
USA	−0.1360

Source: Van Doorslaer *et al.* (1997).

In all countries *IH* is negative, indicating pro-poor inequality in health. The greatest income-related health inequality is in the USA, followed by the UK. Subsequent analyses by the authors revealed that income-related inequality in health was positively associated with income inequality. Exceptions were Sweden and the UK. In the case of Sweden there was lower than expected income-related health inequality given the level of inequality in income. The opposite was true for the UK.

different members of society to be weighted differently from one another in order to ensure equitable distribution (see Tsuchiya and Williams, 2001). These weights could, for example, be used in economic evaluation as an explicit way of addressing distributional issues. Economic evaluation and its role in informing resource allocation decisions are considered in Part II.

SUMMARY

1. Equity is an important policy objective in almost every health care system. However, what is actually meant by equity might well differ across countries. The precise meaning and importance of it will depend on factors such as cultural beliefs and attitudes.

2. There are two main areas of health care in which issues of equity (or fairness) are likely to arise: finance and distribution.

3. A useful distinction can be made between horizontal and vertical equity. Horizontal equity refers to the equal treatment of equals. Vertical equity refers to the unequal treatment of unequals.

4. Equity in the finance of health care has focused on whether there is vertical equity in the finance of health care. This considers the extent to which individuals with unequal ability to pay for health care make appropriately unequal payments. This is usually measured by the extent to which the health care financing system is progressive, regressive or proportional, which refers to whether payments for health care rise or fall as a proportion of income as income rises. The progressivity of health care financing systems is usually measured using progressivity indices.

5. There usually exists within most health care systems a concern that health care is distributed in an equitable way. An important question is what is the distribuendum? That is, what is it that we want to distribute fairly? Three plausible candidates are health care, health and utility.

6. Some aims that are commonly mooted by economists to achieve equity are utilitarianism, equal health, equal expenditure, equal use, equal access, maximin, and the fair innings.

7. The measurement of equity in distribution tends to focus on horizontal inequity in use, which considers the extent to which individuals with the same need for health care have the same use of health care services, and in measuring health inequalities.

Part II

Economic Evaluation in Health Care

Chapter 8

Welfarist and Non-Welfarist Foundations of Economic Evaluation

8.1 THE NORMATIVE ECONOMICS FOUNDATIONS OF ECONOMIC EVALUATION

In Chapter 1, we drew a distinction between positive economics and normative economics. The former is descriptive or predictive in nature: economic analysis describes trends in economic variables and by generating testable hypotheses about the relationships between them explains and predicts further trends. However, many of the questions that health economics seeks to address are also concerned with making judgements about the relative desirability of alternative ways of delivering health and health care. Part II of this book is concerned with how economics is used to evaluate the benefits and costs of alternative uses of resources in the health care sector.

Economic evaluation describes a broad set of analytical approaches used to describe and compare the benefits and costs of competing uses of resources. It is normative in two respects. Most obviously, to conclude that one treatment option is better value for money than another, having weighed up both the benefits and costs, is either explicitly or implicitly prescriptive. Although economists can occasionally be seen actively to promote or oppose a particular option, most emphasise that their role is to provide evidence to *inform* decisions, rather than to *make* them. Restricting the role of the economist to describing the benefits and costs of alternatives does not, however, avoid value judgements. Although the methods of economic evaluation we describe in Chapters 9–12 are highly technical, involving sophisticated modelling and statistical procedures, underlying this quantitative toolkit are views on what constitutes a cost, what is of benefit and how these things are to be valued.

The theory and practice of economic evaluation is therefore inescapably normative in nature. Economic evaluation is crucially concerned with how benefits are to be measured and valued – and the economist's notion of cost is the *value* of other opportunities forgone. Further, given that increasing the benefits enjoyed by one person or persons involves sacrificing benefits to other persons, conclusions about the desirability of any given option invokes value judgements about the extent to which such trade-offs are acceptable and desirable.

The aim of this chapter is to explain the value judgements that underpin the principles and practice of economic evaluation; to show the role these play in providing the theoretical foundations of economic evaluation methods, and to assess critically their defensibility as a basis for social choices.

Although normative economics is often, in the mainstream economics literature, taken as synonymous with welfare economics (for example, Boadway and Bruce, 1984; Johansson, 1991), here we distinguish between two normative economics approaches – welfarism and non-welfarism – which are evident in the practice of economic evaluation of health care. The term 'welfarist' was first used by Sen (1977) as a means of distinguishing the traditional normative economics approach to social choices from contemporary critical non-welfarist positions on it (see Section 8.9). We conclude the chapter by considering whether these normative positions can be reconciled, and by re-iterating the implications of the analyst's normative position for the science of economic evaluation.

8.2 WELFARE ECONOMICS

Welfare economics, or *welfarism*, is generally defined as the systematic analysis of the social desirability of any set of arrangements, for example a state of the world or allocation of resources, solely in terms of the utility obtained by individuals.

Welfare economics is the principal normative tradition in economics. Its aim is to devise a set of rules – essentially, value judgements – that can be used to achieve a logical and consistent ranking of all alternative social states, for example how scarce health care resources are allocated, between which we might choose. Of course, there are many ways in which this might be achieved: we could delegate decision making to politicians, and rely upon their judgements about what is best for society, or an autocrat could make these choices on society's behalf. The distinctive approach taken by welfare economics in assessing the relative desirability of states is traditionally characterised by the following three arguments.

First, welfare economics is based entirely on individualism: the only relevant information in making social choices is the views of the individuals affected by those choices. Individuals – consumers or households – are deemed to be the best judges of their own welfare, and to behave in a manner that is utility maximising. The effects of social choices are therefore considered to be most appropriately measured by considering the impact on individuals *as they see it themselves*. This impact is captured by changes in their utility, any given state of the world being considered is assessed in terms of individuals' evaluations of whether it makes them better, worse or equally well off as in other states of the world. In welfare economics, social welfare – a measure of the well-being of society as a whole – is therefore exclusively a product of the utilities of individual members of society. Judgements by others, for example experts such as health care professionals, and paternalistic views of what is good for people are deemed irrelevant.

Secondly, given its basis in consumer choice theory, welfare economics is consequentialist – it traditionally only takes into account the outcomes for individuals, in terms of their consumption of specific types and quantities of goods and services and the consequent utility obtained. The utility associated with the consumption of goods and services is considered neutral to the process, be it a market, political or other process, of choosing or receiving those goods. Utility is generated only from consumption – our own consumption and, where there are caring externalities, the consumption of others whom we care about.

Thirdly, given that the objective of welfare economics is to devise a decision rule that allows us completely and consistently to rank all states of the world, and that this ranking is to be based strictly on the consequences, in utility terms, for each individual, the principal challenge in welfare economics is to propose a defensible basis for aggregating individuals' preferences. Inevitably, we confront situations where the relative desirability of states depends upon what sort of trade-offs between individuals' utilities we deem acceptable. There is no objective way of dealing with such trade-offs. The basic judgement used in welfare economics, and its defining feature as a normative framework for social choice, is the Pareto principle.

8.3 THE PARETO PRINCIPLE

Since a value judgement is necessary, it seems reasonable to suggest that the best value judgement to use is that which would command widest support – that is, one with which most of us would agree. A value judgement with this characteristic is described as *weak* because the view that it represents is relatively uncontentious. The value judgement that lies at the heart of welfare economics was proposed by Vilfredo Pareto in 1906 (Busino, 1987).

Paretian concepts are especially important to economic evaluation and resource allocation decisions, because they provide a basis for judging a given state of affairs to be optimal or not and for ranking states relative to each other by reference to the utility obtained by individuals in each state. The theoretical basis of Paretian analysis is consumer choice theory (see Chapter 2). This requires that each person can consider a set of states of the world – effectively, bundles of goods – and consistently rank them, meaning that they have stable and transitive preferences. A goal of Paretian analysis, and indeed of welfare economics generally, is to aggregate these individual preferences to produce a social welfare ordering (SWO) – a complete and consistent ranking of all possible states in terms of their social desirability.

As well as defining optimality, Paretian analysis provides a set of related concepts that are important in judgements about social welfare, such as the notion of Pareto improvements. For example, a change in the state of the world that increases the utility of *all* affected people is a *weak Pareto improvement*. A change in the state of the world that increases the utility of at least one person, and does not decrease the utility of anyone else is a *strong Pareto improvement*. Paretian concepts play a crucial role in economics – for example, they provide a means of judging efficiency in production (as we saw in Chapter 3) and provide the basis for the conclusion that competitive markets generate socially optimal outcomes (as we saw in Chapter 5).

Figure 8.1 illustrates the Pareto principle, using a geometric representation of the possibilities for allocating a fixed total quantity of two goods, X and Y, between two people, A and B, known as an *Edgeworth box* (or sometimes as an *Edgeworth–Bowley box*). This is constructed from the indifference curve maps of two individuals, as introduced in Chapter 2, where the walls of the box are the axes for individuals A and B, respectively. Both persons are shown simultaneously, by rotating the indifference map of person B 180° onto that of person A. The length of the X-axis shows us the total quantity of good X available; the length of the Y-axis shows us the total quantity of good Y available. Each and every point within the box is a feasible allocation of these quantities of the two goods between the two people. Choose any point within this box: it represents a unique allocation of quantities of goods X and Y between person A and person B. For example, at point g, person A receives X_1 units of good X and Y_1 units of good Y. The quantity of X received by person B at point g is whatever is left over, that is the difference between the total quantity of good X available and that consumed by person A (X_1); similarly for good Y. Associated with every point within the space defined by the walls of the Edgeworth box is an indifference curve for both person A and person B. This shows us the utility they each experience from

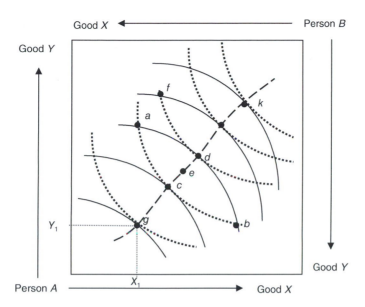

Good X ← Person B

Good Y

f
a
k
d
e
c
g b

Y_1

Good Y

Person A → X_1 Good X

● **Figure 8.1 The Pareto principle demonstrated using an Edgeworth box.**

consuming the exact bundle of goods X and Y represented by that point. Points lying to the north-east in this box will be preferred, that is ranked more highly, by person A than points lying in the south-west, as they are associated with higher utility; the opposite applies to person B.

The Pareto principle offers a means of identifying which of these points can be considered *socially* better than another, by reference to the utility of each person. Examples of each of the following Paretian concepts are provided in Box 8.1.

If, by shifting from one point to another, *both* persons' utility is increased, this is a *weak* Pareto improvement. We would say such a change is a good thing using the Paretian value judgement, and the latter point is therefore Pareto superior to the former. The 'weak' refers to the unobjectionable value judgement invoked in deciding that the new resource allocation is better than the initial one. Who would disagree, given that both people are better off?

If, by shifting from one point to another, one person is made better off, and the other person is *no worse off*, that is they remain on the same level of utility, this is a *strong* Pareto improvement. We would conclude that this change is also a good thing, and that the latter point is Pareto superior to the former. The word 'strong' alerts us to the somewhat stronger value judgement involved.

Box 8.1 Using the Pareto principle to rank alternative allocations of goods

Figure 8.1 shows a fixed quantity of two goods X and Y to be allocated between two people. For simplicity, imagine that this is a pure exchange economy – for example a room containing two people, and a given number of units of good X and good Y. Starting from any allocation of these goods between them, such as that shown by point a, the persons can change what goods they have by choosing to exchange the goods with the other person. What can we say about the overall social welfare arising from the alternative allocations of goods that might arise in this situation? One might have an ethical view on this: egalitarians, for example, might argue that the only correct allocation is that each person gets exactly half each of the quantities of X and Y. The welfare economics approach to judging social welfare, by contrast, focuses on the utility each individual enjoys from the consumption of these two goods. If, for example, one of these persons happened to have very strong preferences for good X and the other for good Y, then an equal allocation of the goods is clearly not going to maximise either their individual or joint welfare.

If we start at point a, it is possible for voluntary exchange to take place between the two persons such that we shift to point b. Both persons A and B are on the same indifference curve at a as at b – that is, both persons A and B experience exactly the same level of utility at a as they do at b. Because each of them would be just as well off after as before this reallocation, points a and b are *Pareto indifferent*. In terms of overall social welfare, the two points are identical and would be ranked equally.

Starting again from point a, reallocating goods between persons A and B such that we shift to point e would enable *both* people to shift onto an indifference curve farther from their origin – that is, both of them experience higher utility as a result of this new allocation of goods. This is a *weak Pareto improvement*. In terms of social welfare, e is therefore Pareto superior to point a.

Starting again from point a, reallocating goods between person A and B such that we shift to point c is a *strong Pareto improvement*: person A is on the same indifference curve at c as at a, but person B has shifted to a higher level of utility. One person is better off and the other is no worse off. In terms of overall social welfare, c is also Pareto superior to a.

Regardless of what the starting point is, Pareto improvements will always be possible, so long as there is a different marginal rate of substitution of x for y

$(MRS_{x,y})$ for different people. Points where the slopes of each person's indifference curves are equal, that is, where $MRS_{x,y} = MRS_{x,y}$, are *Pareto efficient* or *Pareto optimal*. In Figure 8.1, there are multiple Pareto optimal allocations – these have been connected with a broken line, known as a *contract curve*. Once one has arrived at a Pareto optimal allocation of goods, further exchanges of goods can only improve one person's utility by *reducing* the utility of the other. Such changes are *Pareto non-comparable*. It is not possible, using the Pareto principle, to rank states of the world in which one person is made better off and the other made worse off. To do this requires us to invoke a stronger value judgement.

Once all such improvements have been exhausted, we have reached an allocation of goods which is Pareto efficient or Pareto optimal. However, this is not a unique point; there are many possible Pareto optimal allocations. It is easy to spot Pareto optimal allocations in an Edgeworth box. In Figure 8.1, these are the points at which the two individuals' indifference curves are tangent to each other. At such points, the $MRS_{X,Y}$ – the slope of the indifference curve – is identical for both persons. Recall from Chapter 2 that the $MRS_{X,Y}$ might also be thought of in terms of the ratio of MU_x/MU_y. Thus, wherever this ratio is different between people, the addition to satisfaction that is derived from the consumption of X relative to Y is different between each person. The implication is that, wherever this ratio is different between people, there will be scope to improve the utility of at least one person, without reducing that of another, simply by reallocating the endowments of goods X and Y between them.

Hence, an allocation of goods is Pareto optimal if an increase in one person's utility can only be achieved by reducing the utility of at least one other person.

While a weak value judgement, the Paretian approach to social ranking of states is nevertheless a judgement – it cannot be *disproved*, but we might *disapprove of* it. For example, what if the richest person in society were able to increase their utility, while the poor continued to have the same level of utility as before: is this change a good thing? Although a Pareto improvement, this would conflict with both egalitarian and Rawlsian perspectives on equity (see Chapter 7). Similarly, a government policy that reduces poverty may be highly desirable, but if it involves a sacrifice by the rich, no matter how small, it will not be a Pareto improvement (Hammond, 1996).

Further, some Pareto optimal points represent wildly uneven allocations of goods between the two people and, more importantly from the welfarist perspective, very different levels of utility. Pareto optimal points close to A's origin (for example, point g in Figure 8.1) indicate low levels of utility for A, and high levels of utility for person

B; Pareto optimal points close to B's origin (for example, point k) indicate low utility for B and high utility for A. The Pareto principle itself offers us no means of comparing these allocations with each other.

An important limitation of the Pareto principle is, therefore, that it does not provide any means of ranking Pareto optimal states, and that it is neutral to the kinds of distributional concerns that we discussed in Chapter 7. As Tsuchiya and Williams (2001) note, 'A "Pareto improvement" is not concerned with who is better off, or about the relative size of people's gains, but only that there are no losers.'

Box 8.1 demonstrates that what constitutes a Pareto improvement depends on what the starting point – the current state of the world – is. Given a point such as a, we can identify a set of points, lying along and within the lens-shaped space defined by the indifference curves for person A and B passing through a, that would yield either strong or weak Pareto improvements, including the points lying along the line between d and c, which are Pareto optimal. But we cannot compare a point such as a with a point such as g, even though g is Pareto optimal and a is not. Thus, the Pareto principle does not allow us to compare any pair of states of the world that involve trade-offs between people's well-being.

This is obviously a rather fundamental problem. The advantage of the Paretian approach is that the value judgement it embodies is relatively weak; and that it involves minimal informational requirements, requiring only that people can rank the options – bundles of commodities – presented to them. But these advantages come at the expense of its being 'useless as a criterion for social choices in many, if not all, real-world situations' (Johansson, 1991). This point is illustrated nicely by a series of columns in the *Journal of Economic Perspectives* in the late 1980s which considered the question 'Are There Pareto Improvements?'. Some contributors concluded there are *no* examples of Pareto improvements in real life, although one economist, Barry Nalebuff, claimed to have found one: allowing a left-hand turn at a red traffic light! (Although even that could be disputed.) Clearly, if welfare economics is to provide a practical guide to resource allocation in health care, where most decisions are not of the free-left-hand-turn variety, it needs to go beyond the Pareto principle.

8.4 POTENTIAL PARETO IMPROVEMENTS

We have pointed out that, as well as being neutral to distributional equity, an important limitation of the Pareto principle is that it can produce only a partial ranking of social states. The Pareto criterion cannot cope with mixed outcomes, where one person's utility is increased but another's decreased. Consequently, with reference to the points in Figure 8.1:

- it cannot rank all non-optimal points against each other, for example points a and f;

- it does not allow us to rank all Pareto non-optimal points against all Pareto optimal points, for example points f and c; and

- it cannot rank Pareto optimal points against each other, for example points d and c.

The second of these problems – the inability to rank all non-optimal allocations vis-à-vis all optimal allocations – can be addressed if we allow an extension of the Pareto principle to situations where there are gains by some, losses by others, and the *possibility* of monetary transfers between them to compensate the losers. Compensation tests were independently proposed by Kaldor (1939) and Hicks (1939); although frequently conflated, they comprise slightly different means of judging the social desirability of two states.

Imagine that we are contemplating a policy that involves one health authority being allocated an additional £3 million by the government, and another losing £2 million. What can welfare economics tell us about the relative desirability of the state of the world brought about by this policy, compared with the *status quo*? Hicks suggests assessing the desirability of the reallocation by the government by examining the extent to which those who lose would be prepared to bribe those who gain not to make the change. If the policy were implemented, the losing health authority would be £2 million worse off, so they will be prepared to spend up to that amount to avoid the policy. In this instance, the gaining health authority will not be prepared to accept the bribe, as it is less than the gain that they stand to make (£3 million): they would be worse off accepting the bribe (£2 million − £3 million = −£1 million). On the basis of these gains and losses, as assessed by the individuals themselves, the policy is judged socially desirable and should go ahead. In Kaldor's version of this compensation test, if those who gain can potentially fully compensate those who lose (£2 million), such that the losers are no worse off (−£2 million + £2 million = £0) and the gainers can still be better off (by £3 million − £2 million = £1 million) than before the policy then, again, the policy is judged to be desirable.

The monetary assessments of benefit and loss referred to in this example are not based on accounting procedures or some objective assessment of benefit and loss. Rather, they are defined in a very specific way that enables us to link utility, which is an intangible concept that is difficult directly to measure, and money, which is easy to measure. Following Hicks (1939), benefit (loss) may be defined as the maximum (minimum) amount of money that must be taken away from (given to) an individual such that they are as well off after the change as before it. (We return to these concepts in Section 8.5, and give a more formal exposition of them.) For those who lose, this represents the monetary compensation they must receive, were the policy to proceed, such that they return to the same level of utility they had *before* the policy. For those who gain, this represents the amount of money that must be taken away from them, were the policy to proceed, such that their utility returns to its pre-policy level.

In essence, the compensation tests simply involve adding up the monetary losses and gains assessed in this manner; if their sum is positive the policy is recommended for implementation, and if negative it is rejected. The compensation tests preserve the spirit of the Pareto principle. If those who gain do so to such an extent that they could hypothetically fully compensate those who lose and still be better off themselves, this is a strong potential Pareto improvement. If those who gain do so to such an extent that they could hypothetically make a payment to the losers which is greater than the amount the losers require as full compensation, and still be better off themselves, then both could be made better off, which is a weak potential Pareto improvement.

Figure 8.2 illustrates the compensation tests using a utility possibilities frontier (UPF). A UPF plots the pairs of individual utility levels associated with any allocation of goods within the Edgeworth box. The labelled points in Figure 8.2 correspond to those in the Edgeworth box of Figure 8.1. Any point off the contract curve in Figure 8.1, such as point *a*, is a non-optimal allocation of goods and will lie inside the frontier in Figure 8.2. Thus, from point *a*, a shift to either *c* or *d* will be a strong Pareto improvement, and a shift to *e* a weak Pareto improvement. Pareto optimal points – those lying along the contract curve in Figure 8.1 – create the frontier. The UPF has a negative slope: from any Pareto optimal allocation of goods, an increase in one person's utility cannot be achieved without making the other person worse off. Given that this analysis does not require a cardinal measure of utility, we cannot impose any requirement for this

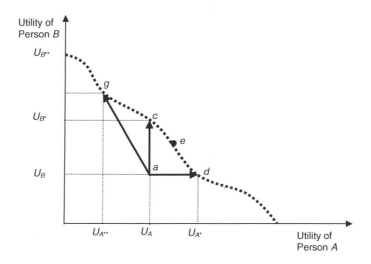

Figure 8.2 **Potential Pareto improvements demonstrated using a utility possibilities frontier.**

function to be strictly convex or concave; thus it is shown here as a non-monotonic, but decreasing, function. The compensation tests enable any point *within* the UPF, for example point *a*, to be ranked against any point *on* the UPF, for example point *g*, that is they address the second type of non-comparability noted earlier. A shift from *a* to *g* does not *in itself* improve social welfare, but the improvement in overall efficiency associated with that change would enable transfers to take place between *A* and *B* such that a movement to a point such as *c* is possible.

There are a number of problems with compensation tests. First, while the compensation tests allow the identification of potential Pareto improvements, the compensation remains potential rather than being realised. The tests require only that compensation be hypothetically possible, but actual money transfers are not required to take place. This is important, because a shift from point *a* to point *g*, which would be deemed socially desirable using the compensation tests, may not in practice be accompanied by compensation for *A*. Implementing this policy without compensation involves a redistribution of wealth or well-being in favour of *B*, at *A*'s expense. The rationale for this, as explained by Boadway and Bruce (1984) is that:

> The purpose of considering hypothetical redistribution is to try and separate the *efficiency* and *equity* aspects of the policy change under consideration. It is argued that whether or not the redistribution is actually carried out is an important but *separate* decision.

Some economists have pointed out that to distinguish between efficiency and equity in this way is somewhat disingenuous, given the expressly normative purpose of welfare economics (for example Little, 1957).

Secondly, compensation may be possible, but may be costly to negotiate and organise. If redistribution is costly, then the identification of potential Pareto improvements that can be achieved by cost-free lump-sum transfers is, arguably, not very helpful in a practical decision-making context.

Thirdly, the use of money as a metric with which to represent the corresponding changes in utility for gainers and losers depends on each unit of this metric (£1) corresponding to equal increments of total utility for each person involved. Imagine a situation where there are identical gains and losses in utility terms, but where those who lose have low incomes and those who gain have high incomes. If we believe that income, like goods, is subject to diminishing marginal utility, the addition to utility obtained from each additional £1 of income is likely to be higher for a low-income person than for a high-income person. The consequence is that the amount of money required fully to compensate the loser for their utility loss from this change will be lower than the amount of money required to compensate the gainer for forgoing the change. Although in terms of utility the gains and losses are identical, the compensation test would deem this policy to be desirable.

Fourthly, there is a theoretical possibility that a change in the state of the world and a reversal of that change might both appear to be socially desirable using the compensation tests. Scitovsky (1941) therefore suggested a qualification, whereby a change in the state of the world is desirable if and only if it is associated with a potential Pareto improvement, and a return to the original state of the world is not.

Finally, while compensation tests allow any non-optimal states to be ranked vis-à-vis any optimal state, they do *not* allow Pareto optimal states to be ranked against each other. The identification of neither Pareto improvements nor potential Pareto improvements is sufficient to obtain a complete and consistent ranking of all states of the world; that is, to obtain an SWO.

8.5 SOCIAL WELFARE FUNCTIONS

The welfare economics approach to social choices might be thought of as a hierarchy of value judgements. Starting with the weakest value judgement, the Pareto criterion can rank many states of the world, but there remain many that cannot be ranked. Further rankings can be obtained using compensation tests, but not for Pareto optimal states. Ranking of alternative Pareto optimal allocations requires us to invoke still stronger value judgements than those represented by the compensation tests.

So far, we have considered the SWO only in ordinal terms, that is, as a social ranking of states of the world. Moreover, it is based upon information on the manner in which individual members of society rank those states. If, however, we had some means of measuring each person's utility, social welfare could also be measured by aggregating these individual utilities in some way. This would allow us to represent the SWO as a social welfare function (SWF), where society's welfare is measured in real numbers as a function of its members' individual utilities. Early economists concerned with these issues, such as Jeremy Bentham and John Stuart Mill, tended to think about utility in very concrete terms that were potentially measurable. Bentham, for example, refers to hypothetical units of measurement called 'hedons', denoting pleasure and deriving from the word 'hedonist'; others have described utility in notional units of 'utils'.

The most general formulation of this is known as the Bergson or Bergson–Samuelson SWF. The level of social welfare (W) associated with any given state of the world (x) is a function of the utility obtained by each individual $U_A, \ldots, U_n$ in that state:

$$W(x) = f(U_{A(x)}, U_{B(x)}, U_{C(x)}, \ldots, U_{n(x)}) \tag{8.1}$$

This is not constrained to have a particular functional form – that is, the mathematical relationships between the variables are left unspecified. Therefore, this SWF does not specify exactly the nature of the trade-offs we are prepared to accept between, for example, U_A and U_B, but it does have some useful properties. First, the only determinants of W are the utilities of individual people – thus, it is a welfarist approach. Secondly, other things being equal, W is increasing in each person's utility, so it is consistent with the Pareto criterion. For example, in Figure 8.3, as the utility of person B increases from U_B to $U_{B'}$ to $U_{B''}$, and the utility of A remains unchanged at U_A, social welfare increases from W_1 to W_2 to W_3. Any curve, such as W_1, shows the various combinations of U_B and U_A that yield identical levels of social welfare and between which society will therefore be indifferent. We would generally expect this curve to have a negative slope: if we increase U_A, U_B must be reduced for society overall to remain just as well off as before. Thus, the SWF can be thought of as society's indifference curve, explicitly showing the manner in which the utility of society's members are aggregated to determine the well-being of society as a whole. Social welfare curves farther from the origin represent higher levels of social welfare.

The Bergson SWF is often drawn, as in Figure 8.3, as convex. This is not a requirement of the Bergson SWF; instead it reflects a particular view about the way that people's utilities are aggregated. Implicitly, inequality in the utility levels obtained by people is regarded as being socially undesirable to some extent, but not completely abhorrent. A convex SWF implies that successive increases in the utility of one person, holding that of others constant, confer diminishing marginal increases in society's welfare. Another way to express this is that the slope of the social welfare function, $-\Delta U_B/\Delta U_A$, which is the amount by which person B's utility must decrease given an increase in person A's utility for social welfare to remain constant, is decreasing.

Assuming that this semi-egalitarian ethic is a reasonable representation of society's preferences over the utilities of its members, the SWO, which is the ultimate goal of

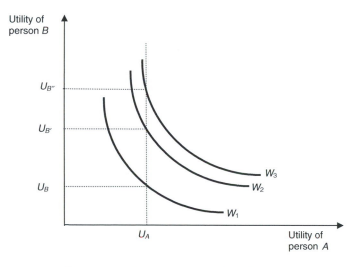

Figure 8.3 The social welfare function.

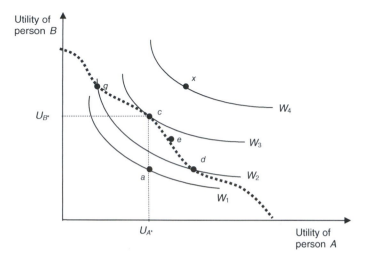

Figure 8.4 The maximisation of social welfare.

welfare economics, can be re-cast as a simple optimisation problem. This is solved by selecting from the UPF the pair of utilities that maximises society's welfare.

This can be seen in Figure 8.4, which combines the UPF introduced in Figure 8.2 with society's preferences over people's utilities, shown by the SWF in Figure 8.3. Points within the UPF, such as a, are not efficient: Pareto improvements are possible by movements to d, c or e. Points such as x are more desirable than any of points c–e, but are not feasible to achieve, given the underlying endowments of resources and existing technology. Points g, c, e and d all lie along the UPF: they are all Pareto optimal and neither the Pareto principle nor compensation tests can rank them. However, given the stronger value judgement captured by the SWF, clearly point c is the best distribution of utility between A and B, as it generates the highest possible level of social welfare (W_3). All of points g, c, e and d are optimal in the Pareto sense, but, according to the SWF, c is the *optimum optimorum* – the best of the best. At this point, the utilities of persons A and B are U_{A^*} and U_{B^*} respectively. This is also referred to as the 'bliss point' or, in Pareto's own language, as the point of 'maximum ophelimity'.

Given that the SWF encapsulates society's view about the trade-offs between people's utility that are acceptable, exactly what shape it is depends entirely on our views on equity and distributive justice. Utilitarians, as we saw in Chapter 7, advocate an ethical position whereby states of the world deemed most desirable are those which generate 'the greatest good for the greatest number', that is they maximise the sum of the utilities of members of society. This yields an SWF given by

$$W = (U_A + U_B + \ldots + U_n) \tag{8.2}$$

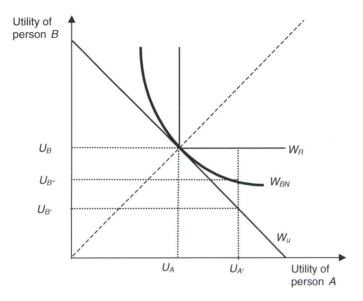

● **Figure 8.5 Utilitarian, Bernoulli-Nash and Rawlsian social welfare functions.**

Given that the utilitarian's measure of the social welfare in any given state is simply the sum of individual utilities, this implies a 1:1 relationship between an increase in utility of one person and the decrease in another's required for social welfare to remain unchanged. The slope of the welfare curves for a strict utilitarian are therefore constant and always equal to −1. In Figure 8.5, the utilitarian welfare function is shown by W_u. An increase in A's utility from U_A to $U_{A'}$ requires an *identical* reduction in B's utility from U_B to $U_{B'}$ in order for social welfare to remain constant. The utilitarian position clearly requires utility to be both measurable and interpersonally comparable, in order for such assessments to be possible.

This SWF is egalitarian in the sense that every person's utility is weighted equally. However, society might want to weight some people's utilities higher or lower than others. In this case, we have a generalised or weighted utilitarian SWF:

$$W = (a_A U_A + a_B U_B + \ldots + a_n U_n) \tag{8.3}$$

where a_i is the welfare weight that society attributes to person i. As with strict utilitarianism, weighted utilitarianism requires utility to be cardinally measurable and interpersonally comparable. The welfare curve is again linear, but with a slope equal to the ratio of the weights, that is $-a_A/a_B$.

What we referred to above, in reference to Figure 8.3, as a semi-egalitarian ethic implies that an increase in A's utility from U_A to $U_{A'}$ requires a smaller reduction in B's utility, in comparison with the utilitarian SWF, from U_B to $U_{B''}$, in order for social welfare to remain constant. This concave social welfare function, the properties of which we have already described, is sometimes referred to as the Bernoulli-Nash SWF. It represents social welfare as the product of individuals' utility functions:

$$W = (U_A \times U_B \times \ldots \times U_n) \tag{8.4}$$

This function, shown in Figure 8.5 as W_{BN}, in effect places a lower weight on the utility of those with high levels of utility. The state of the world selected by maximising it is also known as a Nash solution, because it can be derived from the bargaining theory of John Nash. It reflects what may be viewed as a fair rule by players in a bargaining game (see Section 4.3.6). It is the only rule that satisfies all of these four axioms: no interpersonal utility comparisons; independence of irrelevant alternatives; symmetrical treatment of all players; and the strong Pareto criterion.

An alternative to these is the maximin SWF, where society's welfare is measured by the minimum utility level, that is, the level obtained by its worst-off member:

$$W = \min(U_A, U_B, \ldots, U_n) \tag{8.5}$$

Often referred to as the Rawlsian SWF, following Rawls' (1971) *Theory of Justice*, the implied welfare curves are shown by W_R in Figure 8.5. Given any initial unequal distribution of utility in favour of one person, an increase in the utility of that person will increase society's welfare up to the point where utilities are strictly equal. Beyond that point, further increases in that person's utility will not increase social welfare – only equal increases in utility for both individuals will do so. For example, an increase in A's utility from U_A to $U_{A'}$ leaves W unchanged – because $U_A = U_B$, the increase in A's utility confers no improvement in social welfare, so no reduction in B's utility is required for social welfare to remain constant. The Rawlsian SWF in Figure 8.5 thus treats the utility of person A and person B as perfect complements in the SWF. It is also called the Maximin SWF, because the social choices suggested by such a SWF would involve maximising the position of the worst-off person.

Each of these SWFs rests upon strong value judgements. In essence, an SWF is an explicit statement of ethical beliefs about what is socially good and optimal.

While these are the specific functional forms commonly found in the literature, there clearly exists a wide range of other, distinctive ethical positions and divergent views on what constitutes social equity. Many of these – for example Nozick's (1974) *Theory of Entitlement*, in the libertarian tradition, and Roemer's (1998) writing on *Equality of Opportunity* – cannot be captured as SWFs because the views they present pertain to the fairness of the *process* by which various distributions of goods or utility arise, whereas welfarism restricts its consideration to the *consequences* in terms of individuals' utility, and is neutral to the process by which those are achieved. Thus, although the particular shape and functional form of the SWF must reflect a particular ethical stance, not every ethical stance is capable of being rendered as an SWF. Furthermore, which SWFs are candidates for making social choices is, in practice, constrained by the extent to which we can measure and compare individuals' utility.

8.6 MEASURABILITY AND COMPARABILITY OF UTILITY

Imagine that we had at our disposal a dependable measuring rod for utility that gave us valid measures of change in any one person's utility and that each number on that measuring rod represented the same level of utility across all individuals. Further imagine that we could agree on our ethical position as a society, so we can construct an SWF to aggregate those utilities. Also imagine that we all agreed that welfarism is the right way to make social choices: for any given decision all we are concerned with is the effect of the quantities of goods and services consumed and their consequences for individual utilities. In these circumstances, every social decision could be made by feeding the corresponding utilities into the SWF. The SWO is complete and consistent, and the decisions that maximise welfare would be readily obtained.

The real world is, of course, rather different. In practice, attempts to construct SWFs are constrained by our ability to measure utility. In the absence of a cardinal measure of utility, it might only be possible to measure individuals' preferences on an ordinal scale – and such assessments of utility may not be comparable between individuals.

For cases where information on individuals' preferences is restricted to their ranking of states, Arrow (1951) reported an extraordinary finding. A complete and consistent SWO can only be achieved if we allow one arbitrarily chosen person's preferences to dominate every choice – this person is sometimes called a *dictator*, though this is not meant in the pejorative real-world sense. If we rule out the dictatorship option on the grounds that it is an undesirable way to make social choices, then Arrow's result is that it is impossible to produce a complete and consistent SWO. Arrow called this a 'possibility theorem', but it is usually referred to as *Arrow's impossibility theorem*, because that is a more useful description. Of course, in the unlikely case where all members of a society had *exactly* the same preferences, a social ranking would simply be the ranking common to all of them – in accordance with the weak Pareto criterion. However, in any situation where people's preferences conflict, so that they have differ-ent rankings of states, these cannot be reconciled to produce a consistent *social* ranking. The simplest illustration of the problem, which was used by Arrow in his 1972 Nobel Prize acceptance speech, is provided by a majority voting system.

Imagine that there are three states of the world: x, y and z, which voters are asked to rank. One-third of the voters (group 1) rank these states x, y, z: that is, x is their first, most preferred choice, followed by y, and z is their least preferred option. One-third of the voters (group 2) have the ranking y, z, x; and one-third (group 3) have the ranking z, x, y.

Now consider the ranking of the states generated by a majority vote. Two-thirds of the voters (group 1 and group 3) prefer x to y, outweighing group 2's preferences. And the majority of the voters (group 1 and group 2) prefer y to z, outweighing group 3's preferences. Given that the majority prefers x to y, and the majority also prefer y to z, one might therefore logically expect that the majority prefers x to z. Instead, and paradoxically, the majority (group 2 and group 3) prefers z to x. The social ordering of these states generated by the majority vote is intransitive, that is to say logically inconsistent. While this majority vote example provides something of the flavour of the theorem, it is not a proof of it.

Arrow (1972) concludes: 'The philosophical and distributive implications of the paradox of social choice are still not clear. Certainly, there is no simple way out.'

How might we get around Arrow's finding? One way would be to improve the information available for making social choices – effectively, to develop the cardinal measures of utility that Bentham and Mill once imagined possible. Sen (1970) demonstrated that even if cardinal measures were invented that were meaningful representations of any one given individual's utility, unless these are interpersonally comparable, the dictatorship result persists. Interestingly, health economics is unique among economics subdisciplines in that it has devoted considerable efforts to the development and use of measures of *health-related* utility that are both cardinal *and* interpersonally comparable. This research poses considerable challenges; we discuss the theory and methods in detail in Chapter 10. Another option is to relax the requirements of welfarism – for example, to allow arguments other than individual utility to influence social decision making. We turn to these non-welfarist and extra-welfarist approaches in Section 8.9.

8.7 THE APPLICATION OF WELFARE ECONOMICS

The welfare economics theory we have described so far provides the principal theoretical foundations for economic evaluation. In this section we show how this theory translates into the practice of cost–benefit analysis, which is defined formally in the next chapter. In a practical exercise, decision makers cannot directly observe or compare the individual utilities that are central to the welfare economics approach. Thus, the application of welfare economics relies on the use of money as a proxy for utility.

We introduced the notion of compensating payments in Section 8.5 in relation to Hicks's compensation tests; here we provide a more formal exposition, drawing on Johansson (1995). The basic framework for welfare economics, as we have emphasised, is consumer choice theory: each person is assumed to maximise their utility. They have a limited after-tax income, y, that they wish to spend on n different goods, the consumed quantities of which are denoted by $x = (x_1, x_2, \ldots, x_n)$. Each of these n goods has an associated price denoted by $p = (p_1, p_2, \ldots, p_n)$. The objective is to maximise their utility, subject to their income. Their utility (U) is a function both of the goods they consume (x) and their health status, denoted by z, which we assume can be measured as a single number on a 0–1 scale. Formally, the utility function is given by

$$U = U(x, z) \tag{8.6}$$

and the maximisation problem is

$$\text{Maximise } U = U(x, z) \text{ subject to } p \times x \leq y \tag{8.7}$$

Using this framework we can construct measures of welfare change using money as the metric for comparison. Note that by including health status z in the utility function we can quantify welfare changes arising from a change in health status, which in turn might arise from health care. Hicks (1939) proposed two distinct means of using money to measure changes in utility: the compensating variation (CV) and the equivalent variation (EV). Each can be applied to the assessment of either gains or losses, as summarised in Table 8.1.

In essence, the CV approach seeks monetary amounts that represent the impact on a person of any given change considered *ex post*, relative to their *initial* levels of utility. The EV approach seeks monetary amounts that represent the impact on a person of

Table 8.1 Compensating and equivalent variations for gains and losses

	For a gain arising from a change in the state of the world:	For a loss arising from a change in the state of the world:
CV	The amount of income that would have to be *taken away* from an individual *following* this change, in order that they return to their *original* level of utility	The amount of money that must be *given* to the individual *following* this change, in order that they return to their *original* level of utility
EV	The amount of income that would have to be given to the individual *before* this change, that would increase their utility to the *new* (higher) levels they would obtain were the policy to proceed	The amount of money that would have to be taken away from the individual *before* this change that would give a reduction in their utility to the *new* (lower) level they would experience if the policy were to proceed

Note: These concepts are related to changes in health, and corresponding measures of willingness to accept and willingness to pay, in Chapter 10.

any given change considered *ex ante*, relative to the *new* levels of utility that the change is anticipated to bring. Chapter 10 will explain the practical methods and research instruments used by economists to elicit measures of CV and EV; here we focus on their theoretical rationale and derivation.

To estimate these two money measures of a change in health we need to construct the *indirect utility function*. We know from equation (8.7) that x is constrained by the person's income and prices, that is:

$$x = x(p, y) \tag{8.8}$$

Substituting (8.8) into equation (8.6) yields an expression for the indirect utility function:

$$V = U[x(p, y), z] = V(p, y, z) \tag{8.9}$$

This states that indirect utility, denoted by V, is a function of prices (p), post-tax income (y) and health status (z).

A change in health status, such as might result from receiving health care, will change the person's utility. The change in utility (ΔV) following a change in health status is given by

$$\Delta V = V(p, y, z_1) - V(p, y, z_0) \tag{8.10}$$

where subscript 0 denotes the person's initial level of health (state 0) and subscript 1 denotes the person's final level of health (state 1). Prices and income are assumed to remain constant. ΔV is positive if $z_1 > z_0$, that is, if health status is improved. We want to value in monetary terms the change in utility (ΔV) arising from a change in health.

If health improves, the CV is the maximum amount of money that can be taken from the person after that improvement, leaving them just as well off as they were before the improvement:

$$V(p, y - CV, z_1) = V(p, y, z_0) = U_0 \tag{8.11}$$

This is called the *willingness to pay* for an improvement in health. U_0 is the person's level of utility before the improvement in health (in state 0). If health deteriorates, CV is the minimum amount of money that must be given to the person to compensate for their loss in health.

With a potential improvement in health, the EV is the minimum amount of money that must be given to a person to make them as well off as they would have been after the improvement in health:

$$V(p, y + EV, z_0) = V(p, y, z_1) = U_1 \qquad (8.12)$$

This is called the *willingness to accept* for not receiving an improvement in health. U_1 is the person level of utility after the health improvement (in state 1). If health deteriorates, EV is the maximum amount of money the person is willing to pay to prevent the deterioration.

Note that the CV for a given *improvement* in health is equal to the EV associated with the exactly opposite *deterioration* in health.

These measures of CV and EV provide us with an observable measure of the value of changes in health status reflecting corresponding changes in a person's utility. However, the use of these measures in social decision making requires a means of aggregating them to construct a measure of social welfare (W). A generalised utilitarian social welfare function would be one where social welfare in state i, (W_i) is given by

$$W_i = \sum_{j=1}^{H} a_j V_{ij}(p, y, z) \qquad (8.13)$$

where a_j is the constant welfare weight that society attributes to person j, V is the level of utility experienced by person j in state i, which is a function of p, y and z, and there are H people in society.

Imagine that there is a health care programme that increases the health status (z) of people who receive it but also decreases the health status of other people who do not receive it, because it reduces the quantity of other types of health care programmes available to them. We want to offer a recommendation about whether this programme should be introduced. In a welfarist framework this involves determining whether or not social welfare increases with a move from state 0 to state 1, that is, whether or not ΔW, the change in social welfare, is positive or negative. ΔW is given by

$$\Delta W = W_1 - W_0 = \sum_{j=1}^{H} a_j V_{1j}(p, y, z_1) - \sum_{j=1}^{H} a_j V_{0j}(p, y, z_0) \qquad (8.14)$$

If it is positive, the recommendation is to proceed with this programme; if it is negative, the recommendation is not to proceed.

Unfortunately, the change in social welfare is unobservable. There is no way of directly observing the sign and magnitude of ΔW. However, we can attempt indirectly to capture the nature of the social welfare change by using the measures of CV and/or EV described above. By modifying slightly equations (8.11) and (8.12), we obtain the following:

$$CV: \quad V_{1j}(p, y - CV, z_1) = V_{0j}(p, y, z_0) \tag{8.15}$$

$$EV: \quad V_{0j}(p, y + EV, z_0) = V_{1j}(p, y, z_1) \tag{8.16}$$

We concentrate on CV here, but the following applies equally to EV. Substituting equation (8.15) into equation (8.14) yields

$$\Delta W = \sum_{j=1}^{H} a_j V_{1j}(p, y, z_1) - \sum_{j=1}^{H} a_j V_{1j}(p, y - CV, z_1) = \sum_{j=1}^{H} a_j v_j CV_j \tag{8.17}$$

where v_j is the marginal utility of income of individual j, or

$$v_j = \frac{\partial V_j(p, y, z)}{\partial y_j} \tag{8.18}$$

From the above, it is clear that CV and EV provide us with *part* of the information necessary to determine whether or not a project that improves people's health will lead to an improvement in social welfare. However, it is also clear, for example from equation (8.17), that knowing the CV and EV alone is not all that is required to make an assessment. What we also require is information on a_j, the welfare weight that society places on each person and v_j, the marginal utility of income of person j. Multiplying a_j, by v_j gives us the *marginal social utility of income* for each person.

We require information on a_j, because, as we have already discussed, we cannot achieve an SWO without the decision maker, for example the government, making value judgements about the way in which trade-offs between people are to be handled. The welfare weights are value judgements – essentially, statements of ethics – that are used to describe the relative importance the decision maker puts on welfare changes obtained by different people in the move from state 0 to state 1 and which are to be included in the aggregation process.

The marginal utility of income, shown in equation (8.18), tells us the rate at which a change in income (y) for each person is translated into a change in their utility (V). This explains how money measures of the change in health (CV or EV) convert into a change in utility. Unfortunately, this is unlikely to be constant across individuals. As we have already noted, it is generally argued that there is a diminishing marginal utility of income: as people become richer, successive increases in income yield smaller additions to total utility.

To understand the importance of these concepts, consider the following example. Imagine a society with two individuals, Hugh and Stephen. A health care programme is introduced which benefits Hugh, because he receives it and it increases his health status, but is detrimental to Stephen, because introducing it means that other health care programmes from which Stephen obtained some benefits have been curtailed. We elicit from Hugh and Stephen their CV for the new health care programme and we have also somehow obtained estimates of a and v:

	Hugh	Stephen
CV	+10	−5
a	1	2
v	1	1.5

The sum of these CVs (10 + −5 = 5) is positive so, using a simple compensation test criterion, the new health care programme should be implemented. However, the value for a tells us that society places a greater weight on Stephen's welfare. Additionally Stephen's marginal utility of income is greater than Hugh's. Under these assumptions, the change in welfare from the health care programme is actually negative ($\Delta W = -5$), and therefore the programme should not be implemented. The health care programme, because of its detrimental effect on Stephen, actually reduces social welfare. This example highlights the perils in inferring conclusions about the desirability of a project from simply summing up money measures of changes in utility.

The problem is that the marginal social utility of income is generally unobservable. Therefore, the problem remains that it is difficult to assess the desirability of a change in social states whereby some people are made better off and others are made worse off. Unless one is prepared to adopt some rough and approximate approach it is not possible accurately to aggregate welfare changes across people from money measures of changes in health. For convenience, it is commonly assumed in cost–benefit analyses of health care programmes that equal weight should be given to welfare changes for people and that the marginal utility of income across people is constant. That such strong assumptions are used in the application of welfare economics underlines the importance of caution both in the interpretation of results and in making recommendations.

8.8 NON-WELFARISM

We have so far in this chapter given an overview of the welfare economics foundations of economic evaluation. It is evident that there remain unresolved difficulties in the ability of welfare economics to provide a comprehensive guide to decision making and, in particular, to address the issue that lies at the heart of social choices: the means by which conflicts in preferences and trade-offs between people are to be managed. In this section we expand on the limitations and critiques of welfarism that relate specifically to decisions regarding health care, and discuss the attempts to develop alternative non-welfarist normative frameworks to guide economic evaluation.

Non-welfarism is any normative framework for social decision making that rejects welfarism. There is no single theoretical non-welfarist paradigm; non-welfarism is consistent with a diverse set of theoretical perspectives and propositions.

Welfare economics is often asserted to be the theoretically correct approach to social choices and decision making. Its alleged superiority arises from its basis in the axioms of microeconomic theory, in particular consumer choice theory, and because its central tenets are systematically described and its conclusions derived formally. By contrast, non-welfarist approaches are sometimes dismissed as comprising a 'practical, but not very well formulated collection of rules of thumb' (see Tsuchiya and Williams, 2003). The arguments against using welfare economics as a basis for economic evaluation of health care are as follows.

The Underlying Paradigm of Rational Choice and Utility Maximising Behaviour is Irrelevant to Health and Health Care Behaviours

Welfare economics is viewed by some as 'less relevant to the particular context and background of health care resource allocation, where the objectives of the players do not entirely agree with those upheld by standard theory' (Tsuchiya and Williams, 2001).

Thus, one of welfare economics' main strengths – its basis in microeconomic theory – is disputed in the health sector. The assumptions and models that are used to represent consumer behaviour might be argued to be less relevant to, or at least to provide poor predictions of, individual behaviour with respect to health and health care. These concerns are captured nicely by Culyer (1991), who argued that the implications of welfare economics for policy decisions 'hinge on judgements about the empirical significance of consumer rationality, the 'purity' of the agency relationship, the nature of any externalities, the extent of adverse selection, moral hazard, supplier-induced demand, unnecessary premium loading under insurance, and the empirical validity of the neoclassical behavioural model that, in its normative version, is welfarism's centrepiece'. Given that market failures in health care are such that most health care systems reject the use of markets as the sole means of funding health care (see Chapter 5), is it appropriate to rely on market theories of consumer behaviour and value to provide the basis for allocating resources in non-market settings?

Welfarism Assumes Social Welfare is Determined only by Utility from Commodities

Critics, for example Mooney and Russell (2003), assert that welfare economics is too restrictive in its approach to social choices because its assessment is based traditionally only on individuals' utility from consumption. It seems reasonable to suggest that things other than individual utility from consumption might matter in social decision making – and that therefore welfare economics is simply too limited in scope to deal with factors we know to be important.

However, although much of welfare economics does indeed model social choices in this manner, this may be for expositional simplicity or parsimony in modelling rather than from necessity; welfarism is capable of accommodating any source of individual utility. Indeed it is possible to point to contributions to the welfare economics literature that depart from the simple focus on the individual's utility from their consumption. For example, Culyer (Culyer, 1976) uses a welfare economics framework to analyse the effects of 'caring externalities', that is where utility is a function both of one's own consumption *and* the consumption of others one cares about; see Chapter 5 for a more detailed exposition. Further, Culyer (1991) points to a long tradition of attempts to incorporate non-individualistic approaches into the standard welfare economics framework. This dates back to Bergson's original paper (of 1938) on the SWF, which included unspecified terms in the social welfare function that could be used to represent things other than individual utility that might matter in social choices. It also includes Culyer's own work, which attempted to incorporate Musgrave's notion of merit goods into an orthodox welfare economics framework (Culyer, 1971).

Similarly if, as suggested in Chapter 2 the demand for health care is a derived demand, that is the increase in utility arises from the improvement in health rather than the consumption of health care per se, its benefits are nevertheless able to be represented by effects on utility (Birch and Donaldson, 2003). All the derived demand relationship implies is that it is health, rather than health *care*, which is the source of utility; that utility is therefore a function both of the consumption of goods and services *and* health; and that, as demonstrated by Johansson (1995) and described in Section 8.7, this should be reflected in the SWF. Allowing health to determine utility is entirely possible within a welfare economics framework.

Welfare Economics' Basis in Individualism Excludes Community Values

Regardless of whether utility is permitted to arise only from commodities, or from other sources, the underlying framework of welfare economics is nevertheless firmly rooted in the notion that individuals are utility maximisers. This precludes the idea that individuals might voluntarily be interested in contributing to some common good, which lowers their own utility. Sen (1977) describes this type of behaviour as 'counterpreferential' – for example our obligations and commitments to others. Thus the utilitarian ethic of welfare economics cannot cope with things such as a commitment to community values and community well-being (Mooney and Russell, 2003).

Utility is Fundamentally Flawed as a Measure of Individual Well-being

Perhaps the strongest challenge to welfare economics arises from questions about the ability of its basic building-block – utility – meaningfully to capture well-being. The most compelling and well-known arguments on these issues are made by Sen (1985). His basic assertion is that individuals differ with respect to their ability to convert commodities into well-being. Sen argued that utility has two main problems: physical condition neglect and valuation neglect. A person who suffers from physical condition neglect 'can still be high up in the scale of happiness and desire fulfilment if he or she has learned to have "realistic" desires and to take pleasure in small mercies'. Valuation neglect arises because 'valuing is not the same thing as desiring and the strength of desire is influenced by considerations of realism in one's circumstances'. Measuring social welfare with respect to individual utilities will therefore be misleading, because individuals' assessment of their well-being and utility are affected by their characteristics as people.

Sen described two aspects to these characteristics: *functionings* (what an individual manages to be) and *capabilities* (the freedoms that an individual has to make choices). Because these characteristics are potentially important influences on individuals' assessments of well-being, information on them should be admitted into the process of comparing social states. This is known as *extra-welfarism* – terms extra to utility are included in the SWF. It does not exclude individual utilities from judgements about social welfare, as in non-welfarism, but supplements these with additional information about each state, for example preferences regarding the process by which goods are chosen or consumed, or characteristics of each individual.

Sen's extra-welfarist approach to social choices has received particular attention in relation to choices in the health sector and has, arguably, been developed more in relation to health care decisions than in any other realm of social decision-making. Drawing on the arguments of Sen, Culyer (1989, 1991) advocated a general notion of 'characteristics of people' as pertinent to decisions about health care. The characteristics argued to be potentially relevant to social choices include a broad set of factors: individuals' 'genetic endowment of health, their relative deprivation independently of the absolute consumption of commodities or the characteristics of commodities; their moral "worth" and "deservingness"; whether or not they are in pain, or stigmatised by society'. Other characteristics could include the nature of relationships between people; for example 'the quality of friendships; community support for an individual when in need; social isolation; or changes in them, such as becoming (as distinct from being) a cripple' (Culyer, 1991).

Significantly, only some of these characteristics of people will be 'deemed relevant' (Culyer, 1991); the selection of relevant characteristics, from the menu above, is asserted to be 'related to the concept of need'. Given that the health characteristics are relevant because they are a way of describing deprivation, health care commodities are needed because they can help relieve that deprivation; in other words, health care is a means to an end. Essentially, Culyer extended Sen's very broad notion of particular characteristics to even more general notions of characteristics, but then narrowed the focus to one particular characteristic pertinent to decision-making in health care: *health* (Culyer, 1991). So, the extra-welfarist position that has emerged is that health is included in the SWF. This does not necessarily imply that utility is cast aside – both sets of information can inform social choices. This suggests the following SWF:

$$W = f(U_A, H_A, U_B, H_B, \ldots, U_n, H_n) \tag{8.19}$$

The difference between this and the SWFs described in equations (8.1) to (8.5) is that health may be included, alongside other commodities, as an argument in individuals' utility functions, but social welfare is determined strictly from utilities. In equation (8.19), health enters the social welfare function *directly*, as an additional argument. Health is included not because it is a source of utility, but because it describes a characteristic of people argued to be of importance to decisions about how to allocate health care resources.

McGuire (2001) speculated that, given an SWF such as this, it might be possible to impose Pareto optimality as a normative goal on the goods sector and a competing maximand on the health sector – most obviously, the maximisation of health. There are two complications in this approach. First, utility levels and health levels are unlikely to be independent. Secondly, resources used in the health sector will be drawn from the goods sector. Given these interdependencies between health and utility, identification of an overall optimal resource allocation will be theoretically challenging – and remains to be addressed.

As we have described it, the term extra-welfarism makes sense – it implies there is something extra being taken into account alongside utility. However, in practice extra-welfarism has come to be associated with a very specific interpretation of the broad possibilities inherent in Sen's position. The set of techniques of economic evaluation which constitute *applied* extra-welfarism use health not to *supplement* utility but to *substitute* for it. That is, these economic evaluation approaches focus entirely on the maximisation of health – and this has been to the exclusion of non-health-related utility, such as that derived from the process of care rather than its outcome. The benefits of health care programmes are measured and valued as changes in *health*. Thus both welfarism and extra-welfarism have been subject to the criticism that they ignore preferences over processes that are valued in themselves rather than being instrumental to some outcome, either improved utility in welfare economics or improved health in extra-welfarism (Mooney and Russell, 2003).

Given that, in practice, extra-welfarism has come to be synonymous with the maximisation of health, it is interesting to consider how this position arose. Where did health as a maximand come from? The relevant passages from Culyer's influential (1991) paper set out the rationale in terms of need, as described above. But Culyer did not see health as completely ousting welfare; one possibility is that the focus on health emerged as a pragmatic response to methodological challenges in evaluation, as the theory of extra-welfarism itself does not justify it. Further, a problem with Culyer's rationale for selecting health as the only relevant characteristic of people is that it relies upon some external judgement about what is deemed relevant – and the sources of these external judgements, and on what authority they are based, are unclear.

It is important to note that what has become the orthodox approach to economic evaluation under extra-welfarism has emerged through practice rather than being *required* by it as a normative framework. This includes not just the focus on health, but also the rejection of individualism: the values attached to health are those of the community, not of the individual recipients of treatment.

It is tempting, given that the normative framework for extra-welfarism in health care was first set out in Culyer's writings in the 1990s, to view extra welfarism as an *ex post* rationalisation for practical techniques of economic evaluation that had been applied since the late 1960s and were incompatible with traditional welfarist approaches.

The distinction between non-welfarism and extra-welfarism is rather tenuous and possibly overdrawn. For example, Tsuchiya and Williams (2001) reject the term extra-welfarism and categorise all competing normative approaches as being essentially non-welfarist. And while non-welfarism might be interpreted as an approach whereby information on utilities is rejected in favour of something else – health – it then seems odd that many non-welfarists strongly advocate the use of utility-based measures, such as standard gamble (see Chapter 10), as the means by which health is measured and valued (Parkin and Devlin, 2006). Finally, it is interesting to note that, given that these extra-welfarist or non-welfarist approaches arise from Sen's critique of social choices based on *utility*, Sen has also recently argued that making social choices about health care by relying on measures of self-reported *health* might be extremely misleading for similar reasons (Sen, 2002). We return to issues of measuring and valuing the outcomes from health care in Chapter 10.

8.9 IS THERE A LINK BETWEEN WELFARISM AND NON-WELFARISM?

Given that economic evaluation in health care has come to be dominated by applications of extra-welfarism, there has a growing body of research investigating the extent to which such evaluations, based on the maximisation of health approach, will be equivalent to or consistent with economic evaluations following the welfarist tradition (Johanesson, 1995; Birch and Donaldson, 2003; Dolan and Edlin, 2002).

There are two crucial issues. The first is the extent to which the measures of health that are used – which we describe in detail in Chapter 10 – might be considered *in themselves* to constitute measures of utility. The second is whether or not the allocation of resources achieved using the principle of maximising health is compatible with a Pareto optimal allocation of resources in the economy more generally. The consensus is that very restrictive conditions need to be met if this equivalence is to be established. How one interprets this depends very much on whether one views the issue from a welfarist or a non-welfarist perspective. For example, Tsuchiya and Williams (2001) comment that 'if the objective is to work within a welfarist framework, then this is bad news . . . however, for non-welfarists, whose objective is not to reproduce the results of standard welfarist full-scale cost benefit analysis, this demonstration of non-equivalence is a great relief!'.

We return to these issues in Chapter 12 after establishing the concepts and methods of economic evaluation in detail in Chapters 9–11.

8.10 CONCLUSION

Economic evaluation cannot be undertaken in a value-free manner. The appropriate value judgements to use for this purpose are a matter of some contention, with equally strong advocates for both welfarist and non-welfarist positions and no assurance that they are consistent or can be reconciled. These are non-trivial issues, with important implications for the way in which we approach the allocation of scarce resources in health care. There remains no consensus on the basic questions: What are we trying to maximise? How do we weigh up one person's loss with another's gain?

How, then, is economic evaluation to proceed? One solution is to take a pragmatic approach. Rather than searching for an elusive one-size fits all theoretical gold standard, Tsuchiya and Williams (2001) argue that the purpose of economic evaluation is to help people make specific decisions, and that therefore the policy context should determine the approach to be used in evaluation. However, this conclusion is itself a reflection of the authors' own extra-welfarist position.

Given the lack of consensus, economists have a duty to be explicit about the value judgements they adopt in their analysis, and to communicate clearly to decision makers the effect of value judgements on both the results from economic analysis and the recommendations either stated or implied in them. As Fuchs (1998) states:

> Economics is 'the science of means, not of ends' . . . [I]t can tell us the consequences of various alternatives, but it cannot make those choices for us. These limitations will be with us always, for economics can never replace morals or ethics.

SUMMARY

1. Economic evaluation describes a broad set of analytical approaches used to describe and compare the benefits and costs of competing uses of resources.

2. Welfare economics (or welfarism) is the systematic analysis of the social desirability of any set of arrangements (for example, a state of the world, or resource allocation) solely in terms of the utility obtained by individuals. Welfarism is based on individualism and consequentialism.

3. A basic value judgement used in welfare economics is the Pareto principle. A change in the state of the world that increases the utility of all affected individuals is a weak Pareto improvement. A change in the state of the world that increases the utility of at least one individual, and does not decrease the utility of any other individual is a strong Pareto improvement. A state of the world in which no feasible Pareto improvement is possible is Pareto efficient or Pareto optimal. A state is Pareto optimal if an increase in one person's utility can only be achieved by reducing the utility of at least one other person.

4. It is not possible, using the Pareto principle, to rank states of the world where one person is made better off and the other made worse off. To do so requires us to invoke a stronger value judgement. This problem is called Pareto non-comparability.

5. One consequence of Pareto non-comparability is that the Pareto principle is unable to rank all Pareto non-optimal points against all Pareto optimal points. Compensation tests, such as those derived by Kaldor and by Hicks, can be used in these cases.

6. A complete social welfare ordering might be obtained using social welfare functions (SWFs), which provide a direct way of aggregating individual utilities to obtain a value for social welfare. Common SWFs are the Bergson (or Bergson–Samuelson) SWF, the utilitarian and generalised utilitarian SWFs, the Rawls (or maximin) SWF and the Nash SWF.

7. SWFs can be combined with utility possibility frontiers (UPFs) to identify the combination of individual utilities that will maximise social welfare (the bliss point).

8. Different SWFs rely on different assumptions concerning the measurability and comparability of individual utility. If utility is only measurable on an ordinal scale and if it is non-comparable, then the Arrow possibility theorem states that a complete and consistent social welfare ordering may only be obtained with a dictatorship. If we rule dictatorship as being an

undesirable way to make social choices, then Arrow's result is that any attempt to produce a complete and consistent SWO is impossible.

9. Decision makers cannot directly observe or compare the individual utilities that are central to welfare economics. Thus, the application of welfare economics relies on the use of money as a proxy for utility. Two money measures of changes in utility are the compensating variation (CV) and the equivalent variation (EV).

10. The CV and EV can be aggregated to determine whether a policy has a positive or negative effect on social welfare. This requires additional information on the form of the SWF, the welfare weight that society places on each individual and the marginal utility of income.

11. Criticisms of welfarism in health care are that the underlying paradigm of rational choice and utility-maximising behaviour is irrelevant to health and health care behaviours; that welfarism assumes that social welfare is determined only by utility from commodities; that welfare economics' basis in individualism excludes community values; and that utility is fundamentally flawed as a measure of individual well-being.

12. Non-welfarism is any normative framework for social decision making that rejects welfarism. There is no single theoretical non-welfarist paradigm; non-welfarism is consistent with a diverse set of theoretical perspectives and propositions.

13. Extra-welfarism can be defined as any approach to social choice that admits arguments other than individual utilities into the social welfare function. It does not necessarily exclude individual utilities from judgements about social welfare, as in non-welfarism, but supplements these with additional information about each state, for example preferences regarding the process by which goods are chosen or consumed or characteristics of each individual. In health care an obvious supplement is health.

Principles of Economic Evaluation in Health Care

9.1 WHAT IS ECONOMIC EVALUATION?

Economic analysis helps us to understand the world by describing and explaining economic behaviour. One of the main reasons why this is valuable is that it provides information that will be of help to people in making decisions about the allocation of scarce resources. Economic evaluation (or economic appraisal) is specifically about the provision of such information. It seeks to create, in the context of non-market provision of goods and services, information to inform choices; information that in other areas of the economy would be generated by the interplay of market forces. It is a structured approach to help decision makers choose between alternative ways of using resources.

Chapter 8 introduced economic evaluation using a highly theoretical approach, to emphasise that it has a strong intellectual basis. However, economic evaluation is quintessentially an applied technique, arguably the main practical contribution that economics makes to decision making in health services; the rest of Part II deals with how evaluation is carried out in practice. This chapter forms a bridge between the two, by setting out the principles derived from the theory that guide the practice.

The general term used for this sort of analysis in economics is *cost–benefit analysis* (CBA), and this term remains the most accurate and useful way of describing it. Its basis is the common-sense notion that a decision about whether or not to do something should depend on a weighing up of its advantages and disadvantages – that is, comparing its benefits with its costs. From an economics perspective, this means comparing like with like, because benefits and costs are closely related concepts. Costs measure the value of scarce resources used in terms of opportunity costs, which are the benefits that could otherwise be obtained with those resources. Cost–benefit analysis is therefore simply a comparison of the benefits of one use of scarce resources with those from another. This approach and the systematic way of thinking that it promotes are at least as important as the techniques of economic evaluation.

The original purpose of cost–benefit analysis, which remains the focus of its application in most non-market areas of the economy, is *investment appraisal*. This specifically aims to mimic the investment decisions that would be taken if a large-scale capital project were undertaken in a private market, except that the context is public rather than private. It has therefore been used for many years to appraise such public sector projects as dams, bridges, reservoirs, motorways and airports. It is a straightforward extension to apply the same techniques to hospitals and other health facilities, and to large-scale capital investments such as diagnostic imaging and information technology systems.

However, the predominant use of economic evaluation in health care is not for such large-scale capital projects and indeed its most widespread use is not for investment at all. Rather, it is used to provide information on which products – health care interventions – should be provided by health services for consumption by patients. This has led to the development of a distinctive set of techniques, which have been strongly influenced by the existence of established non-economics techniques used in the evaluation of health care interventions. From the economics point of view, health care is just a special case; but from the medical point of view, economics is just an additional evaluative technique.

Simply providing information on costs and benefits is in itself not evaluative. Rather, in economic evaluation this information is structured in such a way as to enable alternative uses of resources to be judged. There are many criteria that might be used for such judgements. Many of these are important, but are not especially economics based – for example, whether or not the use of resources is ethical and respects human dignity. The criteria that are the focus of economic analysis are efficiency and equity; economic evaluation in health care should in theory regard these as equally important, but in practice efficiency is dealt with far more often and with greater attention to precise numerical estimates.

In private health care markets, efficiency is largely left to market forces, with the assumption that, in a competitive market, profit-making health care organisations have incentives to minimise costs and provide the services that their patients desire. In publicly provided health programmes, market forces might be weak or there might be none at all. Economic evaluation is largely concerned with measuring efficiency in areas where there is public involvement and there are no markets to generate the kind of information – for example, prices and profits – that enable us to judge this. However, it is also likely that public services have different goals from private services. For example, public health organisations might wish to maximise health rather than profits and might also wish to take into account equity as well as efficiency. Economic evaluation – which is concerned with the public context – must therefore take such wider goals into account.

9.2 THE ECONOMICS FOUNDATIONS OF ECONOMIC EVALUATION

9.2.1 Cost–Benefit Analysis

At its simplest, cost–benefit analysis (CBA) is simply an inventory of all costs and benefits, whatever they are and whoever incurs them; this forms a balance sheet in which they are weighed up against each other. This is only possible if all costs and benefits are measured in the same unit; the obvious one is money as the measure of value most used in modern economies. Monetary costs are viewed as a measure of the value of the resources used in an activity; and monetary benefits are viewed as a measure of the value that is placed upon the output of that activity.

It has been recognised that some types of costs and benefits can be measured, but not in terms of money – these are traditionally known as incommensurable items. For example, in evaluating a hospital service, we may have measures of patients' satisfaction with their care in terms of the percentages who are satisfied or not with aspects of it such as standards of cleanliness, but we do not have any measures of the monetary value of changes in satisfaction. Yet other types of costs and benefits may be known or suspected to exist but cannot be quantified at all – traditionally these are known as intangibles. For example, dealing with mental illness in the community rather than in institutions may promote a sense of independence among patients, which is clearly a benefit but is hard to quantify.

The identification of incommensurate and intangible items is context specific and refers to problems of measurement, not to the item itself. Measurement techniques improve. It is increasingly possible to place plausible money values on items once regarded as incommensurate, and many items once regarded as intangible – such as pain and suffering – can now be quantified. For example, subjective feelings such as happiness used to be regarded as entirely intangible, but there is now a large research effort in this area which has quantified this concept (Layard, 2005). Box 9.1 presents a cost–benefit

Box 9.1 A cost–benefit analysis of alternative treatments for mentally ill people

Weisbrod, Test and Stein (1980) analysed information from an experiment that compared traditional hospital-based treatment for people with mental health problems with a community-based alternative. They took a social perspective, including not only costs and benefits to mental health services but also those to a wide range of others including social services, private providers, law-enforcement agencies, and patients and their families. The benefits that could be quantified in terms of money were as shown in the table.

	Hospital-based	Community-based	Difference between groups
Costs			
Direct treatment costs ($)	3138	4798	1660
Indirect treatment costs (for example social services, private medical providers) ($)	2142	1838	−304
Law enforcement costs ($)	409	350	−59
Maintenance costs (social security and voluntary) ($)	1487	1035	−452
Family burden costs (lost earnings and other) ($)	120	72	−48
Total costs ($)	7296	8093	797
Benefits			
Earnings ($)	1168	2364	1196
NET (benefits minus costs)	−6128	−5729	399

Both hospital- and community-based services produced a net loss, but switching from hospital- to community-based care would produce a net benefit. This result was affected by the fact that although the authors had a fuller list of costs and benefits, some of these could not be valued. Non-valued cost items included lost earnings, illness, family illness and stress, burdens on others, illegal activity and mortality. The main non-valued benefits were improvements in patients' mental health.

This study was probably more useful in providing information on the different elements of cost and benefit than in providing an estimate of the net benefit. It was an early CBA in health care and more recent studies would have been able to place values on far more of the items identified in the study but not valued.

analysis comparing hospital and community-based programmes for patients with mental health problems and highlights some of the challenges involved in measuring costs and benefits.

The question of how costs and benefits are to be measured and weighed against each other is obviously a fundamental issue, and indeed forms the main body of work on the topic. The answers to this question are often pragmatic, but they also have very strong guides from theory. However, there are two slightly different intellectual bases for cost–benefit analysis. The first arises from the origins of cost–benefit analysis as a tool used in planning and management of public services. Historically, it was one the key contributions of economics to a multidisciplinary movement (Lyden and Miller, 1972) that also produced Programme Budgeting, which is described in Chapter 12. This tradition, called by Sugden and Williams (1978) the *decision-making approach*, recognises the legitimacy of decision makers appointed by society as the source of many decisions about how costs and benefits are to be measured and weighed. The aim of CBA is to help to maximise the achievement of the decision maker's goals – which is similar to the very general definition of efficiency given in Chapter 1.

The second intellectual basis, which appeared around the same time as the public sector planning movement (Mishan, 1971), regards CBA as applied welfare economics and therefore attempts to operationalise the welfarist analysis discussed in Chapter 8. This provides a very strong guide to issues of measurement and weighing up of different costs and benefits, such as the necessity to, for example, identify all costs as marginal social costs and to employ a social welfare function to aggregate benefits. This tradition, called by Sugden and Williams (1978) the *Paretian approach*, regards economic analysis as providing an independent point of view on public sector decisions, taking the perspective of society as a whole and restricting its interest to efficiency issues. The aim of CBA is to identify Pareto improvements or potential Pareto improvements – which is consistent with the more technical economics definitions of efficiency discussed in Chapters 5 and 8.

What of the non-welfarist approach? It is clearly not entirely consistent with the Paretian approach, since it involves a different notion of what constitutes a benefit. However, non-welfarists regard the definition of what constitutes a benefit as being socially determined, rather than determined by decision makers. It is therefore consistent with the view embodied in the Paretian approach that economic analysis should provide an independent view, based on socially determined objectives, rather than simply serving decision makers who can impose their own objectives. But it could equally be regarded as consistent with a decision-making approach in which the decision maker is an idealised entity who takes a societal perspective, rather than a real one who might in practice have a more restricted view.

The identification of potential Pareto improvements is of course not a simple matter, and in practice neither is the identification of all costs and benefits relevant to any sort of decision maker, real or societal. For that reason, many support economic evaluation as a useful technique even where it falls short of being a full cost–benefit analysis, as it provides at least some useful information. A *partial cost–benefit analysis* usually means that some aspects of cost or benefit have been identified but not valued, and the usefulness of the information depends on whether we believe that if the missing elements were to be valued they would alter the balance of costs and benefits. In real economic evaluations, this is usually dealt with by *sensitivity analysis*, which will be discussed in Chapter 11.

A special case of a partial economic evaluation is where costs are valued but benefits are not. This has a justification on the grounds that it may improve some aspect of efficiency, with other aspects being left to other evaluations. For example, the aim of economic evaluation could be to improve technical efficiency or production allocative efficiency; this *enables* efficiency in both production and consumption to be achieved, but does not *guarantee* it. This justification is of course refuted by the theory of second best, described in Chapter 5, but that theory is best regarded as a warning about overconfidence in making recommendations rather than a view that inaction is best. This kind of partial efficiency is dealt with by a different type of economic evaluation known as cost-effectiveness analysis (CEA).

9.2.2 Cost–Effectiveness Analysis

One rationale for CEA is that whilst costs are usually measured in terms of money, it may be much more difficult to measure benefits that way. Obviously, comparison of costs and benefits that are measured in different units is not straightforward, but a theoretical basis for this can be found in the theory of production efficiency, described in Chapter 3. Recall that the isoquant identifies technically efficient points of production, measured in physical units, and a point where it is at a tangent to an isocost curve is allocatively efficient in production. Cost-effectiveness analysis tries to identify where more benefit can be produced at the same cost or a lower cost can be achieved for the same benefit. The first of these corresponds to a move to the allocatively efficient point from any other point on the same budget line, which must have lower production, and the second from any other point on the same isoquant, which must have higher cost.

However, there are many cases where we may wish to compare alternatives in which neither benefits nor costs are held constant. In this case, a cost-effectiveness ratio (*CER*) – the cost per unit of output or effect – is calculated to compare the alternatives, with the implication that the lower the *CER* the better. However, such ratios must be used with care, as will be discussed below. Box 9.2 shows an example of a cost-effectiveness analysis of a range of family planning services. In this example, the *CER* is expressed in terms of the cost per pregnancy avoided of each option.

Box 9.2 A cost–effectiveness analysis of family planning services

Hughes and McGuire (1996) calculated the cost-effectiveness of different family planning services in the UK. This covered contraceptive methods in family planning clinics and surgical sterilisation, both female and male (vasectomy), in hospital. They compared the direct costs of provision with the number of pregnancies avoided relative to no method and presented the following data tabulated below.

	Cost per user per year (£)	Pregnancies avoided per user per year	Cost per pregnancy avoided (£)
Family planning clinic			
Oral	111.43	0.82	135.89
Diaphragm	112.20	0.67	167.46
IUD	45.93*	0.83	55.34
Spermicide	118.95	0.64	163.94
Injection	123.71	0.85	146.05
Implant	82.53*	0.85	97.09
Condom	64.29	0.73	88.07
Hospital			
Sterilization	18.50**	0.85	21.77
Vasectomy	15.51**	0.85	18.25

*Discounted over 5 years; **discounted over lifetime of protection.

It will be apparent that the aim of this analysis cannot be to recommend which method is most cost-effective and should therefore always be chosen. Many other issues must be taken into account in choosing a family planning method; for example, it makes no sense to offer an IUD to a male user. Whether or not the method is reversible is important, and something useful can be concluded about that: if the user is taking a lifetime decision to have no or no more children, then hospital-based irreversible sterilisation methods are cost-effective, being less than half the cost per pregnancy avoided than the cheapest non-surgical method.

Notice that, unless the best alternative is always to have no family planning at all, these are not incremental cost-effectiveness ratios (ICERs) – see Section 9.5.4. If any of the clinic-based methods could be chosen for any user, then the cost and effectiveness data show that IUD dominates all methods apart from injection and implant, and implant dominates injection, so that most of the methods do not have an *ICER*. The *ICER* for implants is £1830, which is an order of magnitude greater than the *CER* of IUD compared with no family planning. Of course it is unlikely that there would be such a free choice. If there is a restricted choice in individual circumstances between some of these methods, then it is possible to calculate their relative cost-effectiveness from these data.

Hughes and McGuire also calculated these costs taking into account savings to the National Health Services in costs of spontaneous abortion, abortion and birth. In each case the savings outweighed the costs – so every method dominated the option of no family planning.

In summary, CBA seeks to answer whether or not a particular output is worth the cost. CEA seeks to answer the question of which among two or more alternatives provides the most output for a given cost, or the lowest cost for a given output. CBA therefore asks whether or not we should do things, while CEA asks what is the best way to do things that are worth doing. Although this sounds straightforward, the practice of economic evaluation makes it less so, particularly concerning CEA.

9.3 ECONOMIC EVALUATION APPLIED TO HEALTH CARE PROGRAMMES

Many of these concepts and labels concerning efficiency and economic evaluation have become modified in their application to the economic evaluation of health care interventions. This has largely been the result of a programme of sustained research initiated by Drummond (1980), which has led to many refinements (Drummond *et al.*, 2005). This work began with the aim of classifying existing economic evaluations and continued, via improving reporting standards, to offering guidance about the conduct of evaluation using consistent methods. These modifications have been extremely useful and are largely compatible with orthodox economic theories of cost–benefit analysis, but as used in practice they have occasionally been the source of some confusion and dispute, examples of which are discussed below. As noted earlier, they have been strongly influenced by non-economic evaluation techniques and have also increasingly been influenced by concepts arising from *decision analysis* – to be discussed below – and statistical considerations.

The major preoccupation of economic evaluation in health care has been measurement of costs and benefits – what should be measured and how it should be measured – rather than the aims of the analysis. Although this focus is obviously essential in enabling applied economic analysis, it has had the unfortunate consequence that techniques such as CBA and CEA are, as we will see, defined by measurement rather than economic theory. This potentially leads to problems in interpreting and using results from such studies, since there is no guide from theory as to how we should do that.

Recall that the production and cost functions, analysed in Chapter 3, relate inputs to outputs and define the efficiency aspects of the relationship; economic evaluation essentially attempts to quantify them. If inputs and outputs are measured in 'physical' units, then we are dealing with technical efficiency. If inputs are valued and outputs remain in physical units, we have a cost function and we are dealing with production allocative efficiency, and therefore with CEA. If both inputs and outputs are valued, then we are dealing with overall allocative efficiency and therefore CBA. This measurement principle for classification of types of economic evaluation forms a valuable link between economic theory and measurement.

The literature on economic evaluation in health care does not use this measurement principle. It largely uses the term CBA to mean any comparison of costs with benefits where both are measured in money, on the pragmatic grounds that money is the only plausible measure of economic value in modern economies, rather than being defined by its aims. Similarly, CEA is used to mean any comparison of costs and benefits where benefits are measured in units other than money; it is not usually based on the theory of production and is not restricted to comparisons of alternatives that have the same cost or level of output. In fact, much of the economic evaluation literature gives the label *cost-minimisation analysis* to what was traditionally called CEA, and specifically restricts the term CEA to choices between alternatives that have similar types of effects but differing levels of effect and costs. CEA is also occasionally described as an evaluation of technical efficiency, but that is incorrect both in theory and in normal practice.

It can be difficult to specify what the appropriate measure of effect is in CEA. For example, suppose we have a comparison that involves a treatment that prevents heart disease. In one in every 20 cases of disease the person suffers a heart attack; half of those who suffer a heart attack die, which leads on average to a loss of 5 years of life. Suppose that the treatment costs £50 000 to prevent 20 cases. The *CER* could be defined as

- £2500 per case prevented;
- £50 000 per heart attack prevented;
- £100 000 per death averted; or
- £20 000 per life year saved.

In comparisons between interventions that deal with the same illness, it may not matter which of these is chosen, but care is still required to ensure that whichever measure of effect is chosen does not mislead or bias the analysis – for example, if one intervention is better at preventing non-fatal heart attacks but is worse at preventing fatal attacks, the choice of effect measure will be crucial. A more difficult issue is raised if it is recognised that the main output of health care interventions is changes in health itself, recalling that the aim of CEA is to increase output with given costs or lower costs for the same output. It follows that the measure of effect should be one which can be used for all types of illnesses and all types of health care.

The issues that arise in constructing health measures for use in economic evaluation are considered in more detail in Chapter 10. However, such indicators are usually measures of the *value* of health, although not usually expressed in money terms. As a result, a third important type of economic evaluation has arisen, called *cost–utility analysis* (CUA). This label has been given in recognition of the fact that economists often use the word utility to mean value but, as we will discuss in Chapter 10, the precise meaning of this is the subject of some dispute. In addition, the health measure usually used in CUA is gains in *quality adjusted life years* (QALYs); this will again be discussed in detail in the next chapter, but it is essentially a composite measure of gains in life expectancy and health-related quality of life. Box 9.3 shows an example of a CUA of a programme that allowed patients who require intravenous feeding to have this at home rather than in hospital.

Viewed in this way, CUA is an extended and very useful form of CEA that can be used to judge which health care interventions should be undertaken within a given health budget. However, drawing on the measurement principle discussed earlier, CUA is often regarded as a simplified form of CBA because of its valued-output basis; it requires only a money value to be placed on effects to be able to judge whether or not health interventions should be undertaken, irrespective of the budget available. This issue has led to considerable dispute about the status of CUA – is it extended CEA or restricted CBA?

Because of the particular way in which CEA has been applied in health economics, both CEA and CUA in practice usually produce estimates of the observed cost of achieving different levels of output. The difference between the two is that CEA relates to the output of particular types of health care and CUA to the output of health care as a whole, so neither is a full social CBA that takes account of the wider economy as well. However, both could be interpreted as partial CBA or form part of a full CBA. So a plausible answer is that CUA is *both* extended CEA *and* restricted CBA.

9.4 DECISION RULES FOR COST–BENEFIT ANALYSIS

The purpose of economic evaluation is to provide information to make decisions in a structured way. An important part of that structure is to state what those decisions

Box 9.3 A cost–utility analysis of home parenteral nutrition

Detsky *et al.* (1986) looked at options for providing intravenous nutrients to patients who are not able to feed by other means. It compared a home parenteral nutrition (HPN) programme with total parenteral nutrition (TPN) in hospital for patients with acute and chronic conditions and a no-TPN option for acute patients only. The incremental costs and health care outcomes per patient were as tabulated.

	HPN vs. Hospital TPN		HPN vs. No TPN	
	Incremental cost ($)	QALYs gained	Incremental cost ($)	QALYs gained
Acute	−166 880	2.2	154 378	2.9
Chronic	67 429	4.0		
All	−19 232	3.3	99 596	3.6

HPN therefore dominated care hospital for acute conditions and for acute and chronic taken together, as it had both reduced costs and increased benefit. Incremental costs per QALY gained for HPN were calculated as $51 830 compared with the no-TPN option for acute conditions, $16 790 compared to hospital care for chronic conditions and $27 375 compared with the no-TPN option for both acute and chronic conditions.

These findings seem to be rather mixed concerning HPN and to be capable of some further analysis of the differences between acute and chronic conditions. There is also a question whether the *CER* for acute care is acceptable or not. However, the authors concentrated on the dominance of HPN over hospital-based TPN to conclude that it is in fact cost-effective to provide it.

should be, given a particular balance of costs and benefits. These are known as *decision rules*: if we find that the costs and benefits have a particular pattern, then we should take a particular decision. Some of these rules are very simple and obvious; others are extremely complicated.

The simplest rule is the basic one for cost–benefit analysis. If the sum of the benefits of an activity is greater than the sum of its costs, then on efficiency grounds the activity should be undertaken; if costs are higher, it should not; and if they are equal it does not matter either way. Alternative ways of expressing this, which mean exactly the same thing, are that the activity should be undertaken if its *net benefit* – the difference between benefits and costs – is positive or that its *benefit/cost ratio* is greater than 1. As will be explained in Chapter 11, because costs and benefits are often incurred over time, the net benefit criterion is actually usually expressed as a *net present value*, which is the difference between all benefits and costs at all times, expressed in today's values.

This decision rule assumes that any activity that has a net benefit *can* be done. But this may not be true if only some activities can be done and there are imperfect capital markets to provide the necessary investment. For example, it may be that on cost–benefit grounds a health authority ought to build new premises for all of its general practices, new clinics for all of its community services and substantially upgrade all of its hospitals. However, it may have only limited funds available in any year to do that. As a result, it has to choose between its different investments.

If only one activity can be undertaken, then the rule is again obvious: choose the activity with the highest net benefit. Otherwise, decision making becomes far more complex. This problem is a failure of the assumption that costs fully represent opportunity costs, and account needs to be taken of the fact that the opportunity cost of each activity is that others cannot be undertaken. The aim will be to produce the greatest excess of benefits over costs from all of the projects that have the potential to produce net benefits. Unfortunately, that cannot usually be determined by a simple rule such as ranking in order of net benefit or benefit/cost ratio; but there are mathematical methods that may make it possible to find a solution that gives the optimum combination of activities.

9.5 DECISION RULES FOR COST-EFFECTIVENESS AND COST–UTILITY ANALYSIS

Because CEA does not give a direct comparison between the value of effects and costs, decision rules are far more complex than for CBA and are bounded by restrictions on their applicability. The problem arises when the alternatives being appraised do not have equal costs or benefits, but instead there is a trade-off: the greater benefit that one of the alternatives has is achieved at a higher cost. The key problem is how that trade-off is to be represented, and how it can then be interpreted; essentially, encapsulating cost-effectiveness in a single index that can unambiguously interpreted for decision-making purposes. Three approaches to this have been developed: cost-effectiveness ratios; the net benefit approach; and the probabilistic approach.

9.5.1 Ratio Measures

The cost-effectiveness ratio (CER) – the cost per unit of output or effect – is the most popular measure of an activity's cost-effectiveness, with the implication that the lower the CER the better. Given an activity (a health care intervention or treatment), a and its best alternative b, with costs C_a and C_b and effects E_a and E_b, the CER for activity a is

$$CER = \frac{(C_a - C_b)}{(E_a - E_b)} \tag{9.1}$$

or

$$CER = \frac{\Delta C}{\Delta E} \tag{9.2}$$

The numerator of the CER is sometimes called the incremental cost of a relative to b and the denominator is the incremental effect.

9.5.2 The Cost–Effectiveness Plane

A useful way of showing the decision rules that apply to the CER is the *cost-effectiveness plane* (Black, 1990), shown in Figure 9.1. This diagram shows the costs and the effects of an activity compared to some alternative, with costs on the north–south axis and effects on the east–west axis. The two lines indicate zero additional costs and zero additional effects, respectively; north of the zero additional cost line, costs are higher and to the south lower; east of the zero additional effect line, effects are higher and to the west lower. These lines divide all possible cost and effect combinations into four quadrants. To the north-west, costs are higher and effects are lower, so the activity is worse in all dimensions and is said to be *dominated* by its alternatives and should not be used on efficiency grounds. To the south-east, costs are lower and effects are greater, so the activity *dominates* its alternatives and should be used on efficiency grounds. In the other two quadrants, either greater effectiveness is gained at a higher cost, as in the north-east quadrant, or a reduction in costs is achieved at the expense of lower effects, as in the south-west quadrant. In these two quadrants, whether or not the activity should be undertaken on efficiency grounds depends on the trade-off between costs and effects.

The CER of an activity can be represented on this diagram as the slope of a line from the origin, which represents the costs and effects of the alternative, to its cost/effect combination. Two such lines are demonstrated, one in the south-west and one in the north-east; these have been depicted as rays, emphasising that all points on each line represent the same CER. These CERs are positive; those in the other two quadrants are negative.

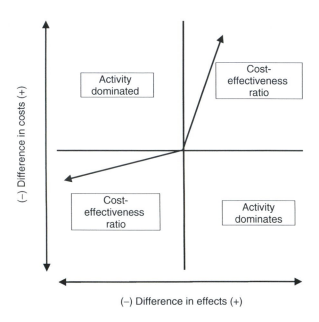

Figure 9.1 The cost-effectiveness plane.

What are the decision rules for the south-west and north-east quadrants? Without extra information on the acceptable size of the trade-off between effects and costs, we cannot say that any activities within them should be undertaken. It is tempting to conclude that if two activities have different *CER*s then the one with the lowest *CER* is more cost-effective and should be chosen. However, this is not necessarily the case. Strictly, *CER*s can be used to compare alternatives only if these can be scaled up or down to achieve the same costs or effects, without affecting the *CER*. In terms of production relationships, this requires there to be constant returns to scale and no indivisibilities.

These problems are even greater if the *CER* is based on CUA – strictly speaking, whenever the same measure of effectiveness is generic to all activities – because the scope of comparisons is then much wider. In this case, the same problems apply as with benefit/cost ratios: if it is not possible to undertake all activities, choosing them in order of *CER* from lowest to highest may not produce the combination of activities that produces the highest output from the available funds. However, as with benefit/cost ratios, it is in principle possible to determine from a complete set of cost and effect data the optimum combination of activities to maximise the improvements in health from a given health care budget or to minimise the total cost of achieving a particular level of health.

9.5.3 The Ceiling Ratio and Acceptability

Although cost-effectiveness analysis can be very useful in a variety of uses, its essential inability to help in the kind of choices that cost–benefit analysis allows – an absolute recommendation for a particular activity rather than one contingent on a comparison with alternatives – has proved such a strong limitation that means have been sought to overcome it. The key to this has been the *cost-effectiveness threshold* or *ceiling ratio*, which is essentially a level of the *CER* that any intervention must meet if it is to be regarded as cost-effective. It can also be interpreted as the decision maker's willingness to pay for a unit of effectiveness.

The decision rule is then straightforward. If the activity is more effective but higher cost, then for it to be cost-effective its *CER* must be less than the ceiling ratio, R_c, that is:

If $R_c > \Delta C/\Delta E$, the activity is cost-effective.

If $R_c < \Delta C/\Delta E$, the activity is not cost-effective.

If the activity is cheaper but less effective, then the decision rule is reversed:

If $R_c < \Delta C/\Delta E$, the activity is cost-effective.

If $R_c > \Delta C/\Delta E$, the activity is not cost-effective.

This issue is often referred to as *acceptability*, meaning that the activity is acceptable on cost-effectiveness grounds. It can be depicted using the cost-effectiveness plane, as in Figure 9.2. The four quadrants are replaced by a simple dichotomy – is the activity above the line, in which case it is not acceptable, or below the line, in which case it is? Within these halves, the only distinction, which is suppressed, is whether the activity would always be acceptable or unacceptable or its acceptability is contingent on the size of the ceiling ratio.

One of the problems with this kind of approach is that it is no longer consistent with the conventional aim of CEA. Except under special conditions, it is not consistent with output maximisation constrained by a budget. This emphasises further the issue of whether CEA and CUA are really reduced versions of CBA or are to be accepted as suitable only for a restricted range of decisions.

9.5.4 The Incremental Cost–Effectiveness Ratio

So far, we have discussed the *CER* with respect to a comparison of an activity with an alternative, without stating what that comparator is except that it should be the *best* alternative. It is useful to distinguish between a comparator that is essentially 'do nothing about the problem with which the activity deals and which incurs no costs or benefits' and one that is 'another way of doing something about that problem'. The

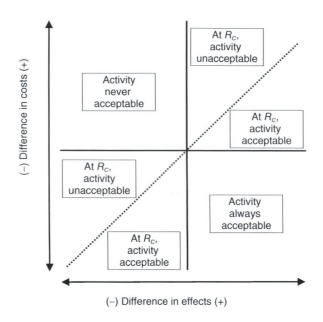

Figure 9.2 Cost-effectiveness acceptability.

CER that arises from the second of these is sometimes called an *incremental cost-effectiveness ratio* (*ICER*) and again there are arguments about the circumstances in which these two comparators should be used, assuming that they are different. However, in most cases the *ICER* is the correct measure to use.

An argument for using the *ICER* is as follows. Suppose that we have a screening programme that can be implemented using one test or two sequential tests. Because of the nature of tests, the first will pick up most of the cases of interest and the second will pick up fewer cases. In this case, the first test detects 10 cases and the second 2, so the one-test screen yields 10 cases and the two-test screen yields 12 cases. The cost of each test is the same, whether it is done singly or sequentially, so carrying out two tests costs almost twice as much in total as carrying out one test, the only reduction being due to not screening those cases found in the first test. In this case, the total costs are £100 000 and £80 000, respectively, so the two-test screen costs £180 000. If we calculate the *CER* for the one-test screen against 'do nothing', it is £10 000 per case detected. If we calculate the same *CER* for the two-test screen, it is £15 000 per case detected. If the ceiling ratio is £30 000 per case detected, the two-test screen, although it does not have as favourable a *CER* as the one-test screen, is still at an acceptable level.

However, the proper way to view the two-test screen is, fairly obviously, that it is a one-test screen with an additional test. The extra cost of the second test converting the one-test screen to a two-test screen is £80 000 and the extra benefit is two cases; the *ICER* is therefore £40 000, which is well in excess of the ceiling ratio. The two-test screen is not cost-effective. The *CER* of the two-test screen against 'do nothing' is an average of the *CER*s of the first test and the second test and is clearly misleading.

Even where there is, strictly speaking, no averaging involved, the *ICER* usually gives more useful information. Suppose that we have two interventions for a particular disease: drugs and surgery. Currently, surgery is performed at a cost of £100 000 and patients live on average 5 years longer as a result. The *CER* is therefore £20 000 per life year gained. The drug costs £210 000 and on average patients live 7 years longer. The *CER* is therefore £30 000. Comparing the two directly in an incremental analysis of drugs relative to surgery, the drug costs an additional £110 000 and gains two additional life years, giving an *ICER* of £55 000. We are using a ceiling ratio of £40 000 per life year gained. Should the drug be provided? The *ICER* gives the correct conclusion that it should not.

What if, for a different illness, there is a drug that has no alternative but has exactly the same costs and benefits as the one that the *ICER* suggested should be rejected? This second drug would be accepted, which on the face of it seems illogical. But it is simply because there is no more cost-effective way of treating patients with the second illness, while there is for the first.

A problem is that if only the *ICER* is evaluated, it must be assumed that the alternative used in the comparator is itself cost-effective; if it is not, the *ICER* may mislead. Suppose in the example above that the cost of surgery was £250 000 and the drug cost was £280 000. The *ICER* for the drug is £30 000/2, giving an acceptable £15 000. However, evaluated against no treatment, the *CER*s are £50 000 for surgery and £40 000 for the drug, neither of which is acceptable. The *ICER* and apparent cost-effectiveness of the drug is an artefact of the inefficiency of the surgical treatment currently used. The optimal solution would be to provide neither.

It is common in economic evaluations to compare more than two mutually exclusive alternatives. In this case the decision rules become even more complicated. Box 9.4 describes a study by Garber and Solomon (1999) which illustrates the correct procedure for comparison of alternative health care programmes, where each patient in the defined population will receive only one of the alternative treatments. The correct procedure is as follows.

1. Rank the options in order of increasing cost.
2. Eliminate options for which another option is cheaper and more effective, known as *simple dominance*.
3. Eliminate options where a combination of two other options is cheaper and more effective, known as *extended dominance*.

Box 9.4 Diagnosis of coronary artery disease

Garber and Solomon (1999) conducted a literature review and meta-analysis to estimate the accuracy of six diagnostic tests for coronary heart disease. They calculated the costs and health effects of alternative diagnostic strategies for patients at intermediate risk (25–75%) of coronary disease over 30 years. Their estimates for one patient group were as tabulated.

Intervention	Cost ($)	Effect (QALYs)	Incremental cost ($)	Incremental effect	ICER ($/QALY)
Exercise	39 815	14.119	Baseline for comparison		
Echocardiography	39 835	14.125	20	0.006	3 333
PTI	39 964	14.125	Dominated		
SPECT	40 510	14.132	675	0.007	96 429
Angiography	41 101	14.370	591	0.005	118 200
PET	41 551	14.134	Dominated		

Angiography dominates PET because it is cheaper and more effective. Similarly, PTI is dominated by Echocardiography. The *ICER*s for the remaining options are calculated with respect to the next cheapest option in each case: thus Echocardiography is compared with Exercise, SPECT with Echocardiography and Angiography with SPECT. The choice between these remaining options depends on the ceiling ratio for the *ICER*.

4. Calculate the incremental cost and incremental effect of each remaining option with respect to the previous option in the list.

5. Calculate *ICER*s for the remaining options.

In summary, *CER*s are valuable indicators of cost-effectiveness but they do need careful handling and are prone to misuse, particularly with an inappropriate choice of comparator. A further issue, which will be discussed in Chapter 11, is that the *CER* has many undesirable mathematical and statistical properties that add to the difficulties of using it.

9.5.5 Net Benefits

With all of the problems attached to *CER*s, it is not surprising that there have been challenges to their dominance. The most prominent of these is the *net-benefit approach* (Stinnett and Mullahy, 1998), which essentially restores the original concept of a cost–benefit analysis without the necessity of imposing a welfarist framework. Strangely, this was not mainly because of the theoretical problems of the *CER* but because of the undesirable mathematical and statistical properties referred to. The aim of this approach is to obtain a single number that is not a ratio. Recall that the *CER* is defined as

$$CER = \frac{\Delta C}{\Delta E} \qquad (9.3)$$

where ΔC is in £ and ΔE is not. The net benefit of an activity is defined as

$$\text{Net benefit} = \Delta E - \Delta C \qquad (9.4)$$

where ΔC and ΔE are in the same units

In order to convert costs and effects to the same units, the net benefit approach relies on the use of the ceiling ratio (R_c) as an implicit value that is attached to a unit of effect. R_c can therefore be used as an exchange rate factor between costs and effects; it can be used to convert costs to the same units as effects, or effects to the same units as costs. If effects are converted, this results in *monetary net benefit* (*MNB*), defined as

$$MNB = R_c \times \Delta E - \Delta C \qquad (9.5)$$

If costs are converted, this results in *health net benefit* (*HNB*), defined as

$$HNB = \Delta E - \frac{\Delta C}{R_c} \qquad (9.6)$$

The decision rule is then straightforward. For MNB:

If $R_c \times \Delta E - \Delta C > 0$, the activity is cost-effective.

And for HNB:

If $\Delta E - \Delta C/R_c > 0$, treatment is cost-effective.

The question is, however, which R_c should be used? If an organisation sets a specific value for this, then there is no problem. However, if we do not have such a value it is necessary to report the net benefit for each value of R_c. Figure 9.3 illustrates this for both MNB and HNB. The activity is cost-effective if R_c is above £10 000 per unit of effectiveness.

Of course, this gives exactly the same results as using *CER*s for a given level of R_c. It is also arguable that this is in effect CBA, although not of course of the full Paretian variety. On all of these grounds, the net benefit approach has considerable merits;

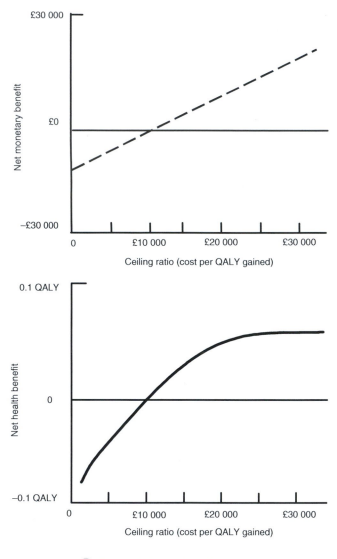

Figure 9.3 Net benefit curves.

further consideration of these in the context of statistical approaches to CEA will be discussed in Chapter 11.

9.5.6 Probabilistic Approaches

Another response to the difficult properties of the *CER* is the cost-effectiveness acceptability curve (CEAC) (van Hout *et al.*, 1994). This again makes use of the ceiling ratio

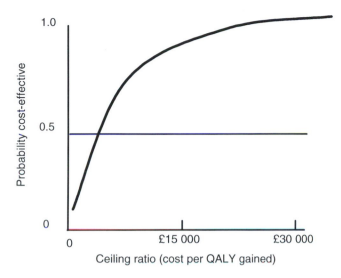

Figure 9.4 Cost-effectiveness acceptability curve.

and the concept of acceptability described earlier. A full treatment of this is given in Chapter 11; here we note only the essentials with respect to decision rules. The *CER* is retained as the measure of cost-effectiveness and this is compared with a ceiling ratio. However, the *CER* is no longer regarded as a number that is observed with certainty, but as a variable whose mean is observed. That mean can take different values depending on the sample of observations on which it is based, leading to the idea that with a given R_c we can only state the *probability* that the activity is cost-effective. This probability will be different for different levels of R_c. This can be represented as in Figure 9.4.

The CEAC has the merit of allowing uncertainty to be expressed while retaining the familiar concept of a *CER*. But although the CEAC is an interesting concept, it is difficult to know how decision makers are supposed to use it. As yet there is no guide to how to read and use a CEAC, and not enough experience of its use. We will return to this in Chapter 11, showing how in practice it is constructed.

9.5.7 Decision Analysis

A framework for investigating treatment decisions that lends itself to economic evaluation is *decision analysis*. This technique, which will be discussed in more detail in Chapter 11, constructs a model of decision making as a sequential process that may have several different outcomes depending on choices that are made and the results of uncertain events. The technique uses the probabilities of the uncertain events and the values attached to different outcomes to determine the best set of decisions, or 'strategy'.

What this adds to the issue of decision rules is that the values attached to costs, benefits, net benefits and *CERs* are *expected values*, rather than values that can be calculated with certainty. This is entirely reasonable given the uncertainty attached to medical outcomes.

9.6 EQUITY IN ECONOMIC EVALUATION

Despite the acceptance by most economists that the equity implications of decisions may be as important as efficiency issues, there is little in the way of formal evaluation of equity and nothing like the standardised quantitative routines that have been developed for efficiency measurement. However, there are some very important equity issues. The reason is that efficiency evaluations deal only with the amounts of resources used and the outputs achieved with them, not how these are distributed between different people, either individuals or groups in society. Most obviously, as was discussed in Chapter 8, a potential Pareto improvement may involve net gainers and net losers but does not require compensation to be paid from the first of these to the second. It also does not distinguish between programmes that redistribute benefits from the relatively poor to the relatively rich or from the rich to the poor, from the relatively sick to the relatively healthy or from the healthy to the sick, or that are neutral with respect to these groups. Even a proposed Pareto improvement may require analysis of distributional effects if a goal in society is to change the distribution of costs and benefits in some way, for example to achieve greater equality in health at the expense of overall levels of health.

As an example of this in health care, the most commonly-used practice in CUA is to use the QALY and moreover to assume that each QALY is worth the same irrespective of who gains it and by what route. This is utilitarian in practice if not by design. Similarly, CBA in practice focuses on sums of benefits compared to sums of costs, not on the distribution of these between people with different characteristics. It also does not usually take account of whether society places different weights on benefits experienced by different people; for example, there is evidence that many people would prefer health services to put a higher priority on improving the health of younger rather than older people (Tsuchiya *et al.*, 2003).

Such distributional issues were discussed in Chapters 7 and 8 and will be considered in more detail in Chapter 12, including the issue of equity and QALYs. In the next chapter we focus on methods for measuring and valuing health care output.

SUMMARY

1. Economic evaluation is a structured approach to help decision makers choose between alternative ways of using resources. It is largely concerned with measuring efficiency in areas where there is public involvement and there are no market-based measures available to judge this. The general term used for this in economics is cost–benefit analysis (CBA), which is used in investment appraisal.

2. Cost–benefit analysis involves constructing an inventory of all costs and benefits of an alternative, whatever they are and whoever incurs them; this forms a balance sheet in which they are weighed against each other. This is only possible if all costs and benefits are measured in the same unit; the obvious one is money as the measure of value most used in modern economies.

3. Cost-effectiveness analysis (CEA) is a partial form of cost–benefit analysis. The rationale for CEA is that while costs are usually measured in terms of money, it may be much more difficult to measure benefits that way. In health economics, cost-effectiveness analysis tries to identify where more health benefit can be produced at the same cost, or where a lower cost can be achieved for the same health benefit. A theoretical basis for this can be found in the theory of production efficiency.

4. Cost–utility analysis (CUA) is a form of economic evaluation in which health benefits are usually measured in terms of quality adjusted life years (QALYs). These are a composite measure of gains in life expectancy and health-related quality of life.

5. In cost–benefit analysis the main decision rule is to undertake an activity if the sum of the benefits is greater than the sum of the costs or, equivalently, if the net benefit is positive. If only one activity with a positive net benefit can be undertaken (for example, if there are limited available funds), then the appropriate rule is to choose the activity with the highest net benefit.

6. In CEA (and CUA) a direct comparison between the value of effects and costs is not possible. The cost-effectiveness ratio (CER) measures the incremental cost of an activity relative to its best alternative divided by the incremental effect. The CER is used in decision making; it is compared to a ceiling ratio, which is a level of the CER that any intervention must meet if it is to be regarded as cost-effective.

7. CERs can be presented graphically on a cost-effectiveness plane, which shows the costs and the effects of an activity compared to some alternative, with costs on the north–south axis and effects on the east–west axis.

8. It is important to measure the *CER* correctly as a comparison with the best alternative rather than some other alternative. Because the costs and effects are incremental to the best alternative, it is often known as an incremental cost-effectiveness ratio (*ICER*).

9. *CER*s can be converted into monetary net benefit and health net benefit measures, using the ceiling ratio to convert incremental costs to incremental benefits or vice versa.

10. Cost-effectiveness acceptability curves account for statistical uncertainty in the *CER* and uncertainty in the ceiling ratio by presenting the probability that an intervention is cost-effective for different levels of the ceiling ratio.

11. Equity issues – the way in which health and health gains are distributed among peoples – are as important as efficiency concerns, yet theory and methods for addressing these within the practice of economic evaluation remain underdevrloped.

Chapter 10

Measuring and Valuing Health Care Output

10.1 INTRODUCTION

In Chapter 3, we discussed how the output of health care can be defined either as the amount of care provided or the health that results from it. As before, we will regard both of these as valid concepts of output. Our focus in this chapter is how each type of output can be measured, with a particular focus on the use of these measures in economic evaluation. As mentioned in Chapter 9, we will also have a special interest in how output can be valued, rather than simply counted.

In most areas of economics, output measurement is relatively straightforward and valuing that output usually poses no real conceptual difficulties. For example, in the private sector pharmaceutical manufacturing industry, output can be measured in physical terms, such as the quantity of drugs produced, and in value terms as the market value of drugs produced. But when a health professional uses these products to treat a particular illness, output measurement becomes more difficult. What is the measure of quantity? Is it numbers of treatments or improvements in health? How are these to be valued? As discussed in Chapter 5, the economic conditions under which health care is usually traded, involving widespread third-party funding arrangements and subsidies, are unusual and may mean that the market may not generate information from which measures of value can be calculated for health care services and treatments. And health improvements cannot be directly sold in a market at all.

10.2 MONETARY VALUATIONS OF HEALTH CARE BENEFITS

In Chapter 8, the concepts of *equivalent variation*, *compensating variation*, *willingness to pay* and *willingness to accept* were introduced as means of measuring welfare changes as a result of changes in resource allocation. These compensation tests are the most usual means of measuring welfare changes in economics, and have money as their natural unit of value. They are the basis of the benefit side of cost–benefit analysis, providing estimates of changes in *consumer surplus*, the difference between what people pay and are willing to pay. In applying these theoretical concepts to the practical measurement of benefits, there are two broad approaches, known as *revealed preference* and *stated preference*.

10.2.1 Revealed Preference

Revealed preference (RP) refers to valuations of goods and services that can be inferred from real choices that are made in the everyday world. It is based on the theory that the choices that people make arise from a comparison of the benefits of alternatives with their opportunity costs. Individuals assess these benefits in accordance with their preferences. The choices that people make therefore reveal their preferences. For example, if we observe that someone will not purchase a dental check-up for £20 but will do so for £10, we can infer that the value that they place upon a dental check-up lies between £10 and £20. If we were able to vary prices between these two limits and observe their choices, we would be able to make a more precise estimate of this value, their maximum willingness to pay for a check-up.

Usually, however, we are concerned with estimating the value of a good or service not to one person but to everyone who might consume it. We are more interested in what is demanded by all consumers at different prices. If patients attach different values to a dental check-up, then different numbers of them will choose to pay for one at different prices – which is, of course, the basis of the demand curve. Their average valuation of a dental check-up – their average willingness to pay – can be inferred from a market demand curve using the same reasoning as for individuals' demand curves.

One problem with using RP is that in cost–benefit analysis we are most often interested in markets where there are no prices directly charged or where prices do not reflect values. For example, health care is often free at the point of consumption or highly subsidised, which poses obvious difficulties for estimating a demand curve. Moreover, if we are interested in obtaining the value of health improvements, as opposed to the value of health services, then we cannot use RP directly as that commodity is not directly traded and has no market. However, there is another way of obtaining RP valuations, which is to search for other ways in which people make trade-offs between money and health care or health. Within this, there are two distinct methods, which have different justifications.

The first method is based on the observation that people may have to incur a number of different costs to obtain a good or service, not just its purchase price at the point of consumption. For example, even if a visit to a general practitioner is free, people may incur monetary outlays, such as the cost of travel to the surgery, and other opportunity costs, such as the cost of their time. If these user costs have an effect on demand similar to that we would observe with a purchase price, then it may be possible to derive a demand curve and to infer valuations from that.

The second method is based on the possibility that even if there is no direct market for a good or service, its benefits can be inferred from other markets in which those benefits are also assessed. If we are interested in measuring the value of changes in health as part of an assessment of the benefits of health care, it might be impossible to do that if health care is provided free. However, it may be possible to observe choices in markets where alterations in health are one of the outcomes, for example by observing wage differentials in labour markets between highly risky and less-risky jobs (Viscusi, 2004), or by examining individual consumption decisions for goods that reduce the risk of ill health. The valuations of health that those choices reveal could then be used in an economic evaluation of health care. For example, suppose we are prepared to pay an extra £5000 for a car with additional safety features that reduce our probability of death from a road traffic accident by 0.001. This indicates that the value of a life is £5000/0.001 = £5 000 000.

10.2.2 Stated Preference

Stated preference (SP) valuations are derived from surveys or experiments, which are often loosely known in health economics as willingness-to-pay (WTP) studies. These may simply ask people to give values directly, or infer them indirectly by, for example, offering people hypothetical choices and observing their responses. SP relies on the assumptions that the values that people state are really those that underlie their choices in the everyday world, and that the choices that they make within the survey are those that they would make if they were really faced with the alternatives offered. Unlike RP, the validity of which is based on economic reasoning, the main theoretical basis of SP is psychological and this makes SP controversial. An extreme view, associated with Austrian economics, is that only choices in the market have relevance to economic analysis; valuations derived from psychological experiments may be of interest but refer to an entirely different phenomenon from that which is relevant to economics. However, most economists seem to agree that it is acceptable to use SP techniques, as long as they are consistent with the aims of economic analysis.

Alternatives include surveys that are basically referendums on the issues. Others include simulated markets, in which the goods are actually provided under experimental conditions – for a health care example, see Bhatia and Fox-Rushby (2003). However, the most widely recognised technique is the *contingent valuation method* (CVM). This refers to the valuation of a good or service, the measurement of value being contingent on the description of the hypothetical market that is given to respondents.

In health economics, stated preference techniques have been used both for the measurement of the value of *health care* and for the valuation of *health*. Applications to health are considered separately below and here we concentrate on the application of contingent valuation to health *care*. Moreover, we will concentrate on contingent valuation studies in which respondents are asked for their *willingness to pay* for health care. In Section 10.8, we will discuss some alternatives to this in the context of valuations of health.

The most important issue in contingent valuation is ensuring that the values that are obtained from it are credible to those whose actions will be informed by any evaluation that uses them. The respondents must understand the market scenarios that are presented to them and find them plausible and meaningful. Otherwise, they will have no idea how to respond to the questions that are asked of them and may even not attempt to give serious answers to them. Among the elements regarded as essential are descriptions, in sufficient detail to be understandable, plausible and meaningful, of the nature of the good or service that respondents would receive, how they would obtain it and how they would pay for it. The last of these, to be credible, must allow respondents to believe that they might actually be asked to do so. Other important features are to ensure that the sample used is representative of everyone who might be affected; that the exercise could be undertaken equally well by all of them; and that the purpose of the study is explained, again so that they provide serious and thoughtful responses. However, the information provided must be the minimum possible, to avoid respondents being overburdened, and in particular must contain nothing irrelevant that might distract respondents.

SP techniques have been refined so that there are best practice guidelines available for conducting contingent valuation studies; for example, Pearce and Özdemiroglu (2002). Within health care, there are no universally accepted approaches to CVM studies, but Gafni (1991) has published a very strongly argued set of guidelines, which include the following elements.

- People cannot plan to consume health care, so their willingness to pay should be expressed as an insurance premium that must be paid so that the service is available if they need it. Furthermore, the scenario should state the probability that they will need it.

- Treatment effects should also be explained in probabilistic terms – the probability of success or failure.

- The willingness to pay of all members of the relevant population is required, so the survey should have a representative sample.

There are number of well-known problems with contingent valuation studies that arise from the artificial nature of the choices that respondents have to make. We assume that in making choices in real life what matters to consumers is the trade-off between the benefits of the good being bought and its cost; their choice may of course be influenced by the environment in which they make the choice, but that is part of the market. In an experiment or survey, the respondent may still behave as a rational consumer, but the environment in which they make choices will be not be a market; their choices may be influenced by utility derived from interactions with researchers rather than providers. In fact, we might expect rational consumers to behave in such a way, offering answers to questions that are strategic. For example, if they believe that they will be asked to pay for the good at some future time and that the study's results will be used to set prices, they have an incentive to state a lower WTP than they would really pay. Alternatively, if they believe that they will not be asked to pay and the study will simply be used to decide on whether or not the good or service should be provided free, they have an incentive to overstate their WTP.

Other problems may arise from respondents being unable to share the researchers' aims. For example, if they do not know or care about their WTP for something that they have never had to pay for or even encountered before, they may resort to a face-saving strategy that will please the researcher. For example, it may be embarrassing to reveal that they in fact know, understand or care little or nothing about something that is clearly of importance, and therefore guess at high WTP. They may seek guidance from interviewers, who must avoid giving any implied cues. Finally, there are a number of problems in making the market scenario realistic; for example, that if someone states that their WTP is £500, they understand that this will reduce their real income by that amount, and they will have £500 less to spend on other things.

Willingness to pay questions can be expressed in different ways, which may deal with some of these problems or possibly cause them! Box 10.1 shows two examples of how WTP questions have been asked, which illustrates some of the issues that researchers have to face.

Box 10.2 shows three ways in which researchers have asked respondents to record their answers. The most obvious is simply to let respondents choose whatever value they want, known as *open-ended* or *continuous* responses. The problem with this is that this is far removed from the way that most people on most occasions are asked to behave in most markets. Faced with such an unfamiliar task, people may give random or completely unrealistic responses. The second method is a *payment scale*, where respondents are given a range of choices. This overcomes the problem of open-endedness, but at the cost of giving cues to the respondent on the size of WTP that

Box 10.1 Willingness to pay questionnaires – questions

Here are two examples of willingness to pay questions:

EXAMPLE 1: BONE SCANS (DONALDSON, THOMAS AND TORGERSON, 1997)

We want to know how much women value the bone scan. A way of finding out the value of things, like the bone scan, is to ask what people would pay for it. Of course, the bone scan is free and will stay free. But imagine you lived in a country where you had to pay for the scan.

Before you answer, think about the scan you have just had. Also, remember the results of the scan will help you and your doctor to decide whether you need help to keep your bones in order.

What is the most that you would pay to have the scan?

EXAMPLE 2: IN-VITRO FERTILISATION (IVF) (RYAN, 1997)

In this section I am concerned with how you **value** IVF treatment.

One way to do this is to find out what the maximum amount of money is that you would be willing to pay for each IVF attempt that you have. **You will not have to pay the amount you state. This is just a way of finding out how strongly you feel about IVF.**

Would you be willing to pay £2000 for your **current** attempt at IVF? If you are not currently undergoing IVF, would you be willing to pay £2000 for your next attempt at IVF?

Remember that any money that you spend on IVF will not be available for you to spend on other things.

These UK examples demonstrate well some of the problems that willingness-to-pay studies have and some ways of solving them. A particular problem in the UK is that researchers are not ethically allowed to imply that services that are currently free might in the future be charged for, which makes describing the context very difficult. Both examples attempt to explain what the task is about by describing it as a way of finding out how much people value things. The first example does try to describe the market context by reference to another country, but this has to be qualified, making it clear that it is an entirely imaginary scenario, by emphasising that the current position is the real market. The second does not attempt to describe any market context in which payment would be made, and in fact uses boldface emphasis to make sure that the context is one of no payment.

The first example tries further to make the context real by asking respondents to think about the benefits that they will derive from the service. The second attempts to ensure that respondents treat the prices as if they were real, by reminding them that expenditure means a reduction in consumption of other goods and services.

Box 10.2 Willingness-to-pay questionnaires – responses

The following are different ways in which respondents can record their willingness to pay.

OPEN-ENDED (DONALDSON, 1997)

Please write your amount in the space below

£_____

CLOSED-ENDED (RYAN, 1997)

So would you be willing to pay £2000? (Please tick appropriate box.)

Yes ☐
No ☐

PAYMENT SCALE

Put a ✓ next to the amounts that you are sure you **would** pay.
Put an ✗ next to the amounts that you are sure you **would not** pay.
Put a O around the maximum amount that you are sure you would be prepared to pay

£0	£30	£55	£80
£5	£35	£60	£85
£10	£40	£65	£90
£15	£45	£70	£95
£25	£50	£75	£100

If £100+ please write in the exact amount　　£_____

These methods have advantages and disadvantages in terms of people's ability to offer responses to them. One way to judge them is according to guidelines that have been produced for best practice in contingent valuation. One of these is that the market and the means of payment should seem plausible. How do these methods measure up to this criterion?

The open-ended method has the merit of simplicity, but it is difficult to justify because it would be unusual to find a market in which one would simply state a price and expect to receive the good or service whatever value was stated. The closed-ended scale is more easily recognisable as relevant to markets that have a fixed price for the good or, if this is regarded as an initial bid, as a market in which haggling takes place between buyer and seller. The payment scale method is a variant of this, relevant to markets where there is haggling, except of course that the respondent is expected to 'reveal their hand' all at once, while the seller reveals nothing at all.

will be considered sensible by the researchers. A variant of this, designed to make the task closer to the way that some markets operate is *iterative bidding*, which can really only be used in an interview. Respondents are given an initial price, and asked whether they would be willing to pay it or not. Depending on their choice, the price will be raised or lowered and their decision again recorded. This continues until they are unable to decide. The third method illustrated is *closed-ended*, also known as *discrete choice* or *binary choice*, where respondents are given only a single value that they must choose to accept or reject. Different values are presented randomly to different people in a sample and WTP values are estimated from the average responses from the sample as a whole.

A recent addition to techniques of stated preference is *conjoint analysis* (CA), which has its roots in market research. CA does not necessarily provide a monetary valuation element, but may do so, and it is common to find this in most health care applications. CA is based on a theory of demand originally suggested by Lancaster (1971), which views goods and services as bundles of characteristics or *attributes*, and it is people's preferences for those attributes that determine the overall preferences for a good. For example, dental care may have positive attributes, such as relief from pain and increased ability to eat, and negative attributes, such as discomfort of treatment and a fee. In CA, respondents are given scenarios that are made up of different levels of attributes. For example, one scenario might offer complete relief of pain but no improved ability to eat with a pain-free treatment that costs £300. Another may offer some relief of pain, improved ability to eat, slight discomfort of treatment and a cost of £100. Depending on the exact approach taken, respondents may be asked to rank these or rate them, but the most popular approach is to offer a choice between pairs of scenarios. If the scenarios are carefully chosen and there is a large enough sample of respondents, relative valuations of the different attributes can be estimated for the group as a whole using variants of statistical regression known as discrete response models. If cost is included, it may be possible to estimate WTP for a good with a given set of attributes. Box 10.3 gives an example of the types of scenarios that may be compared in CA in health economics.

Box 10.3 Discrete choice conjoint analysis questionnaire (Ryan, 1999)

SCENARIO 1

	Clinic A	Clinic B
Attitudes of staff towards you	Good	Bad
Chance of taking home a baby	25%	35%
Continuity of contact with same staff	No	Yes
Time on waiting list for IVF attempt	18 months	18 months
Cost to you of IVF attempt	£1500	£3000
Follow-up support	No	No

	Prefer Clinic A	Prefer Clinic B
Which Clinic would you prefer (*tick one box only*)?		

10.3 THE MEASUREMENT OF HEALTH OUTCOMES

Although the measurement of benefits in terms of money has considerable advantages from an economic theory point of view, the measurement of benefits in terms of improved health has dominated economic evaluation. This has at least four sources. The first is a recognition that plausible RP measures are rare in the health care market, along with a distrust of SP techniques, which has led to the rejection on practical grounds of money measures. The second is a belief that health care is a special good in which there is widespread rejection of willingness to pay as a criterion for resource allocation, and therefore an objection in principle to the use of monetary measures. The third is a belief that cost–benefit analysis is not a practical tool for analysis but cost-effectiveness analysis is, so that health is a more appropriate measure than money anyway. The fourth is that health measurement is a widespread activity in many social and biomedical disciplines and in particular in evaluations by health care professionals; economic analysis can therefore draw upon many existing sources of data and ideas, have a discourse with other disciplines, and in particular talk a common language with the dominant professional groups in health care.

Health was for many years appropriately measured by extreme health indicators – changes in survival, mortality and life expectancy. These are relatively easy to measure and where health problems are dominated by deadly diseases and premature death it is reasonable to concentrate on them. Moreover, at an aggregate level they are often strongly correlated with general levels of disease. However, as health has improved and health care has become more sophisticated, premature death has become relatively less important than other aspects of ill-health. Clinical indicators of health based on biological markers or other signs and symptoms have become more important, for example changes in blood pressure or the chemical composition of body fluids. Recognition that these indicate only that there is disease, but not necessarily that the disease is having any impact on the patient, leads to interest in patient-oriented indicators. Originally, these were concerned mainly with 'function' – how well the patient was able to undertake activities of various sorts. Such functional indicators have the advantage that they are in principle straight-forward to measure, either by observation of a patient or by questionnaire.

However, it was again recognised that this is a narrow view of the impact of disease on humans and that led to a widely accepted more general concept, that health can be measured by its impact on *quality of life* (QOL). This is a very useful concept, although it suffers from many conceptual difficulties and in particular is much less easy to measure than any of the indicators discussed above.

One of the major conceptual problems with QOL is that it is in principle all-encompassing, and this covers aspects of life not normally considered to be related to health. It is arguable that this is not really a problem in assessing the benefits of health care, since economic evaluation actively seeks to measure all benefits, whatever they are; also, as we noted in Chapter 7, some health-based interventions aim to improve not just health but also other factors affecting welfare. However, those who develop and use health indicators prefer to restrict the scope of their measures to those that they believe are related to health, not simply those that health care affects – often for the pragmatic reason that it is difficult enough to measure a complex concept like health and attempting to measure general QOL is a step too far beyond that. This has led to the concept which dominates health indicators of the kind used in economic evaluation – *health-related quality of life* (HRQOL).

HRQOL sounds like a good solution to conceptual problems, but of course it demands a criterion that will enable us to define what is health related and what is not. This can only reasonably be done by invoking a theory of what health is, and underlying most HRQOL indicators is such a theory, even if it not explicitly stated. Although open to dispute, the following definition offers an excellent example of what is required if an HRQOL measure is to avoid being merely *ad hoc*. Patrick and Erickson (1993) defined HRQOL as

> [T]he value assigned to duration of life as modified by the impairments, functional status, perceptions and social opportunities that are influenced by disease, injury, treatment or policy.

The merits of this definition lie in its clear statement about what is to be counted as health and the reasons for doing that – which, in this case, is to measure *values* and to make sure that these are those than can be changed by heath care. In other words, it is an ideal conceptual definition on which to base assessment of the benefits of health care in the context of economic evaluation. In the next section we will consider this issue in more detail.

This concern with QOL, and in particular with overall QOL, prompts a suggestion that to economists is obvious – do we not already have a measure of this, which we call utility, and is this not the concept that we should be using in economic analyses? This observation has led to some distinctive economics-based contributions to the HRQOL industry, but also to some disputes and confusion, as we shall see.

10.4 MAKING HEALTH STATUS INDICATORS FIT FOR PURPOSE

In Chapter 9, we discussed the origins of economic evaluation of health care as in part deriving from a more general, non-economic, set of evaluative techniques. This is nowhere more obvious than in the measurement of health status. As suggested, health status measurement is a very large topic deriving from a number of different disciplines, including both social and biomedical science. The different approaches that these bring may result in quite different and equally valid health indicators; health is a complex entity and it is unlikely that one approach is superior to any other. Moreover, health indicators are intended for a wide variety of uses, all of which may require a different type of indicator. To give only a few examples, they might be used for research into the causes and consequences of ill-health at either the individual or collective level, monitoring the effect of economic and social phenomena or of government health policies on health or planning health services. An important point in thinking about which health indicator should be used in a particular circumstance is that there is a link between the *purpose* for which the indicator is required and the *way* in which it is measured. As we shall see, the purpose for which health state indicators are used in economic evaluation is quite specific, so it is very straightforward to define the specific requirements for its measurement.

Health indicators are derived from many different sources, using many different measures. For example, measures of mortality in a population may be derived from death certificates, and measures of morbidity from records compiled by health professionals or health care facilities. However, we are mainly concerned here with HRQOL indicators that are based on questionnaires or interview schedules, which we will call *instruments*, that are used with patients or members of the general population, whom we will call *respondents*.

There are some general criteria for judging how good a HRQOL instrument is, mainly based on its *psychometric* properties. (Psychometrics is the branch of psychology that is concerned with measurement of psychological phenomena, in the same way as econometrics concerns the measurement of economic phenomena.) The main criteria are reliability, validity, responsiveness and feasibility. *Reliability* means that the HRQOL instrument produces consistent measurements. A particularly important reliability issue is *test–retest* reliability, where the same instrument applied repeatedly to the same respondent under the same conditions produces the same results. *Validity* means that the instrument measures what it is supposed to measure. Validity can be defined in a number of different ways, including *criterion validity*, which is the extent to which the instrument's results correlate with other measures that are known to be valid; *construct validity*, which is how the instrument's results relate to other variables that are suggested by theory; and *content* or *face validity*, which is simply whether the instrument appears to contain and cover the concept that it is measuring. Validity and reliability are related: an instrument cannot be valid unless it is reliable, but a reliable measure need not be valid.

Responsiveness is a more general social research criterion and in this context it usually means how sensitive the results from the HRQOL instrument are to changes in health.

If people who have a serious illness have the same HRQOL scores as healthy people, we might suspect that the instrument is not very sensitive. *Feasibility* simply means whether or not it is possible to use the instrument. A particularly important issue is how acceptable it is to respondents, since if they cannot or will not complete it there will be many missing data.

These general criteria apply equally to a HRQOL indicator that is to be used for economic evaluation, but what are its special requirements? These derive directly from the need for a quantified measure of the benefits of activities that change health, such as health care and government health policies. This suggests that the following three properties are desirable.

First, it should provide an *unambiguous* measure of benefit. This means that we should be able to tell whether a treatment or policy has made health better or worse, or not affected it at all. Without this property, there is no way to judge how efficiency or equity will change, which is of course the point of economic evaluation. The obvious requirement is therefore for a *single number* that summarises the health change. This is sometimes regarded by critics as resulting from a nerdish desire by economists to reduce everything to numbers, but it should be emphasised that it is derived from what economists want to do, rather than being wanted for its own sake.

The second desirable property is that it should be capable of comparing different possible uses of scarce resources. Again, this is because we are interested in the efficient and equitable use of those resources, and economic evaluation is about deciding which possible uses of them are better than others. This implies that it should be applicable to all kinds of possible treatments and policies and, moreover, should be applicable to all kinds of possible health problems.

The third is that it should be capable of being interpreted in terms of values. This is because the health benefits are to be compared with costs. Costs are essentially a measure of the value that we place on the resources used as inputs, so it is logical that the benefits should be measured as the value of outputs. Of course, not all kinds of economic evaluation require this – in particular cost-effectiveness analysis does not have such a requirement – but it is nevertheless desirable. At the very least, it should be able to say that more is preferred to less.

10.4.1 Generic and Specific Measures

Generic health state instruments are intended to be independent of particular health conditions and interventions and therefore applicable in all circumstances. They therefore in effect deal with the entire concept of what health is, and different generic measures reflect different ways in which health is regarded – that is, particular 'constructs' of health deriving from a particular theory of what health is. For example, we may believe that there are two dominant aspects of ill-health, pain and disability, and these are quite separate. The instrument should therefore cover these two aspects separately. An entirely different instrument would be appropriate if, for example, our theory of health was based on a holistic view in which pain and disability are simply two different manifestations of ill-health, or we believed in the ancient Greek theory of humours. Because of their intended wide applicability, generic instruments may contain elements irrelevant to particular conditions – for example, including pain when a particular condition is not painful. These measures are sometimes intended to be an all-encompassing measure that tells you all you need to know in every circumstance, and sometimes a common minimum data set to be collected with other measures, so that at least some key part can be compared across different illnesses and interventions.

The alternative is a *disease-, condition-, treatment-* or *domain-specific* health state instrument. By disease- or condition-specific, we mean that the measure is intended only for a specific illness; by treatment-specific that it is for a particular type of treatment; and by a domain we mean a particular aspect of health, for example pain. Rather than being derived from a theory of health, as generic measures are, they usually reflect the experience of particular conditions, domains or treatments by patients and health professionals. The advantages of specific questionnaires are said to be that they may have greater acceptability to those who complete them, because people are more interested in their own health. It is also alleged that the indicators derived from them may be more sensitive than generic measures, but the evidence in favour of this is not clear cut.

It follows from our earlier argument that for economic evaluation we will mainly be interested in generic measures. There are many different generic measures, based on standard questionnaires that have been developed by different groups of researchers. In this chapter we will examine in more detail one of these, the EQ-5D (Brooks, 1996), mainly because of its relative simplicity compared with many other instruments. The EQ-5D derives its name from the European group (EuroQol) that originally derived it, but it is now used worldwide. The Health Utilities Index (HUI) originated in Canada but is also used worldwide (Horsman *et al.*, 2003). The Finnish 15D instrument – named for the fact that it has 15 dimensions – is at present mostly used locally but it is widely regarded by researchers as having some desirable properties, though also some problems, one of which will be discussed below (Sintonen, 1981). Similarly of mainly local interest is the Australian Assessment of Quality of Life (AQOL), which is of particular interest because its development was very closely guided by theory; other indicators have used theory as a guide, but have been very heavily influenced by accumulated empirical experience of good practice in health measurement derived from a number of different sources (Hawthorne *et al.*, 1999). Lastly, there is a very widely used instrument, developed in the USA, that has a number of different variants and names given to it but is most widely known as the SF-36, an acronym which means that it is made up of 36 items and is a short form of a larger instrument (Brook *et al.*, 1979). In that form it is also known as the MOS SF-36, referring to the Medical Outcomes Survey that developed it, and the RAND-36, from one of its developers. Of particular importance for economic evaluation – because they have been used to derive health state valuations – are even shorter versions of it, the SF-12 and the SF-6, containing 12 and 6 items each.

Many condition-specific measures are designed only for a specific purpose and are stand-alone, for example the Asthma Quality of Life Questionnaire (AQLQ) (Juniper *et al.*, 1993). Others are actually enhanced generic measures, which have add-on questions specific to the condition, for example the MS-QOL54, which is the SF-36 plus 18 specific questions on issues of particular importance in multiple sclerosis (Vickrey *et al.*, 1995). Several thousand condition-specific and generic instruments currently exist for measuring health; a useful searchable data base of these instruments and the associated research literature is available from Oxford University (http://phi.uhce.ox.ac.uk/).

10.4.2 Profiles and Indices

Earlier, we noted that health is a complex concept and that a key element of that is that most theories of health regard health as *multidimensional*, involving many different dimensions such as pain and disability. Any health state can be described as a combination of different levels of these different dimensions. If the health state measure simply consists of a set of dimensions that have different levels, it is known as a *profile*.

As an illustrative example, suppose that we have a health measure that only involves pain and disability. We might define these dimensions in the way shown in Figure 10.1,

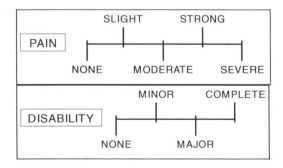

Figure 10.1 Dimensions and levels within a health measurement instrument.

where pain has five levels, ranging from none to severe; disability has four, from none to complete. Within each dimension the levels are ranked, so that we can assume that, for example, severe pain – which is defined to be as bad as pain can be – is worse than strong pain, which is worse than moderate pain, which is worse than slight pain. Any particular health state will involve one level of each dimensions, for example slight pain and minor disability or moderate pain and no disability. In this particular example, there are $5 \times 4 = 20$ possible health states.

Profile measures of health attempt to give an overall picture of health at a particular time, and although levels of health within any dimension can be compared, profiles do not make any comparisons between different dimensions. Important examples of measures that are mainly intended as profiles are the Sickness Impact Profile (Bergner *et al.*, 1981) and the SF-36 mentioned above. In these measures, the measurement within levels goes beyond ranking, assigning a score to each dimension; however, the scores are not comparable between dimensions. Another example is the EQ-5D, which is described in Box 10.4.

Profiles may have strong descriptive value, but the problem from the point of view of economic analysis is that a profile may not be able to identify whether one health state is better than another. Without additional information, we therefore may not be able

Box 10.4 The EQ-5D health-related quality of life classification

The EQ-5D contains five dimensions that describe health-related quality of life, with three levels in each dimension:

Mobility

1. No problems in walking about

2. Some problems in walking about

3. Confined to bed

Self-care

1. No problems with self-care

2. Some problems washing or dressing self

3. Unable to wash or dress self

Usual activities

1. No problems with performing usual activities (e.g. work, study, housework)

2. Some problems with performing usual activities

3. Unable to perform usual activities

Pain and discomfort

1. No pain or discomfort

2. Moderate pain or discomfort

3. Extreme pain or discomfort

Anxiety and depression

1. Not anxious or depressed

2. Moderately anxious or depressed

3. Extremely anxious or depressed

The EQ-5D classification therefore provides a profile of a person's health state. Each of the 243 possible health states can be uniquely identified by a five-digit number, for example '12212' would mean:

No problems in walking about

Some problems washing or dressing self

Some problems with performing usual activities

No pain or discomfort

Moderately anxious or depressed

The EuroQol Group (www.euroqol.org) is currently developing an expanded classification system comprising five levels in each of the five dimensions, yielding $(5^5) = 3125$ health states.

to say whether a change in health state means that health has got better or worse or remained the same. For example, if someone has EQ-5D state 21111, they have some difficulties with mobility but otherwise no problems. We can say that this is better than, say, 22111, because that means that they also have some problems with self-care; however, we cannot say whether this is better than 12111 because they have self-care difficulties *instead of* mobility difficulties. We would only be able to say whether a change from 21111 to 12111 was an improvement or not if we knew how people rated mobility in comparison with self-care.

What is required is an *index*, which is a single number representing the overall level of health. This will allow an unambiguous judgement to be made about whether one state of health is better or worse than another and from an economics point of view this is an essential requirement. As will be discussed below, the numbers may have to have rather stronger properties than simply representing a ranking, because we will want to compare not just health state levels but *changes* in health states. The major disadvantage of an index is that if it is used as the only measure of health it may not provide or may mask important details of health state changes.

An index can be derived as a direct measurement of overall health or can be derived from a profile. The EQ-5D again provides a useful example, as it can be used to provide both types of index, as shown in Box 10.5.

10.4.3 Measuring Health-Related Quality of Life: An Indifference Curve Approach

We can draw together the economics issues involved in constructing an HRQOL indicator using an indifference curve approach, following Culyer, Lavers and Williams (1971). We will use the simple example of a profile given in Figure 10.1. In Figure 10.2 the five levels on the pain dimension are labelled P_0–P_4 and the four levels on the

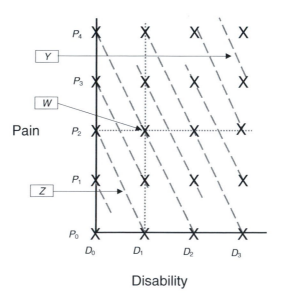

Figure 10.2 Measuring health-related quality of life: profile of ill-health, relative ranking and absolute values.

Box 10.5 Health state indexes and the EQ-5D

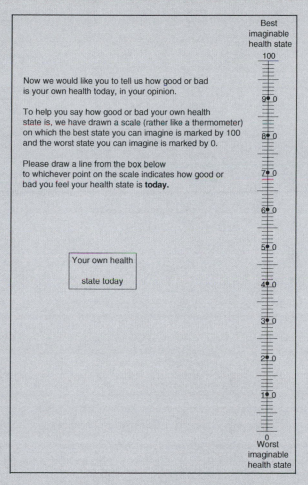

Now we would like you to tell us how good or bad is your own health today, in your opinion.

To help you say how good or bad your own health state is, we have drawn a scale (rather like a thermometer) on which the best state you can imagine is marked by 100 and the worst state you can imagine is marked by 0.

Please draw a line from the box below to whichever point on the scale indicates how good or bad you feel your health state is **today**.

Your own health state today

Best imaginable health state
100
9 0
8 0
7 0
6 0
5 0
4 0
3 0
2 0
1 0
0
Worst imaginable health state

One way to obtain a single number representing a health state is simply to ask for it in that way! The EQ-5D instrument, shown here, provides a way to do this using a visual analogue scale (see text) known as the **EQ-VAS**.

The status of numbers collected in this way is disputed. Although it is reasonable to regard them as representing a ranking, it is not clear if someone rates their health state at one time as 25 and another as 50 that they are twice as healthy on the second occasion, or even that the change from 0 to 25 is the same change in health as 25 to 50.

This index has very good properties in terms of reliability, and can be used in time series to show patterns of fluctuations in health.

An alternative is to convert a profile (see Box 10.4) into an index. The York MVH project did this using a model calculated from data from a survey of 2997 people who completed a TTO exercise (see text) on 43 EQ-5D health states. Each health state was regarded as a combination of attributes, and a regression model was estimated using levels 2 and 3 in each EQ-5D dimension as dummy variables, taking the value of 1 if they exist and 0 otherwise. The resulting model took the form of an additive multi-attribute utility function, although there were two complications: a constant term representing any deviation from full health, giving a value 0.03 below the full health level of 1, and another representing very poor health evidenced by the existence of level 3 in any of the dimensions. The resulting equation was:

$U = 0.97 - 0.066 \times$ Mobility level 2 $- 0.271 \times$ Mobility level 3 $- 0.029 \times$ Self care level 2 $- 0.097 \times$ Self care level 3 $- 0.127 \times$ Usual activities level 2 $- 0.224 \times$ Usual activities level 3 $- 0.144 \times$ Pain & discomfort level 2 $- 0.376 \times$ Pain & discomfort level 3 $- 0.114 \times$ Anxiety & depression level 2 $- 0.259 \times$ Anxiety & depression level 3 $- 0.305 \times$ Any level 3

The index takes values from 0 to 1. Health state 12122, for example would have a value of $0.97 - 0.029 - 0.114 = 0.683$, while health state 32111 would be $0.97 - 0.271 - 0.029 - 0.305 = 0.365$.

For a review of this and other health state valuation research on the EQ-5D, see Szende *et al.*, (2007)

disability dimension are labelled D_0–D_3. Each point X describes a unique health state, in terms of a particular combination of pain and disability. The 20 points together describe every possible health state given this classification system.

In a strict profile measure of health, we cannot compare dimensions, but this does not mean that we cannot compare health states. Health states to the South-West of a point are unambiguously better, for example the point marked W is worse than any of the points in the quadrant marked Z, including those on the dotted lines, which are worse in only one dimension. Health states to the North-East of a point are unambiguously worse, for example point W is better than any of the points in quadrant Y. However, we cannot, without extra information, rank point W compared to any of the points inside the other two quadrants. In this case, health is always worse in one dimension and better in another, and since dimensions are not compared we cannot make an overall judgement. In other words, a profile cannot compare and rank every possible health state.

What is required is an explicit ranking of health states, which can be thought of as deriving from indifference curves that embody the relative weight given to different dimensions and to different levels within dimensions. As a first step, we might regard the dashed lines as representing equal rankings for the points on them. However, from an economics point of view it will be important to attach a number or weight to each line, which quantifies the relative value attached to each point. These weights incorporate relative values both for dimensions and for scale points within dimensions. If we maintain the indifference curve analogy, then these can be thought of as utilities, though in this case only utility derived from aspects of HRQOL and not any other aspect of life.

10.5 THE MEASUREMENT OF HEALTH GAIN

Another way to describe the way in which the benefits of health care are best measured for economic evaluation is that the impact of health interventions should be measured as *health gain*, which is calculated as the difference in health with and without the intervention. This is consistent with the calculation of the incremental effect used as the denominator of the cost-effectiveness ratio (CER), as shown in Chapter 9. Health comprises two dimensions: the level of health experienced at a given point in time and the length of time for which that level of health is experienced. If the level of health is quantified using the concept of HRQOL, we can analyse the health experience of a person as variations in HRQOL over time, representing the prognoses with and without treatment. Figure 10.3 demonstrates this. The lower dashed line represents the path that a person's HRQOL will take following the onset of a particular illness without any health care intervention. If there is an intervention, then the patient's prognosis will alter, and HRQOL will follow the path of the upper dashed line that starts at that point of intervention.

The quantity on the vertical axis is a single number representing HRQOL at a point in time – the ways in which this can be derived are discussed in some detail below. It takes the value 1 for 'full health' – the implication being that this value is as good health as that person can experience. The value 0 is more complicated, as it represents the strange concept of 'no health'. Such a state most obviously exists when there is the absence of life, but it can also be experienced while alive if the health state is very poor. It is not the lowest value that health states can take, however, as it is possible to conceive of health states that are worse than being dead. In fact, there is in principle no lower bound to negative values for health.

The next step is to consider how this can be used to create an overall indicator of health and changes in health. In general, health is regarded as the product of the level of health and the length of time that it is experienced, in other words a measure of fully healthy time. For example, if we have an HRQOL of 0.5 and this is experienced for six days, we have experienced the equivalent of three days of full health. Given curves of the

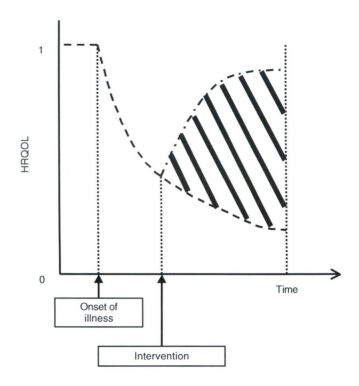

Figure 10.3 **Measuring the health gain from interventions.**

kind shown in Figure 10.3 representing prognosis, the total amount of health experienced with this prognosis will be measured by the area under the curve (AUC). The incremental effect of the intervention is the difference in the AUC with and without the intervention. This is shown by the area with diagonal shading in the figure.

Although this way of viewing the benefits of health changes as the AUC is widely accepted, there is less agreement about the way in which it should actually be calculated. The most commonly used measure is *quality-adjusted life years* (QALYs). This is calculated, in a similar way to the example above, by multiplying the amount of time in a particular health state by the quality of life during that time, summing over all time periods and standardising to a year. An example of how this is done is given in Chapter 11.

An alternative is *healthy year equivalents* (HYEs) (Mehrez and Gafni, 1989). One important critique of QALYs is the implied assumption that quality of life is valued independently of length of life; another is that it does not incorporate uncertainty. For

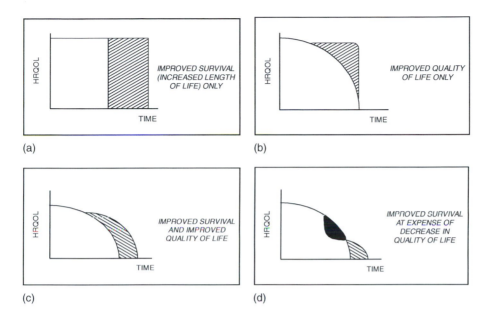

Figure 10.4 Measuring gains from different types of intervention.

these and other reasons, HYEs were devised to calculate directly the AUC. The precise way in which this is done is also shown in Chapter 11.

However the AUC is derived, health gain is calculated by comparing the AUC with and without the intervention. Figure 10.4 demonstrates this for different types of intervention. The area marked by the diagonal shading is the difference in the AUCs of the non-intervention and intervention prognoses. In the context of QALYs, it is a QALY gain, which could form the denominator of a *CER*. In principle it would be possible to estimate this directly rather than by estimating the two separate AUCs and subtracting one from the other.

The resulting health gain measure is extremely versatile, enabling the comparison of health effects that are very different in nature from each other. Figure 10.4 illustrates the range of possibilities. The first graph (a) shows that it can be used to value changes in health that have no impact on quality of life but have changes in length of life. This is in fact the original concept of a QALY, best reflected in its name – there is an increase in life years but these should be weighted by quality of life during those years. For example, most people would value ten years survival without pain more highly than ten years with pain; similarly, they would value survival for ten years in whatever health state – assuming that it was not so bad that being dead was preferable – to five years in that state.

The second graph (b) shows that the AUC measure can be used where there is no change at all in survival but a change in the quality of life during the person's remaining life.

The third graph (c) shows another scenario, where both survival and quality of life are changed. In this case not only is quality of life increased for the time that the person would live without the intervention, survival continues beyond that time.

The final graph (d) is a more complex example illustrating further the versatility of the measure. This example might represent a radical treatment which reduces a person's quality of life but enables them to live longer. In this case, there is a positive health gain deriving from increased survival, measured as an increment of quality of life over the increased length of life, but this must be weighed against the decrement of quality of life over the time that they would live without the intervention. A simple way to evaluate this would be to calculate a net benefit – does the positive area outweigh the negative?

This property, that the AUC measure of health gain can measure very diverse types of effect, and therefore in principle all health care interventions that affect health, is a powerful one which many regard as its chief advantage. However, there is an opposing view, that this demonstrates a fatal weakness in the whole concept because changes in quality of life and in length of life can never be valued on the same scale. In this view, an improvement of 5% in quality of life for 20 years cannot really be equated to one year of extra life; the two cannot even be compared.

A third measure of this type is *disability-adjusted life years* (DALYs) (Fox-Rushby, 2002). DALYs are rather different in that they measure ill-health rather than health. QALYs and HYEs weight years by health, so that the more there are of them the better and the benefits of a health intervention are that QALYs or HYEs are gained. DALYs weight years by ill-health, as measured by disability, so that the fewer there are the better, and a health intervention would be evaluated using reductions in DALYs. DALYs have been heavily promoted by the World Health Organisation and the World Bank for use in developing countries, and their use in the Global Burden of Disease Project is discussed in Chapter 12. Details of how they are calculated are given below.

10.6 NON-MONETARY VALUATION OF HEALTH STATES

We now have a health state indicator that meets almost all of the requirements that we stated earlier. All that remains is to ensure that it implies values. But what does this mean? Value is a quite general term that does have some specific meanings in economics – and in other social sciences – and it is not clear which should have primacy. We are here concerned with non-monetary values, and as suggested earlier, this usually means utilities. But utility itself is not a concept that has a single meaning, and moreover there is no well-defined way of measuring it. Hence there are controversies and disputes about how non-monetary values should be measured and there is no real consensus on the best approach.

It is therefore no surprise that there are several alternative techniques available and in widespread use. What is common to valuation methods is that they are usually based on interviews or questionnaires in which respondents are presented with 'scenarios' that describe a health state. Sometimes these are stylised descriptions based on the way that specific illnesses are experienced by patients; very often they are descriptions of particular health states according to a profile measure, such as the EQ-5D. Using a particular technique, respondents are asked to place a value on one or more health state.

Many of the techniques used to derive index numbers for health states originate from psychometrics, and indeed most were originally developed as part of psychophysics, the study of how people respond to physical stimuli. Techniques include *magnitude estimation*, where people are asked simply to give a direct estimate of size; *paired comparisons*, where people are asked to state which of two alternatives is preferred; and *rating scales*, which are discussed below. Other techniques have more economics-based origins, including *standard gamble* and *time trade-off*, which are discussed below, and the *person trade-off* or *equivalence* method, where people are asked to judge the relative importance of health states in terms of equivalence – the number of people they would like to see cured of them. The following are the most commonly used methods.

10.6.1 Rating Scales, Category Scales and Visual Analogue Scales

These form a distinctive class of health measurement instruments that again originated in psychometric research. Although similar, they have some important distinctions, the labels that are applied to them are not always consistent and there are a number of important variants within them. What is similar about them is that they are a single scale on which respondents mark a point which they believe best represents a health state, either one that is or has been experienced or one that they are asked to imagine. We will not discuss the difference between rating and category scales as they are unclear and not important for our needs. Currently of most importance in economic evaluation is the *visual analogue scale* (VAS), although its role is controversial (Parkin and Devlin, 2006). This usually consists of a single line with verbal and numerical descriptors at each end. Scale markers are often added to the line, and these are sometimes also numbered. Respondents are presented with a set of health states and are asked to rate the desirability of each by placing it at some point on the line on or between the two endpoints.

An example of a visual analogue scale is the EQ-VAS described earlier. The instrument described in Box 10.5, however, was intended for recording a respondent's current health state. There is a variant of this, the EQ-5D VAS, which has a similar design but records respondent's valuations of health state scenarios defined according to the EQ-5D classification system.

10.6.2 The Standard Gamble

The standard gamble was invented specifically to measure von Neumann–Morgenstern (vNM) utility. In its application to health, illustrated in the upper part of Figure 10.5, respondents are given a choice between two alternatives; one (Alternative 1; A_1) is a health state with certainty, (H_1) and the other (Alternative 2; A_2) is a gamble that has two possible outcomes that involve different states of health, H_2 and H_3, with particular probabilities attached to them, $p(H_2)$ and $p(H_3)$. The method relies on the fact that vNM utilities have the property that the expected value of a choice is the value multiplied by its probability. (In fact, vNM utilities can be defined as utilities to which these kind of mathematical manipulations apply.) Since H_1 is offered with certainty, its probability is equal to 1, so its expected value, $EV(A_1)$, is equal to its value, $v(H_1)$. Therefore the choice is between

$$EV(A_1) = v(H_1) \tag{10.1}$$

and

$$EV(A_2) = v(H_2) \times p(H_2) + v(H_3) \times p(H_3) \tag{10.2}$$

Since there are only two alternatives, $p(H_2) + p(H_3) = 1$, which may be equivalently stated as $p(H_3) = 1 - p(H_2)$.

The key assumption made is that people will state their preferences for A_1 and A_2 on the basis of the relative size of their expected values, which are determined by different values of $p(H_3)$ and $p(H_2)$. The respondent will choose A_1 if $EV(A_1) > EV(A_2)$ and A_2 if $EV(A_2) > EV(A_1)$; and if they are indifferent between them, $EV(A_1) = EV(A_2)$. The experiment is intended to vary $p(H_3)$ and $p(H_2)$ in order to identify the point of indifference, which produces a simple equation:

$$v(H_1) = v(H_2) \times p(H_2) + v(H_3) \times [1 - p(H_2)] \tag{10.3}$$

The final step is to solve this equation for the value of H_1 by fixing the values of H_2 and H_3. The usual way to do this is by stating H_2 to be 'full health', whose value is

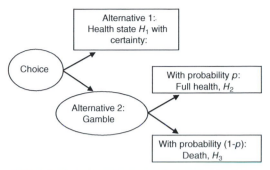

Visual aid used to help respondents with the standard gamble task

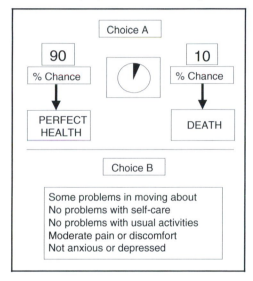

○ **Figure 10.5 The standard gamble method for a chronic health state preferred to death.**

by definition equal to 1, and H_3 to be 'death', whose value is by definition equal to 0. This produces

$$v(H_1) = 1 \times p(H_2) + 0 \times [1 - p(H_2)] \tag{10.4}$$

and therefore

$$v(H_1) = p(H_2) \tag{10.5}$$

The value of a health state is therefore simply equal to the probability accorded to obtaining full health.

The method described here applies only to a chronic health state that is preferred to death. The reason for this is slightly complicated. One of the alternatives within the gamble is death, which is of course permanent but can be viewed as the complete removal of HRQOL for what would otherwise be the person's remaining life span. So, a slightly different set of options is offered for a *temporary* health state in which the worst option can be related to a similar period as that health state. In this case, respondents are offered a choice between a temporary health state H_1 with certainty and a gamble with the possible outcomes of full health with probability p and the worst possible state H_2 with probability $(1 - p)$. If they are indifferent between these, the value of health state H_1 is $p + (1 - p) \times H_2$.

The lower part of Figure 10.5 is a stylised version of the kind of visual aids, or 'props', that are used by interviewers to assist respondents to give answers in an SG survey. These are necessary because what respondents are asked to do is likely to be an unfamiliar task for which they might require different types of explanation as to what they are supposed to do. A particular feature of this is the probability 'wheel' which seeks to demonstrate to respondents the meaning of probability, since that may be particularly difficult for some people to handle. As may be seen, in this stylised example we have presented a health state scenario in terms of an EQ-5D profile.

10.6.3 Time Trade-Off

The time trade-off (TTO) method was originally invented as a way of obtaining von Neumann-Morgenstern utilities that was easier to use than the standard gamble.

There are a number of different ways in which the TTO could be applied, but the most common way is as follows. Respondents are given a choice between two health profiles: a particular health state for a given number of years and full health for a shorter period of time. In effect they are asked to trade between quality of life and length of life. The method tries to establish where they are indifferent between the two by varying the amount spent in full health. The assumption is that, other things being equal, people will choose the option that produces the highest QALY value, where a QALY is simply defined as the product of length of life (LOL) and quality of life (QOL).

$$QALY_i = LOL_i \times QOL_i \qquad (10.6)$$

The upper part of Figure 10.6 demonstrates this. If the respondent is indifferent between two health profiles, A and B, then $QALY_A = QALY_B$, that is

$$LOL_A \times QOL_A = LOL_B \times QOL_B \qquad (10.7)$$

If B is the health state that we wish to value, we can calculate QOL_B by fixing LOL_B to be a particular number of years and by defining A as full health, thereby fixing the value of QOL_A as 1. Therefore,

$$QOL_B = LOL_A/LOL_B \tag{10.8}$$

For example, suppose that one of the alternatives is a particular state of health for 5 years and the respondent states that this is equivalent to 4 years in full health. The value of that health state is $4/5 = 0.8$.

Strictly speaking, this method applies only to a chronic health state preferred to death. For a chronic health state *worse* than death, the following method is often used, as illustrated in the lower part of Figure 10.6. The respondent is offered a choice between

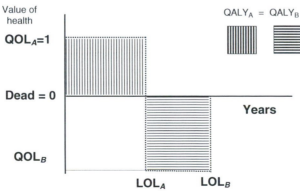

Figure 10.6 The time trade-off method.

(1) LOL_A years of full health plus $(LOL_B - LOL_A)$ years at health state QOL_B, which is worse than being dead, and (2) immediate death. If the respondent is indifferent between these, then the value of QOL_B is $LOL_A/(LOL_A - LOL_B)$, which is a negative number. This is because the first alternative is valued as the sum of the positive and negative areas and the other alternative is valued as 0. If the respondent is indifferent between options, then their total values are equal, so $0 = [1 \times (LOL_A) - QOL_B \times (LOL_B - LOL_A)]$.

10.6.4 How Do We Choose Between These Methods?

It is sometimes asserted that the so-called 'choice-based' measurement techniques, such as SG and TTO, are preferable for economic evaluation studies. Various reasons are given for this, mainly that people will not reveal their true preferences if they are not constrained to behave as they do in real life when expressing them, which is by choosing. However, these theoretical arguments are not as compelling as they might appear. All of the techniques – whether 'choice based' or not – are experimental or survey-based and, while there are good reasons for applying economic behaviour reasoning to revealed preferences, there is less to applying it to stated preference experiments. This is particularly the case in measuring health values or utilities, since there is no real-world trading in them and therefore no plausible experimental replication of a market in which trading takes place. In addition, the use of SG and TTO requires careful consideration. For example, SG results are likely to be affected by the attitude to risk of the respondent (see Chapter 6) and TTO results are likely to be affected by their time preference (see Chapter 11).

Moreover, it will be obvious from our earlier definitions of stated preference (SP) and revealed preference (RP) that all of these techniques are based on SP. However, it is sometimes claimed (by for example Drummond *et al.*, 2005) that methods that *indirectly* provide values, such as SG and TTO, are RP and those that provide them *directly*, such as Magnitude Estimation and VAS, are SP. However, it is clear that this is simply an analogy, since in every case preferences are stated, and the theoretical superiority of RP in terms of having basis in economic theory simply does not apply to indirect measures of values.

It is therefore sometimes argued that theoretical issues are of less importance than practical ones. The latter are largely based on the desirable psychometric properties, discussed earlier, that the data that result may have, plus the efficiency of their collection in terms of the cost of obtaining a sample of a particular size. In these terms, VAS measures are argued to have some advantages over others; however, the TTO is widely seen as an acceptable compromise between simplicity and theoretical rigour.

10.7 MULTI-ATTRIBUTE UTILITY MEASURES

We have noted that economists have been particularly interested in health indicators that can be interpreted as utilities, since that is the standard concept for analysing issues of well-being and quality of life. A particularly important type of indicator, therefore, is one based on what is known as a *multi-attribute utility* (MAU) *function*. Sometimes such indicators are given this title explicitly; in other cases they can rather be interpreted as MAU-based indicators. Some of the measures described earlier fall into this class.

MAU theory is also derived from the Lancaster characteristics theory discussed earlier, in which the good is not health care but health. In a MAU model, utility is derived from health state *attributes*, A_i, which may be thought of as similar to the health state 'dimensions' referred to earlier. The utility function is therefore

$$U = f(A_i) \tag{10.9}$$

In measuring health states, we are interested in particular in two properties of the utility function. One is the conditional utility of each attribute, its effect on utility with the other attributes held constant, which is defined as $\partial U/\partial A_i$. The other is the interaction of each attribute with each other attribute, expressed as the term $A_i A_j$.

Although the functional form can take any shape, a popular and easy assumption is that it is additive, which if there are no interaction terms can be expressed as

$$U = \sum_{i=1}^{n} w_i A_i \tag{10.10}$$

In this case the conditional utilities, w_i, are sometimes referred to as *weights*. This additive function can be made more complex by including interaction terms, for example,

$$U = \sum_{i=1}^{n} w_i A_i + \sum_{i=1}^{n} \sum_{j=1}^{n} w_{ij} A_i A_j \tag{10.11}$$

where w_{ij} is the weight for the interaction term $A_i A_j$. Another widely used function is the multiplicative utility function, usually expressed in log linear format as

$$\log U = \sum_{i=1}^{n} w_i \log A_i \tag{10.12}$$

The EQ-5D can be used within a MAU framework, and some widely used sets of health state valuations have been derived empirically using regression techniques to estimate a MAU model. The best-known of these is the York MVH model, described in Box 10.4. The data on which this is based were obtained from a study in the UK whose protocol and methods have been used extensively in other countries. All of the instruments discussed earlier (EQ-5D, HUI, 15D, AQOL) have MAU theory-based valuations attached to them. The SF-36 does not have a MAU model attached to it, but its even shorter versions, the SF-12 and the SF-6, have had MAU-based valuations estimated in the UK.

An attraction of MAU-based instruments is that in undertaking an assessment of health benefits we do not have to undertake valuation tasks of the kind described in the previous section. All that is required is to ask respondents to record their health state, for example using the EQ-5D descriptive system, and use the pre-scored MAU model, for example the algorithm in Box 10.5, to compute the HRQOL score.

In developing a useful MAU-type instrument, there are trade-offs to be made between their complexity, their descriptive value, their precision and their practicality in actual use. An important issue is the trade-off between the extent to which they are descriptively rich – having many fine gradations of health derived from large numbers of dimensions and large numbers of possible levels within them – and are practical in terms of the ability to place values on the health states. Indicators with a small number of possible states may lack descriptive richness, but may make it plausible for all of them to be valued directly, or at least a large proportion. If there are a very large number of states, an alternative strategy must be used, for example sampling from some health states and extrapolating to others. The EQ-5D is a very simple instrument in these terms, with 245 states, including 'unconscious' and 'dead'; the HUI has around one million, the AQOL one billion and the 15D, which has great descriptive richness, 30 billion.

10.8 THE VALUATION OF HEALTH STATES: WILLINGNESS TO PAY FOR HEALTH CHANGES

We began this chapter by discussing monetary valuation of health care and explained that dissatisfaction with this led economists to non-monetary valuation methods that dealt not with health care itself but with health. However, a middle way between these has been suggested, in which monetary values are derived for health, and stated preference techniques can and have been used as alternatives to the techniques described above in the measurement of health itself.

One possible way to do this is to use a variant of the willingness-to-pay methods described earlier for valuing health care. Of course, these are strictly not contingent valuation methods since there is no market for health itself and hence no possible description of such a market. It would be possible to describe the health care market that is assumed, but there is no imperative to do so and in some cases that might be quite inappropriate. Otherwise, many of the problems and good practices that apply to surveys relating to health care also apply to those relating to health.

As described in Chapter 8, the application of compensating and equivalent variation and of willingness to pay and to accept in the context of health is conventionally rather different from that of evaluating a good or service. This is because health benefits are evaluated with respect to changes in quantities – of health and of income – without reference to changes in prices. Utility is viewed not as a something that people maximise in order to choose combinations of health and income, but as the outcome of such combinations that exist in different states of the world. There are therefore no complicating issues such as income effects.

CV, EV, WTP and willingness to accept (WTA) are defined according to two possible exogenously determined changes in states of the world with respect to health: other things being equal, it will either deteriorate or remain the same. In each case, it is assumed that this state can be altered, so that deterioration can be prevented or an improvement brought about. The different dimensions of benefit measures are therefore as follows.

Compensating variation	Compensation for a health change	
	Health improvement	Take money
	Health deterioration	Give money

Equivalent variation	Compensation for no health change	
	No health improvement	Give money
	No health deterioration	Take money

Willingness to pay (WTP)	Person pays money	To obtain a health improvement or prevent a health deterioration

Willingness to accept (WTA)	Person is given money	To compensate them for a health deterioration or no health improvement

If we assume that the difference between two health states can equivalently be regarded as a decline from the better health state or an improvement from the worst health state, then we have four ways of measuring the value of the change in health.

	Money amount	Effect of money transfer
CV/WTP	Maximum that must be taken away from a person	To leave them as well off as before an improvement in health
Example question: Suppose that a particular health treatment or health policy would improve your health from A to B. What is the most that you would be willing to pay for this?		
EV/WTP	Maximum that must be taken away from a person	To make them as well off as they would have been after a deterioration in health
Example question: Suppose that a particular health treatment or health policy would prevent your health deteriorating from B to A. What is the most that you would be willing to pay for this?		
CV/WTA	Minimum that must be given to a person	To leave them as well off as before a deterioration in health
Example question: Suppose that a particular health treatment or health policy would prevent your health deteriorating from A to B. The government does not provide the treatment or undertake the policy, so your health deteriorates. What is the minimum compensation that you would need to be as well off as if your health had not deteriorated?		
EV/WTA	Minimum that a person must be given	To make them as well off as they would have been after an improvement in health
Example question: Suppose that a particular health treatment or health policy would improve your health from A to B. The government does not provide the treatment or undertake the policy, so your health does not improve. What is the minimum compensation that you would need to be as well off as if your health had improved?		

As an example, a respondent has an income of $£Y_1$ and a quality of life of H_1, which produces a utility of U_1. Other things remaining the same, their health would deteriorate to H_2 but their income would remain at $£Y_1$, which would produce a lower utility of U_2.

They are asked how much they would be willing to pay to prevent deterioration of their QOL to H_2. Strictly speaking, they should be asked to identify the point at which they are exactly compensated by the increase in their health for the loss of income brought about by the payment. Suppose that they were willing to pay $£X_A$;

that would reduce their income to $£(Y_1 - X_A)$. This implies that the utility that they derive from $£Y_1$ and H_2 is the same as from $£(Y_1 - X_A)$ and H_1; that is, U_2. However, they could equally be asked what they would be willing to accept as compensation for the deterioration in their health. Suppose that they were willing to accept $£X_B$, which would increase their income to $£(Y_1 + X_B)$. This implies that the utility that they derive from $£(Y_1 + X_B)$ and H_2 is the same as from $£Y_1$ and H_1; that is U_1.

The following table summarises the different combinations of QOL and income that produces the two different levels of utility.

Utility	U_1		U_2	
QOL	H_1	H_2	H_2	H_1
Income	$£Y_1$	$£(Y_1 + X_B)$	$£Y_1$	$£(Y_1 - X_A)$

The willingness to pay value $£X_A$ is an equivalent variation measure, because it is evaluated with respect to the final utility level U_2, and the willingness to accept value $£X_B$ is a compensating variation measure, because it is evaluated with respect to the initial level of utility. There is no reason why these should be the same, even though they are equally valid measures of the value of the difference between H_1 and H_2. But what of the other two possibilities?

To evaluate these, we must reverse the scenario so that the initial health state is H_2 and the initial income is $£Y_1$ and then ask what they would be willing to pay to improve their health to H_1 or what they would be willing to accept as compensation for remaining at H_2. According to the above table, this would mean that the initial utility was U_2 and therefore that the compensating variation – measured according to the initial utility – must be X_A. This implies that this would be the amount that they would be willing to accept as compensation for remaining at H_2. Using similar reasoning, the equivalent variation, which is the willingness to pay to improve their health to H_1 should be X_B.

In theory therefore, EV/WTP = CV/WTP and CV/WTA = EV/WTA. If a monetary evaluation study is carried out, EV and CV should produce the same value if the same method – WTP or WTA – is used, but it is not necessarily the case that EV measures produced under WTP and WTA will give the same value, and the same is true for CV measures. Looked at another way, although there is no reason why a WTP study should produce the same result as a WTA study, we would expect the values derived from a WTA study to be the same irrespective of whether a CV or EV measure is used, and the same to be true for a WTP study.

Can we say any more about the WTP and WTA values except that they may be different? With a typical good or service, the assumption is that it will form a small element of total consumption, with many other goods that could substitute for it. So, the good or service and income are perfect substitutes, with linear indifference curves, as in the upper digram of Figure 10.7. The change from H_1 to H_2, evaluated keeping U_1 constant, is X_B and keeping U_2 constant it is X_A. As you can verify from the figure, $X_B = X_A$, in other words WTA and WTP should be equal. However, in the case of health, it is arguable that health and wealth are not perfect substitutes; if we then make the usual assumption about the shape of indifference curves, that there is a diminishing marginal

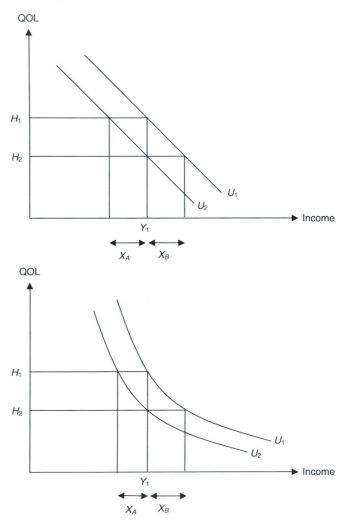

Figure 10.7 Willingness to pay and willingness to accept.

rate of substitution then the indifference curves U_1 and U_2 will be as in the lower diagram of Figure 10.7. As you may again verify, X_B should be greater than X_A – in other words, WTA should be greater than WTP.

In practice, it is usually found that WTA is greater than WTP for a wide range of goods and services, and it is often observed that the discrepancy is greater than can be explained by the existence of substitution effects. An explanation for this is *loss aversion* – people attach a greater value to something that they already have than to something that they can obtain. A bird in the hand is worth two in the bush even if it is certain that the birds in the bush will both end up in the hand.

10.9 THE VALUE OF LIFE

Finally, we look at the placing of monetary values on life itself, with the aim of evaluating either actions that reduce the number of deaths or actions that incidentally increase the number of deaths. Although these do have applications in health care, they are rather more widely found in the evaluation of other health-affecting activities, such as road safety and environmental change. There are in fact, two different traditions in this, one which may be called the *human capital* approach, and the other the value of avoiding premature death.

The human capital approach is a rather old concept of how economics might measure the value of health improving activities, originating in the fact that mortality was the most important outcome of ill-health and was relatively common. The evaluation of public health measures was therefore entirely appropriately evaluated in terms of reductions in numbers of deaths, and its economic value in terms of the money-equivalent value of those lives. In its crudest form, it is the present value of all of a person's contributions to Gross National Product (GNP) over their lifetime. There are of course more sophisticated versions of this, but in its essentials that is what it attempts to measure. It is an entirely appropriate measure to use if the evaluation is solely in terms of what happens to GNP and has a wider justification if maximising GNP is regarded as the correct maximand.

Measuring the value that is placed on the avoidance of premature death was often called in the past the *statistical value of life*. It is more commonly found in the evaluation of projects such as road building, in which the road traffic accident deaths that this will avert should be counted as part of a cost–benefit analysis, or as the major benefit of safety-improving measures. Essentially, it asks what people are willing to pay to avoid a reduction in the *risk* of death. Individuals' WTP values are summed to give a value that they are collectively willing to pay. Typical figures calculated from this give the collective WTP value for a reduction in risk sufficient to prevent one premature death in millions of pounds.

SUMMARY

1. Economic evaluation is concerned in part with how the output of health care can be defined, measured and valued.

2. Monetary valuation of health care benefits can be undertaken using revealed preference (RP) and stated preference (SP) approaches. RP refers to valuations of goods and services that can be inferred from real choices that are made in the everyday world. SP valuations are derived from surveys or experiments, which are often loosely known in health economics as willingness-to-pay (WTP) studies. The most widely recognised SP technique is the contingent valuation method. This refers to the valuation of a good or service, the measurement of value being contingent on the description of the hypothetical market that is given to respondents.

3. A recent addition to techniques of SP is conjoint analysis, which views goods and services as bundles of characteristics or attributes, and it is people's preferences for those attributes that determine the overall preferences for a good.

4. The measurement of benefits in terms of improved health is common in economic evaluation. In particular, the concept of health-related quality of life (HRQOL) has dominated health indicators of the kind used in economic evaluation.

5. Indicators for measuring benefits that are based on questionnaires or interview schedules are called instruments. There are some general criteria for judging how good an instrument is, based on its reliability, validity, responsiveness and feasibility.

6. Instruments can be generic or disease-, condition-, treatment- or domain-specific.

7. If the instrument consists of a set of dimensions that have different levels, it is known as a profile. If the instrument is an index, then it can produce a single number representing the overall level of health.

8. Health can be regarded as the product of the level of health and the length of time that it is experienced, in other words a measure of fully healthy time. If the level of health is quantified using the concept of HRQOL, we can analyse the health experience of a person as variations in HRQOL over time, representing the prognoses with and without treatment.

9. The most commonly used measure that follows this approach is quality-adjusted life years (QALYs). This is calculated by multiplying the amount of time in a particular health state by the quality of life during that time, summing over all time periods and standardising to a year. Alternatives to

QALYs are healthy year equivalents (HYEs) and disability-adjusted life years (DALYs).

10. Non-monetary valuation of health states can be undertaken with a variety of means, including rating scales, category scales and visual analogue scales, the standard gamble and the time trade-off.

11. Multi-attribute utility (MAU) measures can be used to compute the utility associated with different health states. In a MAU model, utility is derived from health state attributes. When estimating MAU models we are interested in the conditional utility of each attribute, which is quantified by the weights given to each attribute and their interactions.

12. An alternative to monetary valuation of health care benefits and the measurement of benefits in terms of improved health is to value the willingness to pay for health changes. This utilises the concepts of compensating and equivalent variation and of willingness to pay and to accept.

13. It is possible to place monetary values on life itself using a human capital approach or using statistical value of life studies.

Chapter 11

Economic Evaluation Methods

11.1 INTRODUCTION

This chapter provides an overview of the way economic evaluation methods are used in the health sector to assess value for money. Whereas Chapters 8 and 9 examined the theory and principles underpinning economic evaluation, our focus here is on the *practice* of economic evaluation – although clearly the theory and principles of economics informs both the evaluator's methodological tool kit and the way results are interpreted in order to draw conclusions about resource allocation.

One way to view economic evaluation is that it is a balance sheet, in which the costs and benefits of the outcomes of decisions are weighed together. It might be thought that the economist's task is simply to fill in that balance sheet and produce summaries of the results, but in practice economic evaluation is much more complicated. An obvious example is that we are usually evaluating non-marketed goods, and because information on costs and benefits are not automatically generated by a market these data must be specially collected or generated. Moreover, the vision of a balance sheet does not reflect the complexity of real-world decision-making, in which there is considerable uncertainty about the actual numerical values that should be attached to costs and benefits. This chapter is about how in practice we obtain and use the data that economic evaluation requires.

11.2 SELECTING THE VIEWPOINT

The motivation for any economic evaluation is a practical question asked in a specific context: Should we fund drugs for all patients with Alzheimer disease, or only for those with moderate to severe forms of that condition? How frequently should mammography screening be done, and for women of what ages? Which is better: an expensive hip prosthesis that lasts longer, or a cheaper version with a greater probability of revision in the future? These are all examples of quite different sorts of questions confronting policy makers and which economic evaluation can inform.

Which method is to be used, even what constitutes a benefit and a cost, and how these are to be valued, depends on *who* is asking these questions, and *why*. Is it patients, lobbying for better health services? A health care provider, for example a hospital, trying to improve its efficiency? A third-party funder, trying to ensure that health care budgets are being used wisely? Or a medical devices company, wanting to market its products? The purpose of the economic evaluation will have a fundamental impact on the viewpoint from which the evaluation is to be performed; and the viewpoint chosen can occasionally have an important effect on the judgement whether something is or is not good value for money. Consider the options listed in Table 11.1. The characteristics of these options, their impacts, and the way in which different sorts of costs and benefits are spread between different parties, mean that in each case the choice about what viewpoint to adopt is likely to have an important influence on the results and conclusions of an economic evaluation.

There is a connection between the choice about perspective and the choice about the preferred method of economic evaluation. For example, cost–benefit analysis (CBA) generally adopts a societal perspective (Mishan, 1971; Dasgupta and Pearce, 1972), in keeping with its foundations in welfare economics, as detailed in Chapter 8. However, in practice CBA is rarely used in the health care sector. The question of perspective is somewhat more complicated in the more common case where cost-effectiveness analysis (CEA) or cost–utility analysis (CUA) are to be used, since benefits and costs are not measured in the same units and how any given perspective is interpreted may be different for the numerator and the denominator of the cost-effectiveness ratio (CER). Gold *et al.* (1996), reporting on the US Washington Panel on CEA, advocated taking a societal perspective on costs. However, they suggested that changes in productivity as a result of improved health – which have a monetary value – should not be offset against health care costs in the denominator as that might result in 'double counting' if the value of improvements in productivity are already factored into the utilities used to calculate QALYs in the numerator. Drummond *et al.* (2005) are less directly prescriptive but suggest that, 'when in doubt, the analyst should always adopt the societal point of view, which is the broadest one and is always relevant'.

An important advantage of the societal perspective on costs in CEA is that it avoids the possibility of identifying as cost effective options that appear so merely because

Table 11.1 Why does perspective matter?

Option	Characteristics	Option	Characteristics
A law making cycle helmets compulsory	Government enacts the legislation and incurs some law enforcement costs, but the vast majority of the costs are borne by cyclists who are compelled to purchase helmets. Hansen and Scuffham (1995)	**compared to** ⇔ Routine addition of fluoride into reticulated water supplies.	Taxpayers bear the cost; all individuals benefit from reduced risk of dental illness, but especially those with lower incomes. Griffin, Jones and Tomar (2001)
An effective treatment for back pain is discovered	Back pain impacts on the use of health services but has a substantial effect on the ability of sufferers to return to work. From a societal viewpoint, improvements in productivity are important, but any reductions in the payment of sickness benefits are merely transfers from one person to another, with no net gain or loss. Changes in benefit payment would therefore not be included, although from the point of view of taxpayers, the reduced costs would be seen as an important benefit. Maniadakis and Gray (2000)	**compared to** ⇔ Screening for breast cancer.	Mammography screening results in early detection and effective treatment of breast cancer; evidence suggests it is most effective in older women. It is generally shown to be cost effective in terms of costs per life-year gained. The improvements in life expectancy and quality of life that are produced are dominated by those whose workforce participation is typically low; productivity gain is not an important benefit of this intervention. Szeto and Devlin (1996)

Table 11.1 *Continued*

Option	Characteristics		Option	Characteristics
At-home treatment or supportive care is substituted for in-hospital care, facilitating early discharge	From the health service point of view, this might be cost-neutral, cost-saving or cost increasing overall. Similarly, transferring services out of hospitals may increase or decrease costs incurred by patients and their caregivers. Many conclusions about the cost-effectiveness of early discharge restrict their perspective to that of the health service, ignoring the costs to families. Dougherty, Soderstrom and Schiffrin (1998) Beech Rudd, Tilling and Wolfe (1999)	compared to ⇦	Inclusion of IVF in health insurance or health system funded cover	A difficulty in the economic evaluation of IVF is that, while it is a health service, the benefits are not improvements to *health-related* quality of life as such, so measures such as QALYs or life years are not appropriate. This suggests CBA would be a more appropriate method; with benefits assessed using willingness to pay, and a social perspective on costs. The problem is that this evidence on value for money is not readily compared to that from other health services. Devlin and Parkin (2003)

they shift costs between sectors or groups. Gerard and Mooney (2003) argue that where benefits are considered in terms of health outcomes, as in CUA, the costs should be restricted to those that have opportunity costs in terms of health outcomes. Another way of thinking about this is that it reflects the decision makers' approach to evaluation and the extra-welfarist foundations of such techniques. That is, if the aim is to maximise health gain from a fixed budget, then arguably only costs that fall within that budget should be taken into account. Applying this argument to the evaluations undertaken by the National Institute for Health and Clinical Excellence (NICE) in the UK, Devlin, Appleby and Parkin (2003) noted that

> A wider perspective on costs would require NICE to extend its remit to optimising resource use in the public sector generally, not just health care, and indeed in the economy as a whole. In other words, an 'über-NICE' would be required to compare all possible uses of society's total resources. Decisions made from this broader perspective might maximise society's welfare but would not maximise health gain from the NHS budget.

Restricting the perspective on costs in CUA and CEA to health service costs is by far the most common practice in published papers. However, as Johannesson (1995) and Byford and Raftery (1998) point out, this approach would lead to an allocation of resources that is not allocatively efficient in the welfarist sense; indeed Johannesson (1995) argues that, taken to the extreme, it would imply that the only costs that should be included are health service costs arising in one fixed-budget period, for example ignoring changes in future costs and resource use.

The issue of what perspective to adopt in economic evaluation also affects the way health benefits are to be measured and valued in CUA. Although the perspective commonly taken in assessing costs in CUA is that of the health service, a social perspective is commonly adopted in the valuation of health outcomes – QALYs are estimated using social values, rather than those of patients (Gold *et al.*, 1996; NICE, 2004). Nevertheless, some guidelines for economic evaluation (for example those of Ramsey *et al.*, (2005) recommend that analysts collect preference weights as part of clinical trials, so that patients' preferences can be incorporated into CUA. This remains controversial, partly because there is evidence of systematic differences between patients' and the general public's valuation of health, particularly for chronic states: those experiencing ill health appear to adjust to it and to attach less disutility to it than those asked to imagine being in those states (Brazier *et al.*, 2005). There is also the question whether the preferences of those who pay rather than those who consume should be used. A further issue concerns whose health is measured: the health outcomes that are measured and valued in CUA are usually, but not always, restricted to the recipients of treatment, rather than directly incorporating spill-over effects on the health-related quality of life of others. We will discuss these issues in more detail in Section 11.3.

Given the contention over the issue of perspective, what practical guidance is available? Brouwer *et al.* (2006b) suggest adopting a two-perspective approach in all routine analyses, presenting one cost-effectiveness ratio based on the health care perspective and another based on the broader societal perspective. They argue that 'the health-care perspective may assist the health-care policymaker better in achieving health-care goals, while the societal perspective indicates whether the local rationality of the narrow health-care perspective is also in line with societal optimality'.

In health care systems where economic evaluation evidence is used as part of a systematic decision-making process, the perspective is, for all intents and purposes, dictated by the stated requirements issued by the government body charged with preparing or considering evidence (for example, NICE, 2004). Byford and Raftery (1998) conclude that 'at the very least, economic evaluations should be explicit about the perspective they adopt. The exclusion of items, whether for practical reasons or as a result of pre-trial assessments, must be made explicit, explained, and discussed in terms of their likely influence on the final results.'

The following sections detail the practical steps involved in identifying, quantifying and valuing resource use and benefits.

11.3 ESTIMATING COSTS

As we emphasised in Chapter 1, resources are limited – with the implication that the devotion of resources to any existing or proposed health care intervention necessarily diverts resources from some alternative use. This notion of opportunity cost is fundamental to the way costing is undertaken in economic evaluation. Costs are, in essence, the value of the resources used. In CBA 'the analyst must be interested in the benefits to be derived from the expenditure in question compared to the benefits that would have been obtained if the money had been used elsewhere' (Dasgupta and Pearce, 1972). This concept, *social opportunity cost*, may also be relevant in CEA or CUA in cases where the analysis adopts a societal perspective (see Section 11.1). In the more common case, where the more restrictive health service perspective is used, opportunity cost still provides the conceptual basis for valuing resource use, but what is forgone is interpreted in a more restricted way: the next best opportunity forgone *within the health sector*.

The basis of economic costing is therefore quite distinct from accounting or financial cost approaches. The process of costing involves three steps: (1) identify and describe the changes, both increases and decreases, in resource use that are associated with the options to be evaluated; (2) quantify, in physical units, those changes in resource use; and (3) value those resources.

Most of the relevant resources, for example disposable rubber gloves, are bought and sold in markets, and prices for these are readily observable. Providing that these markets are competitive, firms will adopt technically efficient production processes to minimise production costs, and competition between firms will ensure that prices reflect well the opportunity cost of these items. This draws on the proof, in welfare economics, of the First Fundamental Theorem of Welfare Economics, which was discussed in Chapter 5: in competitive markets, equilibrium prices of a good exactly equal both the marginal cost of their production *and* the marginal value consumers attach to them. Under these circumstances, economic costing is relatively straightforward: costs equal the quantity of a resource used multiplied by its price.

In reality, many markets are not fully competitive. For example, the wages paid to doctors may be a reflection of the lobbying power of medical associations or restrictions to licensing, rather than the value of their skills. The prices of drugs may reflect the effect of government regulations on licensing, pricing and intellectual property. Deviations of price from opportunity cost may arise from factors such as imperfect competition created by the inherent characteristics of the marketplace, for example a natural monopoly, or from distortions to markets created by government interventions. Where these are known, prices should be adjusted so that they better reflect opportunity cost. In practice, such adjustments are difficult to make and would rely on good information on the underlying costs of production, which is often not available. Further, where the perspective is that of the health service, there is an argument for not adjusting prices, on the grounds that the prevailing prices, even if inefficient, are *those they must pay* and are relevant to their budget. For example, the fixed prices for Health Related Groups (HRGs) for hospital procedures, set by the UK Department of Health, are highly unlikely to be a reflection of the marginal cost of every UK hospital. However, they are the prices which are used by those who commission services, the Primary Care Trusts (PCTs), and are therefore relevant for use as a basis for costing hospital care from an NHS perspective.

Where prices are used, it is important to consider whether the option being evaluated will, if implemented, result in price changes. This may be particularly important when the option will result in large changes to market conditions. For example, the inclusion of varicella vaccine on the schedule for routine immunisation, compared to its being available for individual purchase, changes both supply and demand conditions. Demand will increase because of the resulting subsidy to consumers; this enables large-scale manufacture and distribution; but the government may effectively become a monopsonist with great power to negotiate prices centrally. Predicting the effects on market prices is extremely difficult, and is best dealt with by incorporating plausible ranges around existing prices in sensitivity analysis, which is considered further in Section 11.6.

Valuing resource use becomes still more difficult in cases where there are *no* markets. This includes the value of patients' time in seeking and receiving care or of caregivers' time in providing informal supportive care. The latter can be an important element of costs and, as we saw in Table 11.1, may be particularly important in the evaluation of health care options that rely on such inputs. Values can be assigned to these resources using the same principle – opportunity costs. A carer's time may be valued at the wage rate where work is forgone, or at the value of leisure forgone. The attribution of values to non-market activities, sometimes called 'shadow pricing', can require heroic assumptions, so evaluations for which these costs are important should undertake a sensitivity analysis of plausible alternative valuations for these resources.

Finally, although the emphasis in economic evaluation is on marginal changes in costs and benefits, the available data frequently relate to *average* costs across patients in a given setting, or across settings. Average cost data have the principal advantage that they are readily available and that they will give an indication of the changes in costs *on average* that will be experienced when results are generalised or transferred to other settings. There are two issues with using average cost data. First, the addition to or reduction in costs from increased or decreased resource use may be higher, lower or the same as the average cost. Unfortunately, knowing what the relationship is between average and marginal cost requires information on the latter – the absence of which is the reason average costs are used! Secondly, average cost data obscure potentially important issues with respect to the technical efficiency of providers. If average costs are derived in one setting, for example a hospital, this assumes that the hospital is using the optimal combination of inputs. If average costs are derived from multiple settings, they will include a variety of underlying production technologies and a variety of underlying levels of production efficiency. Average costs are therefore less than ideal, because they comprise a 'black box' of underlying cost and production decisions. Analysts can add considerable value to their analyses – and aid the transferability of results – by describing and analysing the production technologies that underlie aggregate cost data.

11.3.1 Methods and Data Used in Estimating Costs

Approaches to costing fall into two broad types: macro- or 'top-down' costing, and micro- or 'bottom-up' costing. These are distinguished largely on the basis of the level of disaggregation at which individual resources are measured and valued as separate components.

A top-down approach may involve using pre-existing data on total or average costs and apportioning these in some way to the options being evaluated. Costs are not decomposed into their constituent quantities and prices. In contrast, a bottom-up approach identifies, quantifies and values resources in a disaggregated way, so that each element of costs is estimated individually and they are summed up at the end. The latter provides a greater insight into the health care programme being evaluated and facilitates the reporting of costs as components of quantities and prices – which in turn is a considerable advantage for transferability of findings between settings. For example,

Table 11.2 Categories of resource use in micro-costing

Type of cost	Quantity of resource	Value of resources: prices, imputed prices, or unit costs
Health service		
Staff (by type of staff)	Time	Wages + on-costs
Consumables (e.g. food; medicines; syringes)	Number/amount	Price
Overheads (shared institutional costs)	Proportion of total (or an approximation, e.g. square metres of floor space for the programme)	Proportional allocation
Capital items	Number of uses/proportion of total lifetime uses	Market price/rental value/replacement value
Other services		
For example, social services, ambulance services, voluntary agencies	Amount (as above, for health services)	Price (as above, for health services)
Patients, families and carers		
Time	Hours	Wage rates/imputed values
Out of pocket costs	Amount	Price
Changes in production and earnings	Time	Wage rates

it facilitates re-analysis for different sets of prices that might prevail in different health care settings. It is, however, more time consuming. Table 11.2 shows the types of resource use that might be included in a bottom-up costing, and the manner in which the quantities and values may be dealt with in each.

Costing exercises may draw on a wide range of sources of data. Top-down studies generally rely on secondary data sources, such as routine accounting or management data. At the other extreme, clinical trials can design costing into the research design, so that individual record data of health care resource or patient costs are collected alongside clinical data. These data are amenable to more sophisticated statistical analyses, as will be discussed below.

Patient costs may be obtained via patient and caregiver surveys. These may rely on retrospective recall of costs, or may take the form of patient diaries.

11.3.2 Issues in Costing: Where Do We Draw the Line?

Any new health care programme can have a complex and wide-ranging effect on resource use. In addition to the costs of delivering a service, there are costs that might be offset elsewhere in the system, including knock-on effects for future resource use in the health service or elsewhere. The identification of changes in resources may reveal a very long list of resource implications 'rippling out' from a given programme. However, in practice, it may not be possible for all these costs to be measured and valued in an economic evaluation. Indeed, in some cases the magnitude of resources involved may be quite minor, of little consequence for results, and not worth the analytical effort that would be involved in generating cost data. In those circumstances, 'a good case can be made for excluding particular effects if they are likely to have little impact on the overall results. Pre-trial literature reviews and modelling can help prioritise items of importance' (Knapp and Beecham, 1993). This 'reduced list' method has been demonstrated by Knapp and Beecham (1993) to capture most relevant costs in mental health service evaluations, with the top five most costly services accounting for 94% of the total cost and the next five for only 4%. Byford and Raftery (1998) suggest that caution is required, however, citing a study costing screening for colorectal cancer that found reduced list costing to be less successful (Whynes and Walker, 1995). However, all studies inevitably have to address the issue of where to draw the line in costing. The analyst has a responsibility to carefully justify any subjective decisions about which types of resource use are to be included and which excluded.

11.3.3 Issues in Costing: Should Future Costs and Cost Savings Be Factored into Analyses?

Health care programmes can affect both length and quality of life; these in turn interact with both current and future health care use, relating both to the condition of interest and to other conditions. Weinstein and Stason (1977) argue that the cost of 'saving' life in one way should include the future costs to the health service of death from *other* causes. The basis for this argument is that preventing premature death yields a benefit, captured in the denominator of a *CER*, but also a cost of the health services that would otherwise not have been consumed. Potentially, this argument would also extend to other sorts of non-health-care costs. Should a smoking cessation programme factor in the increased health, pension, residential care and other costs associated with extending the lives of smokers?

Moskowitz (1987) argues against this, suggesting that 'this argument is inexhaustible and philosophically difficult to justify. If carried to the extreme, it would lead us to abandon all medical care. This would be the ultimate cost effective strategy.' In practice, different analysts respond to this issue in different ways: examples may be found of economic evaluations of mammography screening that do (Gravelle *et al*, 1982) and do not (Szeto and Devlin, 1996) incorporate future health care costs. Methodological differences of this sort reduce the ability to make valid comparisons between results. A cogent argument against the inclusion of future costs is that these relate to specific programmes or treatments which *in themselves* ought properly to be the subject of economic evaluation.

In practical terms, this issue is a matter of researcher discretion, similar to the wider issues already noted concerning the appropriate boundaries for costs to be considered in an evaluation. Pragmatically, costs in the distant future, once discounted, may tend not to exert much influence on results (see Section 11.5), in which case the issue is largely irrelevant.

11.3.4 Issues in Costing: What If Cost Data Are Sourced from Different Time Periods?

A common issue in evaluation is that some cost or price data pertain to one, recent period, and other costs or prices relate to other, earlier periods. It is important to ensure that, where any cost data relate to different years, these are inflation-adjusted prior to analysis. This is because the purchasing power of a pound, or any currency, changes through time and therefore a pound in one year does not mean the same thing as a pound in another year. Even where this is not an issue, *all* studies should report the year and currency in which their results are reported (for example '2004 Australian dollars') as this facilitates the transferability of results from that setting to others.

In the remainder of the chapter, we will assume that any costs are reported in comparable, inflation-adjusted currency units. In Section 11.5 we will discuss a completely separate issue: whether we should *value* future costs and benefits differently from those in the present.

11.4 THE MEASUREMENT OF HEALTH GAIN

Chapter 10 described the theory and practice of the measurement of health, and described how in principle we can use the resulting data to measure the gains in health from health care interventions. Here we outline how in practice these health gains can be measured. The most widely used measure in economic evaluation is QALYs, but we also consider two other possible measures of health gain: one healthy year equivalents (HYEs), because of its theoretical interest and the other, disability-adjusted life years (DALYs), because it is very widely used for economic analysis in developing countries and may be of increasing importance in economic evaluation studies in such countries.

11.4.1 Measuring Quality-Adjusted Life Year (QALY) Gains

In Chapter 10, we described QALYs as being an area under the curve (AUC) measure, and illustrated this as a continuous function relating HRQOL to time. In practice, health state measurement is not so precise as to allow the detail that such a function would require, and the ways in which illnesses progress are not as neat. The usual way in which QALYs are calculated is by means of assessment at discrete points over time. In the intervals between these points, HRQOL is assumed to be constant, although

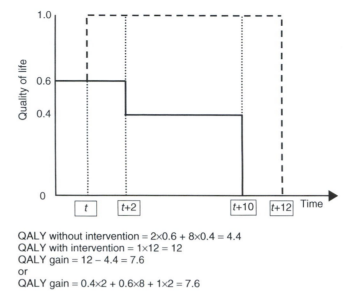

QALY without intervention = 2×0.6 + 8×0.4 = 4.4
QALY with intervention = 1×12 = 12
QALY gain = 12 − 4.4 = 7.6
or
QALY gain = 0.4×2 + 0.6×8 + 1×2 = 7.6

Figure 11.1 Measuring QALY gains: discrete point calculations.

there are occasionally some slightly more sophisticated assumptions such as a linear increase or decrease, or smoothed estimators between two fixed points.

Figure 11.1 illustrates this with a hypothetical example. The patient has at time t a health state valued at 0.6. If they have no treatment, their health will follow the solid line; it will deteriorate after 2 years (time $t + 2$) to 0.4 and then remain at that level until death 8 years later (time $t + 10$). If they do have treatment, shown by the dashed line, then their health state will immediately rise to full health, valued at 1.0, and remain at that level until death 12 years later ($t + 12$).

The QALY gain, used in the denominator of the CER, can be calculated in two equivalent ways. First, we can calculate the total QALYs with and without the treatment and subtract the latter from the former. Without the treatment, the patient has 2 years at 0.6, which is 1.2 QALYs, plus 8 years at 0.4, which is 3.2 QALYs, making a total of 4.4 QALYs. With the treatment, the patient has 12 years at full health, which is 12 QALYs. The gain is therefore 7.6 QALYs. Alternatively, we can calculate the QALY gain directly. The first 2 years have a QOL improvement from 0.6 to 1, which is 0.4, giving a QALY gain of 0.8; the next 8 years have a QOL improvement from 0.4 to 1, which is 0.6, giving a QALY gain of 4.8; the final 2 years are additional years at full health, which is 2 QALYs gained. This gives a total of 7.6 QALYs gained, as before.

It is in fact rare to find data in the real world that are as specific as this, as the natural history of diseases – that is, the details of how they progress over time in individuals – is a very complex topic, requiring data that are hard to collect and analyse. For many diseases, the natural history is not known with precision; details relevant to quality of life issues over time are rarely known; it is even rarer for time series information on quality of life itself to be known; and the time intervals at which data are recorded are rarely capable of capturing key points in disease progression but are instead determined by other factors, such as when patients consult a doctor.

This simple QALY model incorporates some assumptions about the relationship between the value assigned to health at particular times and the time itself. First, although values may change over time owing to changes in underlying health, they do not change because of the length of time for which they are experienced. For example, if a health state is given a value of 0.96, then every month spent in it is assumed to be worth 0.08 QALYs and every year in that state is worth 0.96 QALYs. This assumption is known as *constant proportionality*. It is quite plausible, however, that time and value are not independent in this way; for example, strong pain may be tolerable for short periods, but not for very long – this is known as *maximum endurable time*. In theory it would be possible to obtain valuations for health states that relate to different durations, but this would require a lot of information that, to date, has not been practical to collect, so the assumption of constant proportionality is usually made on the grounds that it provides a reasonable approximation.

Secondly, the model assumes that QALYs are valued equally, whenever they are gained or lost, so that an improvement of 1 QALY spread over the next 5 years is valued equally to no improvement in the next 5 years but an improvement of 1 QALY spread over the following 5 years. Again, this may not be true, since in general people prefer to have benefits sooner rather than later, and in the context of QALY losses they may prefer to have them later rather than sooner. This can be, and is, dealt with by discounting, which is considered in more detail in Section 11.5, but as we will see it is controversial.

Finally, the periods of time in QALY estimates refer to periods of people's lives and therefore in effect also describe the progress of illness as their age changes. Any changes in underlying illness due to age can again easily be incorporated in this model, but it may also be that *values* are different at different ages. This makes matters far more complicated, though it can be taken into account by attaching different weights to different ages. But this is again controversial, especially since it is sometimes, as discussed in Chapter 7, asserted that values attached to older people's health should be lower. We will discuss it further in Chapter 12.

11.4.2 Measuring Healthy Year Equivalents (HYEs)

HYEs attempt to incorporate what are seen by its proponents as two key features of health state values: that they should represent utilities and that they should place life-years and health within the same metric. It is proposed that this is achieved using a two-stage procedure involving an initial assessment of the utility of a health state, followed by conversion of the utility into an equivalent number of healthy years of life. A specific proposal is that an assumption is made that respondents' utilities conform to von Neumann–Morgenstern (vNM) axioms and therefore the first stage uses a standard gamble of the usual kind, in which alternatives are a particular health state for a given number of years, and a gamble in which the outcomes are full health for the same number of years and death. As usual, the aim is to find the probabilities attached to the gamble that will produce indifference with the health state. However, rather than using the implied health state values themselves, a second stage is undertaken in which the gamble with the probabilities that have been found is valued using a time trade-off against full health. The number of years of full health that is found to be equivalent to the gamble is the HYE value.

Proponents of HYEs claim that they meet the requirements for an economics measure that can be understood by others who require cost-effectiveness information, while QALYs do not (Gafni and Birch, 1993). However, HYEs have also been criticised (Buckingham, 1993; Culyer and Wagstaff, 1993), partly because of theoretical shortcomings and partly because of practical considerations. Theoretical considerations include that under the assumptions that are incorporated in the two-stage procedure the result must be identical to the results of a simple time trade-off, and any observed differences that might result will be due to the use of uncertainty and differences in the mechanics of the procedures, rather than reflecting a more accurate assessment of values. The main practical consideration is that the proposed method is very complex and there are doubts whether it is feasible to undertake large-scale research using it.

11.4.3 Measuring Disability-Adjusted Life Years (DALYs)

DALYs were developed by the World Health Organisation (WHO) and the World Bank (WB) as a health indicator that would be relatively easily measured in a wide variety of countries, especially those with lower incomes and therefore lower health care budgets and unsophisticated health information systems. They were seen as an improvement on using mortality alone and, by including disability, which was seen as being more easily measured than quality of life, they promoted the measurement of morbidity. Essentially, the DALY is a measure of population ill-health that combines information on the time that people live with a disability and the time that they lose to premature mortality. The aim is therefore to reduce DALYs.

Disability is measured with respect to functional status only, on a scale that ranges from 0, which is perfect functional health to 1, which is as bad as disability can be. Mortality is measured by comparison to what is regarded as the maximum life expectancy that humans can expect to have – which currently is that of women in Japan.

The standard procedure with DALYs is to map them to particular diseases. Discounting – see the next section – at a rate of 5% is standard. The values that are applied to health states are established by a person trade-off (PTO) valuation of health states by international experts in public health.

DALYs have been subjected to some severe criticisms as part of a general critique of the WHO/WB Global Burden of Disease project. These are considered in Chapter 12.

11.5 DISCOUNTING

11.5.1 The Rationale for Discounting Monetary Costs and Benefits

Economic evaluation involves a comparison of the benefits and costs of two or more options. These options may differ not only with respect to the overall *magnitude* of costs and benefits but also with respect to their *timing*. Consider the following options:

- A screening programme for the early detection of sexually transmitted disease, chlamydia, incurs costs in the current time period, while the benefits in terms of the prevention of infertility will not be evident until some time in the future.

- Cataract surgery incurs costs now but also produces immediate benefits in terms of improved vision, which persist through time.

- Heart transplantation incurs costs now and produces immediate benefits, but also requires a substantial ongoing annual cost for the remainder of the recipient's life, in the form of drugs to prevent the rejection of transplanted organs.

Each of these treatments has a quite different time profile of costs and benefits. This is relevant to economic evaluation because people are not indifferent to the timing of costs and benefits: we generally prefer to postpone costs and to enjoy benefits now. In other words, the value we attach to the benefit or cost reduces over time.

This phenomenon – known as positive time preference – is also argued to be relevant to social choices. Consider the following thought experiment. As a health care funder for your region, you are given an additional budget of £10 000 to spend on health care, which must be spent entirely on one of two government priorities, disease 1 and disease 2. With disease 1, the extra £10 000 incurred now will yield an extra 10 QALYs now. With disease 2, the same costs incurred now will yield an extra 10 QALYs *in 10 years' time*. The interventions are mutually exclusive and, if you do not spend the money, it will be clawed back by the government. Which would you choose?

Most people, it is argued, will prefer to spend the money on disease 1, since the payoff in terms of health gain is immediate. This suggests that there is positive *social time preference* and therefore it is argued that costs and outcomes that occur in the future should be given a lower weight compared to those that occur in the present. This is known as *discounting*; its precise use in evaluation is outlined below.

There are a number of reasons for people, individually and collectively, to have a positive time preference. One reason is that in a growing economy, where individuals will be better off in the future, the idea that people have a diminishing marginal utility of income implies that we will derive more satisfaction from an event now, when we have less income, than in the future, when we will be richer. A second is that individuals have a risk of death and other adverse events, so that we may wish to take account of the possibility that we will not be able to consume in the future. This is not an argument usually made at the societal level, however. A final reason is sometimes called short-sightedness, irrationality or impatience, but from an economics point of view it is a legitimate preference for an individual. It is less clear that it is an acceptable preference for society in general.

There is an alternative argument for discounting in public sector investment decisions, which is known as *social opportunity cost*. The resources invested in public projects, such as a particular health care programme, could have been invested in a private sector project, which would earn a rate of return on the investment. If there is no discounting in the public sector, the rate of return on society's scarce resources will be overvalued compared to their use in the private sector, which may lead to public sector projects being undertaken instead of more socially beneficial private sector projects. To avoid such inefficiency, it is necessary to ensure that public and private projects have a consistent discount rate, sometimes implicit in the private sector, but always explicit in the public sector.

A now-discredited argument is couched in terms of risk and uncertainty. The more distant in time a particular event, the less certain we are that it will occur and if it does how important it will be. We therefore place a higher value on the present, about which we are more certain, and the suggestion is that a *risk premium* should be added to the discount rate. This has long been recognised as a dubious approach (Sugden and Williams, 1978), but government agencies, such as the UK Treasury, have only recently recognised that risk is more appropriately addressed by calculating the *expected* value of future costs and benefits. Indeed, this was an important factor affecting the UK Treasury's revision downwards, in 2003, of the discount rate to be applied in public sector appraisal from 6% to 3.5% (HM Treasury, 2003).

11.5.2 The Discounting Formula

The use of discounting has the effect of giving less weight to future events. Economic evaluation weights future costs and benefits using a *discount rate* (*r*) according to the year in which they accrue, then adds them up and expresses them in *present value* (*PV*) terms. In effect, the discounting formula allows us to calculate, for any given monetary amount in the future (for example £100 in 2 years' time), the amount of money in the current time period (for example £90) such that an individual would be indifferent between them. The discounting formula used is

$$PV = FV \times \frac{1}{(1+r)^t} \qquad (11.1)$$

where PV = present value, FV = future value, r = discount rate, t = time period. The expression $1/(1+r)^t$ is known as the discount factor.

This discounting formula, which is the one conventionally used in economics, assumes a single, constant discount rate and an exponential functional form, as first proposed by Samuelson (1937). The discount rate that is chosen is applied to all time periods but, just as compound interest increases any initial amount invested exponentially, so discounting works to reduce the present value of future amounts. Recently, the emerging economics and psychology literature has given rise to alternatives, such as 'hyperbolic' (Henderson and Bateman, 1995), 'proportional' (Harvey, 1995) and 'slow' discounting (Weitzman, 1994, 1999). Under each of these schemes, the discount rate declines as impacts of the programme occur farther into the future. These alternative models suggest that time preference is better represented as decreasing impatience. For example, if offered the choice between £100 now and £120 in one year's time, most people will choose the immediate £100. However, given the choice between £100 in 5 years and £120 in 6 years most people will choose £120 in 6 years.

The impact on the present value of a project of using proportional instead of standard discounting procedures is quite dramatic: discounting with a constant discount rate of 10% per year values outcomes that occur now to be about 14 000 times more important than outcomes that will occur in 100 years. In contrast, proportional discounting, with an initial discount rate of 10%, values outcomes that occur now to be 11 times more important than outcomes that will occur in 100 years (Harvey, 1995). These alternative approaches remain contentious in economics, not least because the idea of a changing discount rate violates our usual economic assumptions about stability of preferences and gives rise to time inconsistencies. For that reason, the standard discounting formula continues to be used.

The application of discounting is straightforward using spreadsheets, but it is helpful to have a good intuitive understanding of the arithmetic, so a simple example is provided in Box 11.1.

It is usual for discounting to operate on an annual basis. This means that any costs that are incurred within one year from the introduction of a health care programme

Box 11.1 Discounting a future stream of costs

For simplicity, imagine a project which incurs costs of exactly £100 million in the current year and for each of the following four years. In order to estimate the total costs of the programme, and to weigh this up against its benefits, we need to be able to add up these costs. Because they occur in different time periods, we need to discount the future values in order to convert them into present-value equivalents, and then sum them.

The profile of costs through time looks like this:

t_0	t_1	t_2	t_3	t_4
£100	£100	£100	£100	£100

't_0' effectively means 'now' (or anything within the current one-year time horizon, since discounting is usually done on an annual basis); t_1 means 'the year after that', and so on, out to t_4, which is the costs in the fifth year.

We now apply the discounting formula, plugging in the 'r' and the 't'. If the discount rate is 5%, then $r = 0.05$ and 't' is simply the subscripted value for the time periods 0 (now), 1 (next year) and so on, as follows:

t_0	t_1	t_2	t_3	t_4
£100×1/(1 + 0.05)^0	£100×1/(1 + 0.05)^1	£100×1/(1 + 0.05)^2	£100×1/(1 + 0.05)^3	£100×1/(1 + 0.05)^4

Look at what is happening in t_0. The discount factor $1/(1 + 0.05)^0$ is equal to 1, and that means that £100 in t_0 also has a present value of exactly £100 – it is not discounted, because things that happen 'now' are important to us. Now look at t_1. The discount factor is $1/(1 + 0.05)^1$ which equals 0.9524. We now take the £100 in t_1 and multiply it by 0.9524, which gives a figure of £95.24. This is *lower* than £100, because we have discounted it – placed a lower value on it – as it occurs next year, which is less important to us. Working this through for each of the five years yields the following present values:

t_0	t_1	t_2	t_3	t_4
£100 m	£95.2 m	£90.70 m	£86.38 m	£82.27 m

Adding these up yields a present value of £454, compared to the £500 that would be obtained simply by adding up the future amounts without discounting.

> Discounting works to place increasingly less importance on things that happen far out into the future. For example, if the stream of £100 continued until year 10, undiscounted costs would be £1000, but discounted costs would be £810.

are classified as being in the present time period and are therefore not discounted. With regard to the discount formula, such costs are said to occur in year 0 and therefore have a discount factor of 1. The implication is that any health care option that has its incremental costs and effects within the current one year need not be discounted.

11.5.3 The Choice of Discount Rate

The degree of time preference is represented by a discount rate, r. Clearly the choice of discount rate is important, because this will affect the magnitude of costs in an economic evaluation. The larger the value of r, the less weight is given to future events, so the present value of costs incurred in the future is smaller. Conversely, the smaller the value of r, the more weight is given to future events, so the present value of costs incurred in the future is greater.

There is controversy surrounding the choice of discount rate to be used in economic evaluations. In practice, it is usually admissible to select a central best estimate and then to vary this systematically in a sensitivity analysis to determine the impact of the choice on the conclusions of the study. The criteria to use in selecting the base-case value for the discount rate and the range of values for inclusion in sensitivity analysis are that they should be consistent with economic theory; should include any government recommended rates; and should include rates that have been used in other published studies to which the results may be compared or be consistent with current practice.

In general, the baseline discount rate adopted by most economic evaluations of health care programmes within the National Health Service in the UK, including by NICE, is that used by HM Treasury (2003) for appraising investment in public sector projects. At the present time, this discount rate is 3.5%. However, given the sensitivity of the results of an economic evaluation to the choice of discount rate, and the fact that the rate chosen will affect the cost ranking of different projects with different time profiles, it is good practice to calculate costs using a range of discount rates. There is no agreement regarding the best range of discount rates to use for this, though it would be normal to vary the discount rate between 0%, that is, no discounting, and 10%.

11.5.4 Discounting Health Effects

It is generally accepted that future costs should be discounted in an economic evaluation and, in CBA, it is also relatively non-controversial that benefits, in monetary terms, should also be discounted. In contrast, there is considerable debate surrounding the issue of whether to discount health outcomes such as QALYs, and what the appropriate discount rate is.

This debate has arisen for various reasons. A key feature, however, is that health outcomes are not usually expressed in monetary terms: it is generally accepted that a sum of money received in the present is worth more than that same sum of money received in the future, and this is why we discount costs expressed in monetary terms. However, it may be argued that health benefits are not 'tradable' in the same way because at an individual level one cannot 'give up a year of life' now, invest it, and obtain more than a year of life in the future.

The debate therefore concentrates on the issue of whether individuals have a time preference for receiving health benefits now rather than in the future in the same way that they might have a time preference for gaining monetary benefits now rather than later in life. Arguments both for and against this view are plausible, and the issue is currently unresolved.

Since it is usual for discounting to operate on an annual basis, health benefits that have an effect with a duration of less than one year would not normally be discounted anyway. Therefore, the issue of whether or not to discount health benefits only becomes important if the health care programme under consideration produces benefits that last for more than one year.

The effect of not discounting health benefits is to improve the cost-effectiveness of all health care programmes that have benefits beyond the current time period, because not discounting increases the magnitude of the health benefits. But as well as affecting the apparent cost-effectiveness of programmes relative to some benchmark or threshold, the choice of whether to discount will also affect the cost-effectiveness of different health care programmes relative to each other; that is, it may affect the *relative* cost-effectiveness of health care programmes. Discounting health benefits tends to make those health care programmes with benefits realised mostly in the future, such as prevention, less cost-effective relative to those with benefits realised mostly in the present, such as cure.

Most national guidelines for pharmacoeconomic research recommend that both costs and benefits should be discounted, and at the same rate. In 2004, NICE, for example,

Table 11.3 Weinstein and Stason's consistency argument

Programme	Cost	Benefit
A	$10 000 now	1 QALY in 40 years' time
A1	$70 000 in 40 years' time	1 QALY in 40 years' time
A2	$70 000 now	1 QALY now
A3	$10 000 now	1/7th of a QALY now
B	$10 000 now	1 QALY now

changed its recommended discount rate from 6% for costs and 1.5% for effects to 3.5% for both. But there remains considerable debate on this issue (see Brouwer *et al.*, 2006). Theoretical arguments advanced in favour of discounting benefits, and for applying the same rate to both costs and effects, include the consistency argument (Weinstein and Stason, 1977) and the paralysing paradox (Keeler and Cretin, 1983), which we will consider below.

Table 11.3 describes a health care programme A which costs £10 000 now and yields 1 QALY in 40 years' time. Option B costs £10 000 now, and yields 1 QALY now. To argue that health outcomes should not be discounted is equivalent to saying that society is indifferent between A and B. However, because costs *are* discounted, this invokes a consistency problem. Consider A1–A3, each of which is a variant of programme A. In A1, the cost is £70 000 in 40 years' time, the present value of which, where $r = 5\%$, is £10 000 now, so both A and A1 have identical costs. Both have as their benefit 1 QALY in 40 years' time. So A and A1 are equally good value for money. Now consider A2: this is a programme that has £70 000 costs now and gains 1 QALY now. This programme is rather as if we could pull both the future costs and QALYs in A1 from 40 years' time into the current period. Because both costs and benefits are being transformed in this way, the *CER* in A2 is the same as in A1. So, in terms of a social ranking of programmes, A = A1 = A2. Now consider A3. Again, a transformation has been applied: both the benefits and the costs in A2 have been divided by 7, so the *CER* for A3 is identical to A2, and A = A1 = A2 = A3. Note that none of the options A1, A2 or A3 involves discounting QALYs, so the initial proposition that QALYs should not be discounted has been preserved in those variants of A. However, clearly A3 is *not* equal to B. Discounting costs and not discounting effects lead to a logical inconsistency.

A related argument is provided by Keeler and Cretin's (1983) paralysing paradox, illustrated in Table 11.4. Consider a health care programme, option 1, which is assessed in the current time period, t_0. The *CER* obtained by dividing the costs by the QALYs gained may well suggest that option 1 is good value for money. However, in a situation where costs are discounted but not health effects, it would be desirable for the decision maker to delay implementation of that programme until the following year (option 2).

Table 11.4 Keeler and Cretin's paralysing paradox

Programme	Time period		
	t_0	t_1	t_2
Option 1	Costs t_0/QALYS t_0		
Option 2		Costs t_1/QALYS t_0	
Option 3			Costs t_2/QALYs t_0

Considered from the current time period (t_0), option 2 has lower costs, but the same QALYs, and therefore a more favourable *CER*. The decision maker will prefer option 2 to option 1. However, delaying the programme for yet another year – option 3 – reduces costs, and the *CER*, still further. So option 3 > option 2 > option 1. Delaying the programme always improves cost-effectiveness, yielding the prediction that, where costs are discounted but QALYs are not, cost-effective interventions will always be delayed. Turning the proverb on its head: always leave to tomorrow what can be done today!

There have been some important challenges to these theoretical arguments. For example, the Keeler and Cretin finding relies on a set of assumptions that do not reflect reality. In practice, health care funders have time-limited budgets and do not defer decision indefinitely (Parsonage and Neuberger, 1992). van Hout (1998) has argued that the discount rate for health could be based on the expected growth in healthy life expectancy and the diminishing marginal utility related to such additional health, rather than the diminishing marginal value placed on income, as for costs. Gravelle and Smith (2001) argue that if the value of health grows over time, discount rates that are used for costs cannot directly be applied to effects, and should therefore be adjusted downwards.

11.6 MODELLING-BASED ECONOMIC EVALUATION

Earlier, we claimed that economic evaluation is much more complex than filling in and summarising a balance sheet. There are many calculations behind the estimates of costs and benefits, which are embodied in what is called an economic evaluation *model*. In practice, all economic evaluation in health care is now conducted in this way, and there are two reasons for this. One is that economic evaluations are usually based on different sources of data, which have to be linked together. The other is that there are many sources of uncertainty about the numerical information used in an economic evaluation, which will result in uncertainty about its results. In both cases, a formal model will help. We will first discuss the use of multiple data sources. Uncertainty is discussed in detail in Section 11.8, and here we discuss the modelling framework in which uncertainty is examined, called *decision analysis*.

11.6.1 Using Multiple Sources of Data

It is very unlikely that all of the data that are required for an economic evaluation will be generated from a single source. Of course, it is in principle possible to design an experiment that would generate all of the data, but this is in fact rarely done. The reason for this is explained in Section 11.7, where we discuss the use of economic analysis as a part of a clinical trial. So, in practice the information on outcomes is obtained from multiple sources that need to be linked, sometimes in complicated ways, particularly because it is possible that they will not be entirely consistent.

Figure 11.2 illustrates how a simple economic model links data from different sources. It describes a hypothetical CUA of a new treatment for a chronic disease, the objective of which is to obtain an estimate of the treatment's *CER* compared to the alternative, which is the way in which the disease is currently managed by the health care team. This *CER* is located in the box to the far right of the diagram. A simple balance sheet that would enable us to calculate this would contain the data in the two boxes to the left of that – the estimated costs with and without treatment and the estimated utilities with and without the new treatment. However, these data are not observed directly, but must be obtained by calculation from other sources. The data that we actually have are contained in the boxes with straight line borders, and data calculated from them are contained in boxes with wavy borders.

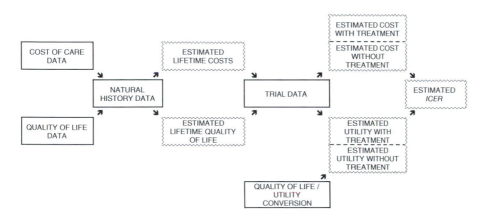

Figure 11.2 Economic evaluation model.

A critical piece of information is a numerical value for the difference that the new treatment makes to costs and benefits. In this case, the source of this information is a clinical trial, that compared the alternatives of the new treatment and existing disease management. This produced an estimate of the treatment effect, the effectiveness of the new treatment compared to existing disease management, contained in the box labelled 'Trial Data'. This information can be applied to data on the cost and benefit outcomes of current management to estimate the costs and benefits of the new treatment, which is what we need to calculate the *CER*.

Unfortunately, we also do not have data on the costs and benefits of existing management, because this would require a study that measured all of the outcomes over the whole time that the patient has the disease – which since it is a chronic disease means the patient's whole lifetime. However we are able to calculate them using other sources of data. We have information on the cost of caring for people with the disease, collected by a survey of a cross-sectional sample of patients. We also have information on the quality of life of patients with the disease, from a different survey. These are contained in the boxes to the far left of Figure 11.2. But they will only be a snapshot of the costs and quality of life of patients, not a profile over the patient's lifetime. So, we use another study, contained in the box labelled 'Natural History Data', that reported on how the disease evolves over time in individuals, and their life expectancy. This detailed information is applied to the yearly cost and quality of life data to give us the lifetime data that we need.

There is a final issue. The quality of life data that were published used a health status instrument in the form of a profile, and we wish to measure benefits in terms of utilities. Fortunately, another survey calculated utilities for every possible health state defined by that instrument, contained in the box labelled 'Quality of Life/Utility Conversion'.

Thus, there are now all of the ingredients that are needed to create the *CER*, and a recipe for combining them. But do we have enough information to make a decision? That may depend on the degree of certainty that we have about the data that have been used. To examine this issue, we need a more formal set of techniques, which go under the general title of *decision analysis*.

11.6.2 Decision Analysis

The main purpose of economic evaluation is to inform decisions about alternative uses of scarce resources. This involves using uncertain information; in practice, although uncertainty can be reduced, it is unlikely that we can remove it entirely. Decision analysis specifically looks at decision making under uncertainty, using theories of probability and of expected utility. It has a set of quantitative techniques that are applied in the following five steps.

1. Structure the problem by constructing a mathematical model of decision making as a series of connected events. This involves identifying decision alternatives, or strategies, listing the possible outcomes of each alternative and specifying the sequence in which the events take place. For example, the decision might be about choosing between medical and surgical treatment for a particular illness. The events will include provision of the treatments and the outcomes will include the impact on the patient's health of the treatment. Some of the events will be certain, for example providing the treatment; others will be uncertain, for example whether or not the patient's health improves as a result.

2. Quantify uncertainty by assigning probabilities to chance events.

3. Quantify preferences by assigning values to all possible outcomes of chance events.

4. Combine uncertainty and preferences to arrive at the best decision by calculating the expected value of each strategy.

5. Perform *sensitivity analysis*, which involves the systematic changing of the assumptions in (1)–(3) to see the impact on (4).

Although not the only decision analysis technique, the most common involves use of a *decision tree*, which is a useful way of envisioning a decision analysis model. Figure 11.3 illustrates a decision tree for a hypothetical example. The tree is made up of *nodes*, which represent events and *branches*, which connect the nodes.

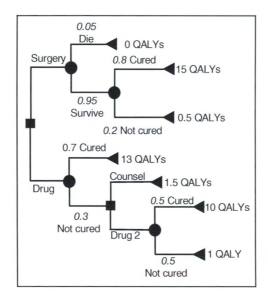

Figure 11.3 Decision tree.

Square nodes are *decision nodes*, which represent decision points controlled by the decision maker. In our example, the initial decision is between medical treatment, leading to a branch labelled 'Drug', and surgical treatment, with a branch labelled 'Surgery'. There is also a second decision, which is contingent on whether or not the first drug provides a cure. If it does not, there is a decision between a second-line drug and counselling to help the patient cope with the decision not to try further treatment. A decision node can have more than one alternative, for example, physiotherapy as well as surgery and the drug, but these must be *mutually exclusive* – the patient cannot have two of these therapies at the same time or all three. If it *is* possible to have more than one, then there should be an explicit alternative – in our example, that would require a third branch, labelled 'Drug and Surgery'.

Circular nodes are *chance nodes* or *probability nodes*, which represent chance occurrences that are not under the control of the decision maker. In our example, there are four chance nodes. The surgery branch has an initial chance node representing the probability that the patient survives the operation. There is then a second-chance node for those patients who do survive, which shows the probability that they are cured or not. The drug branch has an initial chance node showing the probability of cure with the first-line drug, and a second-chance node for those patients who have not been cured by this and have been offered the second-line drug. Each branch leading from a chance node must have a probability attached to it – for example, the probability of cure by surgery is 0.8. Chance nodes can also have more than one outcome, for example 'Improved' as well as 'Cured' and 'Not cured', but again these must be mutually exclusive. They must also be *collectively exhaustive*, which means that they must cover all possible outcomes – hence the probabilities attached to all branches from a node must sum to exactly 1.

Triangular nodes are *terminal nodes*, which represent the final outcome associated with a particular pathway through the decision tree. Each of these must have a value assigned to it. In our example, the values are expressed in terms of QALYs; a patient who has survived surgery and been cured will obtain 15 QALYs, while a patient who was given medical treatment, was not cured by the first drug and then was given counselling will obtain 1.5 QALYs.

The next stage is to calculate the value that each alternative has, by combining the uncertainty and outcome data into what are called *expected values*, which we discussed in Chapter 6 in the context of health insurance. The expected value of an activity which has known risks is the average return when the activity is repeated many times. It is calculated as the sum over all possible outcomes of the probability of the outcome multiplied by the value of the outcome. For example, if an activity X has two outcomes a and b which have probabilities $P(X_1)$ and $P(X_2)$ and values $U(X_1)$ and $U(X_2)$, the expected value of X is

$$E(X) = P(X_1) \times U(X_1) + P(X_2) \times U(X_2) \tag{11.2}$$

More generally:

$$E(X) = \sum_{i=1}^{n} P(X_i) \times U(X_i) \tag{11.3}$$

A way in which this is often done is *folding back* or *pruning* the decision tree, so that separate expected values for all events are revealed. This procedure is undertaken from right to left, working back from the final outcomes, pruning branches of the tree at the decision nodes, and finishing with the original choice. In our example, the first expected value to be calculated is for those who survive surgery; it combines the probability of cure and the QALYs obtained by those who are cured and those who are not cured:

$$EV(\text{survive surgery}) = (0.8 \times 15) + (0.2 \times 0.5) = 12.1$$

Similarly, the expected value for those who have the second drug is

$$EV(\text{Drug 2}) = (0.5 \times 10) + (0.5 \times 1) = 5.5$$

This expected value enables us to make our first decision. The expected value of Drug 2 is greater than the value of counselling. So, we would choose Drug 2 if the patient was not cured by Drug 1.

The next step is to calculate the expected value of surgery. One of the values to be incorporated is no QALYs for those who do not survive, which is one of the final outcomes. However, the other value, for those who do survive, is not a final outcome but is an expected value – EV(survive surgery) calculated above. So the expected value of surgery is

$$EV(\text{Surgery}) = (0.05 \times 0) + (0.95 \times 12.1) = 11.495$$

Similarly, the expected value of medical therapy is made up of a final outcome, if the patient is cured, and an expected value, if the patient is not cured and has the second-line drug:

$$EV(\text{Drug}) = (0.7 \times 13) + (0.3 \times 5.5) = 10.75$$

We now have all of the information required to compare the alternative strategies. The expected value of surgical treatment is greater than that of medical treatment, and if the decision-making criterion is to choose the most beneficial option, then it should be surgery. We are also able to quantify the advantage of surgical treatment:

$$\text{Incremental benefit of surgery} = (11.495 - 10.75) = 0.745 \text{ QALYs}$$

11.6.3 Markov Models

The decision analysis model that we have looked at describes a process in which a fixed sequence of events leads to an outcome and, except that they are sequential, does not involve as an important feature a time dimension. But many real world processes are dynamic – patients are not usually simply cured or not as a result of treatment, they may initially get worse, then improve, perhaps relapse and improve again before they are finally thought of as cured. *Markov models* are a way in which these processes can be structured and analysed.

In health care evaluation, the most common use of Markov models is in analysing the evolution of health states over time for a particular illness. The models assume that patients at any time are in one of a specific number of *Markov states*, in this case health states. Over specific time periods, called *cycles*, they either stay in the same state or move to one of the other states, with a given probability of moving known as a *transition probability*. Figure 11.4 shows a simple example in which there are three possible states: well, sick and dead. There will be an initial distribution of a population between these states; if this is a patient population, all will be in the state 'sick'. During the first cycle, some will become well, some will die and others will remain sick, giving a new distribution. This will be repeated for the second cycle, but there are now two other states that have to be taken into account: if the patients are well, they may remain well, become sick or even die; but those who died during the first cycle cannot of course move from that state – which is known as an *absorbing state*. This can be repeated as many times as required, although in this particular model eventually everyone will end up in the absorbing state, demonstrating Keynes' assertion that in the long run we are all dead.

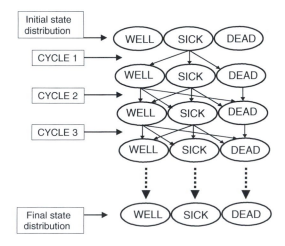

Figure 11.4 Markov cycles.

How the distribution changes over time and how quickly it converges to a final state depends on the size of the probabilities, which are often expressed in the form of a *transition matrix*, such as:

		Finishing state		
		Well	Sick	Dead
Starting state	Well	0.5	0.4	0.1
	Sick	0.2	0.5	0.3
	Dead	0	0	1

If we consider a group of 1000 sick patients, in the first cycle, 500 will remain sick, 200 will become well and 300 will die. In the second cycle, of the 500 who are sick, 250 will remain sick, 100 will become well and 150 will die. Of the 200 who are well, 100 will remain well, giving a total of 200 well people; 80 will become sick, giving a total of 330 sick people; and 20 will die, making 170 total deaths and therefore a total of 470 dead people. This will continue for as many cycles as are required. Table 11.5

Table 11.5 Markov process

Cycle	Well	Sick	Dead	Total	Total utility	Cumulative utility
0	0	1000	0	1000		
1	200	500	300	1000	500	500
2	200	330	470	1000	398	898
3	166	245	589	1000	313	1211
4	132	189	679	1000	245	1456
5	104	147	749	1000	192	1648
6	81	115	804	1000	150	1799
7	64	90	846	1000	118	1917
8	50	71	880	1000	92	2009
9	39	55	906	1000	72	2081
10	31	43	926	1000	56	2138
11	24	34	942	1000	44	2182
12	19	26	955	1000	35	2216
13	15	21	965	1000	27	2243
14	11	16	972	1000	21	2265
15	9	13	978	1000	17	2281
16	7	10	983	1000	13	2294
17	6	8	987	1000	10	2304
18	4	6	990	1000	8	2312
19	3	5	992	1000	6	2319
20	3	4	994	1000	5	2324

shows the distributions for the first 20 cycles. Note that the total always remains the same. In this model, everyone is dead by the 30th cycle.

To make this useful for economic evaluation, we have to add in costs or benefits or both; we will give an example of measuring utilities. For this, we require a utility value for each of the health states. Suppose that the utility assigned to being well is 1, to being dead is 0 and to being sick is 0.6. At the end of the first cycle we will accumulate for that time period $500 \times 0.6 + 200 \times 1 = 500$ utility units; let us assume that a cycle is one year, so that means 500 QALYs. At the end of the second cycle we accumulate a further $330 \times 0.6 + 200 \times 1 = 398$ QALYs, giving a cumulative total of 898 QALYs. The last two columns of Table 11.6 show how QALYs accumulate over time; for simplicity we have ignored the effect of time preference, though this could be taken into account by discounting. Note that most of the QALYs are accumulated in the early years; the total after 30 years is 2340, but 90% of this is gained in the first 10 years.

A simple way in which this can be used to compare alternative treatments is to make an assumption that different treatments will have different transition probabilities and therefore generate different utilities or costs. There are different assumptions that can be made within Markov models – for example that the probabilities or utility values change over cycles – and states and the transitions between them can be made much more sophisticated.

11.7 TRIAL–BASED ECONOMIC EVALUATION

Although from an economics point of view, economic evaluation in health care is just an application of more general cost–benefit techniques, from a health care point of view, cost–benefit and cost-effectiveness analyses are just special kinds of more general health care evaluation. The dominant technique in general health care evaluation is the clinical trial, in which an experiment is carried out under controlled conditions to determine in a scientific way which of a number of possibilities is best. This is promoted for good reason, because its focus is on the *effectiveness* of health care interventions. Other methods of determining effectiveness, such as case records and uncontrolled experiments are open to bias and the consequences of carrying out ineffective, or even harmful, procedures may be great, as will the consequences of not carrying out effective procedures.

As a result, there have been considerable efforts to include economic analysis within trials. In theory, this is reasonable and indeed desirable, since if we can design an experiment that includes all of the data required by economic analysis it may answer the questions that we want to answer in a scientifically rigorous and highly acceptable way. It would also automatically deal with many of the problems of uncertainty about data that modelling has to worry about. In practice, however, this has proved to be very difficult to do. The reasons are partly that there is reluctance by those who undertake clinical trials to include economic data and alter their trial protocol to meet economics considerations; and partly because clinical trials as normally carried out have proved unsuitable as the only source of data for economic evaluations (Buxton et al., 1997; Halpern et al., 1998).

This unsuitability of clinical trials mainly results from their artificial nature. To ensure replicability of results, they are conducted under the equivalent of laboratory conditions, which means that they may not be representative of actual medical practice, which is what economic evaluation is seeking to inform, and may not be widely generalisable. Even the economic data that are collected may not be typical of the wider world. It might be argued that it is possible to conduct a trial that would overcome these problems, and in fact there are trials – called pragmatic trials – that attempt to do this. But such trials have to collect a very large amount of data and collect them for a very long time; they will therefore be very expensive and take a long time to report. Decision making cannot always wait a long time, and in any case given change in health care, such a trial might be looking at an obsolete technology or problem that has changed considerably.

As a result, many argue not only that it is inevitable that real-world clinical trial data will of necessity have to be supplemented by a great deal of economic modelling, but that this is in fact a superior way of conducting economic evaluation. As Halpern et al. (1998) put it, modelling deals with a real-world problem – decision making with imperfect knowledge under uncertainty – and provides timely information. However, it is the case that economic models can and should include data from clinical trials, and if the trial contains relevant economic data then these are a good source of such information.

11.8 DEALING WITH UNCERTAINTY: SENSITIVITY ANALYSIS

We have discussed how decision analysis deals with certain types of uncertainty by assigning probabilities to events within a model. Clinical trials also incorporate uncertainty, since effectiveness results are generally provided as both a mean effect and also a confidence interval. Other aspects of uncertainty are dealt with by *sensitivity analysis*, which is a set of techniques that essentially seek to analyse how sensitive results are to uncertainty. In the context of modelling, it analyses how sensitive results are to changes in the model, for example changes in the structure of the decision tree or in the data that are contained within it.

What do we do if we find that the results are sensitive to changes in assumptions or data? Essentially, we need to improve the data that we have and to reduce the amount of uncertainty. In what follows, we refer to the model that has the best assumed structure and data as the *base case*. The assumptions and data that we wish to test are referred to as *parameters* of the model.

11.8.1 One-Way Sensitivity Analysis

One-way sensitivity analysis means looking at how sensitive results are to changes in one parameter. Figure 11.5 illustrates this, using the example of the alternatives of surgery and drug therapy for a particular illness and the sensitivity of the results to assumptions about the appropriate discount rate. The *CER* for surgery versus drug therapy is measured as the incremental cost per QALY gained:

$$CER = (\text{Cost}_{\text{Surgery}} - \text{Cost}_{\text{Drug}})/(\text{QALYs}_{\text{Surgery}} - \text{QALYs}_{\text{Drug}}) \qquad (11.4)$$

The issue for the decision maker is whether the *CER* is below the ceiling ratio, in which case surgery is the preferred option, or above it, in which case drug therapy is preferred. The solid line shows how *CER* changes as the discount rate changes. It increases as the discount rate increases because, although there are some longer-term follow-up and maintenance costs for surgery, most of its costs are immediate, while the drugs must be

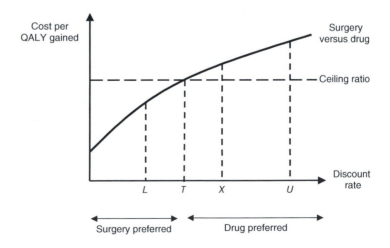

Figure 11.5 One way sensitivity analysis.

taken over a long period. As a result, the incremental cost of surgery rises as the discount rate rises because the cost of the drug option falls; hence the *CER* is increasing.

The point *X* shows the base case value of the discount rate. Drug therapy is preferred because the *CER* is higher than the ceiling ratio, shown by the horizontal dashed line.

If at every possible value of the parameter the decision to accept or reject surgery is the same, then the decision is clear cut and we can confidently state that the decision is not sensitive to the value of the uncertain parameter. In our example, this is not the case. At low levels of the discount rate, surgery is preferred, but as it increases the relative cost-effectiveness changes so that at some point drug therapy is preferred. At the point *T* the *CER* is equal to the ceiling ratio, and a change in the preferred option occurs. This kind of analysis is known as *threshold analysis*. This is not the same usage of this term as in cost-effectiveness threshold, which is another term for the ceiling ratio. *T* is the threshold value for the parameter being varied – in this case the discount rate – between accepting one option and another.

If *T* and *X* are very different, then it is reasonable to say that the results are not sensitive to the values of the parameter; if they are very similar, then they are sensitive. But what do we mean by 'very different' and 'very similar'? A simple way to understand this is to consider what may be called *plausible range*s for the parameter – what may be considered as sensible upper and lower values for it, shown in the figure as *U* and *L*. These could be informed by expert opinions or some other method – a popular method used to be to raise and lower the base case value by some percentage. Where possible, a better approach is to use proper statistical procedures, which will be described below. Whatever the source, given a plausible range *U* to *L* it is easy to tell whether the optimal decision is sensitive to the assumptions underlying the parameter value. If *T* lies within *U–L*, as in the example, it is sensitive; if outside, it is not.

11.8.2 Multi-Way Sensitivity Analysis

It is possible to vary more than one parameter at the same time and view the combined impact on the outcomes. Unfortunately, for more than two or three parameters, this becomes very cumbersome, but it is quite easy to see how this works for two parameters, as in Figure 11.6. The two parameters are the discount rate, as before, and the assumed proportion of patients that experience adverse events with the drug. Obviously, the drug adverse event rate will not affect the surgical option, but the higher it is the higher the cost for the drug option and therefore the better the relative cost-effectiveness of surgery. Each point on the figure shows a different combination of the discount rate and adverse event rate. Some will favour surgery and others drug therapy; the solid line shows all of the combinations where the *CER* of surgery compared to drug therapy is equal to the ceiling ratio – in other words, a threshold line rather than a point.

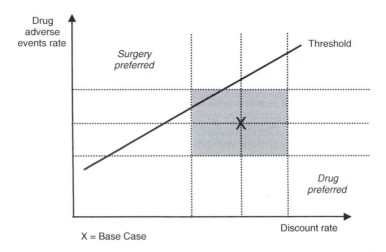

Figure 11.6 Two-way sensitivity analysis.

Plausible ranges may also be defined, and in combination they define an area in which the results are plausible, shown as the grey box. Note that in this case, if we were to look at separate one-way analyses of the parameters, we would conclude that the results were not sensitive to the value of them. This is shown by the lines that pass through the base case X, which in each case cross the threshold outside of the relevant plausible range. However, in combination the results are sensitive to the assumptions, since the threshold line is partly within the plausible region. The reason is that the one-way analyses are evaluated at the base case value for all parameters, but the two analyses are evaluated at all plausible values. One-way analyses can therefore be misleading. In fact, we should investigate the impact of the plausible ranges of *all* parameters in combination.

11.8.3 Statistically–Based Sensitivity Analysis

The problem with 'plausible range' methods is that their basis is often unclear and not testable. Statistical theory gives us a way in which we can quantify uncertainty in a consistent and easily interpretable way, by regarding the base case results as a *point estimate* of cost-effectiveness and sensitivity analysis as providing an *interval estimate*, or confidence interval. When this is done as part of a decision analysis model, it is called *probabilistic sensitivity analysis*, but when it is forms part of a trial-based analysis it is called *stochastic cost-effectiveness analysis*. Many of the analytical tools used in these contexts are very similar, but the concepts and methods underlying them are sometimes rather different.

In stochastic cost-effectiveness analysis we have patient level cost and outcome data from economic analysis alongside clinical trial from which we wish to estimate a confidence interval for the *CER*. Unfortunately, this is problematic because ratios do not have simple probability distributions, and the distribution from which confidence intervals can be calculated has to be approximated. There are a number of possible solutions to this, but the most popular is to employ a statistical technique called *bootstrapping*, where the distribution of *CERs* is generated by repeated sampling from the data.

In the context of modelling, a *CER* distribution can be created using Monte Carlo simulations. This requires a distribution to be assumed, if it is not known, for each of the model's parameters, and samples to be taken from those distributions from which the *CER* is calculated. Repeating this many times builds up an empirical distribution of *CERs* in a similar way to bootstrapping, although the sampling is not from real observations but from simulated observations derived from, in some cases, assumed distributions.

There is, however, a far worse problem with *CERs*. It is quite possible that the distribution of *CERs* may spread over more than one quadrant of the CE plane and the *CER* has discontinuities at the boundaries between different quadrants. In particular, a distribution may include both positive and negative values for the *CER* and these mean such different things that it makes no sense to include them in the same confidence interval.

There are two possible solutions to this, which we introduced in Chapter 9: the net benefits approach and the cost-effectiveness acceptability curve (CEAC), which are both based on a critical ceiling ratio or threshold defining the level of cost-effectiveness that a treatment must achieve to be acceptable. Net benefit is not subject to the problem that the *CER* has, because it is a single number rather than a ratio. It is therefore straightforward to calculate a confidence interval for it.

The CEAC deals with this in a different way, essentially by retaining the *CER* but replacing the concept of a confidence interval. It was invented by van Hout *et al.* (1994) specifically to deal with the problems with CE confidence intervals in the context of clinical trials but has been adapted for use in modelling using probabilistic rather than stochastic CEA. The *CER* distribution enables us to calculate the probability that a treatment is acceptable, given a particular value for the ceiling ratio. Each possible level of the ceiling ratio is plotted against its associated probability, giving the CEAC described in Chapter 9.

SUMMARY

1. The perspective of an economic evaluation is important because it determines which method of economic evaluation is to be used, what constitutes a benefit and a cost, and how these are to be valued. Common viewpoints are that of the health service and that of society as a whole. Researchers should be explicit about the viewpoint they adopt.

2. When estimating costs, the aim is to estimate the value of the resources used in terms of their opportunity costs. The process of economic costing involves three steps: identifying and describing resource use changes; quantifying them in physical units; and valuing them.

3. Approaches to costing fall into two broad types: macro- or 'top-down' costing, and micro- or 'bottom-up' costing, distinguished largely by the level of disaggregation with which individual resources are measured and valued.

4. It is important to ensure that, where any cost data relate to different years, these be inflation-adjusted prior to analysis.

5. Quality-adjusted life years (QALYs) can be measured as the area under a curve relating HRQOL to time. Empirically, calculation of QALYs can be problematic because HRQOL is not measured continuously but at discrete points in time.

6. Healthy year equivalents (HYEs) attempt to incorporate two key features of health state values, representing utilities and placing life years and health within the same metric. A two-stage measurement procedure assesses a health state's utility, then converts it into an equivalent number of healthy life years. Proponents of HYEs claim that they are uniquely suitable for economic evaluation; critics that HYEs have theoretical shortcomings and are impractical.

7. Disability-adjusted life years (DALYs) were developed as a measure of population ill-health that is easily measured in a wide variety of countries, especially those with lower incomes. This was seen as an improvement on using mortality alone, including disability, which is more easily measured than quality of life. DALYs combine information on the time that people live with a disability with the time that they lose to premature mortality.

8. Alternatives in economic evaluation may differ with respect to their timing. Most people put a lower weight on costs and outcomes that occur in the future, so these should be discounted compared to those that occur in the present. Economic evaluation weights yearly costs and benefits using a discount rate and sums them to form a present value.

9. It is generally accepted that future costs should be discounted in an economic evaluation and, in CBA, that benefits should also be discounted. There is a debate about whether or not to discount health outcomes such as QALYs, and what the appropriate discount rate is.

10. There are many calculations behind the estimates of costs and benefits, which are embodied in what is called an economic evaluation model. In practice, all economic evaluation in health care involves modelling of some kind, because economic evaluations are usually based on different sources of data, which have to be linked together, and there are many sources of uncertainty about the numerical information used in an economic evaluation, which will result in uncertainty about its results.

11. The main purpose of economic evaluation is to inform decisions about alternative uses of scarce resources. This involves using uncertain information; in practice, although uncertainty can be reduced, it is unlikely that we can remove it entirely. Decision analysis specifically looks at decision making under uncertainty, using theories of probability and of expected utility.

12. The most common decision analysis technique involves the use of a decision tree, which is a useful way of envisioning a decision analysis model. Markov models are a way in which dynamic real world processes can be modelled.

13. Uncertainty can be dealt with in economic evaluation using sensitivity analysis. One-way sensitivity analysis looks at how sensitive results are to changes in one parameter. Multi-way sensitivity analysis varies more than one parameter at the same time and views the combined impact on the outcomes.

14. Stochastic cost-effectiveness analysis estimates a confidence interval for the CER from patient level cost and outcome data. One method of doing this is to use bootstrapping, where the distribution of CERs is generated by repeated sampling from the data. It is also possible to compute confidence intervals around net benefit measures.

15. An alternative statistical framework to the confidence interval is to use the cost-effectiveness acceptability curve.

Chapter 12

The Use of Economic Evaluation in Decision Making

12.1 THE DECISION–MAKING CONTEXT: WHY IS ECONOMIC EVALUATION USED?

The methods of economic evaluation detailed in Chapters 9–11 were developed to inform resource allocation decisions about health care. We have already considered how methodological issues – such as uncertainty over costs and effects – can be handled in analysis and reported to users. The aim of this chapter is to consider how *in practice* economic evaluation evidence is used in decision making, and to highlight issues that persist in making resource allocation decisions based on value for money.

Two decades ago, studies reported that the growing enthusiasm of economists in undertaking economic evaluation was not matched by use of the resulting information in practice: few decision makers reported using economic evidence in the process of making real-life decisions (Ludbrook and Mooney, 1984; Drummond, 1987). The situation now is markedly different. Economic evaluation is widely and systematically used in a number of developed economies, such as Australia, the UK, New Zealand and Canada; and in under-developed economies aid and development agencies make extensive use of economic evaluation evidence to help target scarce resources to greatest effect (World Bank, 1993). In England and Wales, economic evaluation is used by the National Institute for Health and Clinical Excellence (NICE) in its guidance on the use of new and existing medicines, treatments and procedures within the NHS (see Box 12.1). The

Box 12.1 Decision making using economic evaluation in the UK: the National Institute for Health and Clinical Excellence (NICE)

In England and Wales, the National Institute for Health and Clinical Excellence (NICE) was established in 1999 to address geographic variations in access ('postcode prescribing', see Box 12.2) by providing national-level guidance on the effectiveness and cost-effectiveness of new health technologies in the NHS.

Three centres produce different types of NICE guidance: the Centre for Public Health Excellence deals with the promotion of good public health and the prevention of ill health; the Centre for Clinical Practice deals with the appropriate treatment and care of people with specific diseases and conditions; and the Centre for Health Technology Evaluation deals with the use of new and existing medicines, treatments and procedures based on technology appraisals.

NICE's technology appraisal process involves consideration of both clinical and economic evidence, undertaken in the following stages.

1. The Department of Health (DH) produces a list of provisional appraisal topics.

2. Consultees and commentators are identified, including national organisations and groups representing patients and carers, and bodies representing health professionals, manufacturers and research groups.

3. NICE works with the DH to develop a scope document, which sets out what the appraisal will cover and the questions to be asked. Consultees and commentators can comment on the draft scope.

4. The DH formally refers technology appraisal topics to NICE.

5. NICE commissions an independent academic centre to review published clinical and economic evidence on the technology and prepare an assessment report. This usually includes an economic evaluation of the technology conducted using a set of methodological guidelines. Consultees and commentators are invited to comment on the report.

6. The assessment report and comments on it are drawn together in an evaluation report.

7. An independent appraisal committee considers the evaluation report. It hears evidence from nominated clinical experts, patients and carers before making

its first recommendations in the appraisal consultation document (ACD). Consultees and commentators have four weeks to comment on the ACD. It is made available online so that health professionals and members of the public can comment on it.

8. The independent appraisal committee considers the comments on the ACD, then makes its final recommendations in the final appraisal determination (FAD). The FAD is submitted to NICE for approval. Consultees can appeal against the final recommendations in the FAD.

9. Guidance issued: If there are no appeals, or an appeal is not upheld, the final recommendations are issued as NICE guidance.

Owing to concerns over the time NICE takes to produce its guidance, a new, rapid process for assessing drugs and other treatments to sit alongside its usual process is being introduced. The Single Technology Appraisal (STA) process will produce guidance more quickly on life-saving drugs that have already been licensed and on new medicines close to when they first become available.

NICE wields considerable power with respect to health technology evaluation: in 2002 the implementation of its decisions was made mandatory in the NHS in England and Wales. By August 2006 NICE had published 87 technology appraisals.

motivation for using economic evaluation in decision making generally includes one or more of the following.

(a) To Maximise the Benefits from Health Care Spending

The health care systems in the UK and New Zealand, both of which are publicly funded, fixed-budget systems, use economic evaluation to make national-level decisions about the mix of health care services to fund. In some cases, this is also accompanied by use of economic evaluation at a local or regional level by budget-holders to inform their resource allocation decisions. Of course, how benefit is interpreted differs between jurisdictions – for example, in the UK, benefit is equated with health improvement, preferably measured by QALYs gained (NICE, 2004); but in France, scepticism about theoretical and empirical issues regarding QALYs has led to their *not* being recommended as a basis for social choices, and cost–benefit analysis (CBA) is used instead for decisions about reimbursement of pharmaceuticals (Collège des Èconomistes de la Santé, 2004).

(b) To Overcome Regional Variations in Access

An important motivation behind the establishment of NICE in the UK is to address 'postcode prescribing' – variations in access to health care depending on place of residence (Rawlins and Culyer, 2004; Devlin and Parkin, 2004). In the UK, this is regarded as an equity issue because in a national health care system such variations are difficult to defend. Variations in medical practice across regional and national borders have, however, long been observed and questioned (see, for example, Cooper, 1975). There is an extensive literature on variations in medical practice in the USA (Wennberg and Gittleson, 1982). In Box 12.2 we show how these variations in medical practice care are not just unfair but also inefficient.

Box 12.2 The inefficiency of 'postcode lotteries' in health care

Differences in access to treatments in the NHS frequently give rise to high-profile cases – for example, in 2006 it became evident that women diagnosed with breast cancer in one region of the UK have access to a new drug, Herceptin^{TM}, which women in other regions with similar diagnoses are denied. This and other cases of 'post-code lotteries' for health care give rise to media interest, political pressure and legal challenges to local health care funders, some of which have been successful and have lead to women being granted access to this treatment ('Woman wins battle for breast cancer treatment' *Guardian*, 13 April 2006).

Most of the assertions about postcode rationing in the UK, both by the NHS and by stakeholders, have focused on the implications for equity. Specifically, geographical variations in access violate *horizontal* equity in health care use, which we discussed in Chapter 7: 'like' individuals (clinically) are being treated in an 'unlike' manner (in terms of access to treatment technologies).

Another way of thinking about postcode rationing is that it is *inefficient*. It suggests variations in medical practice that are unjustified by clinical evidence, or by epidemiological or cost differences between regions. Imagine that the health system comprises just three regions, each of which holds different information and views about the value for money of Herceptin. Region 1 believes that, given the cost of procuring Herceptin (approximately £24 000 per patient per year) represented by the marginal cost curve, and given their view of the marginal value of this treatment (shown by MB_1), the optimum use of this drug is Q_0. In contrast, Region 3, facing the same marginal cost of procurement, believes there is considerable marginal value (MB_3) to its patients of accessing this treatment – resulting in Q' treatments being consumed.

WELFARE LOSSES FROM POSTCODE PRESCRIBING

Let us assume that Region 2 is, in fact, correct in its assessment of marginal value, MB_2. Given MB_2, by denying Herceptin to its patients, Region 1 generates a welfare loss shown by area a – too little is being consumed given that the 'true' marginal value is MB_2, not MB_1. Similarly, Region 3, which has recommended Q', generates a welfare loss of area b: too much is consumed, and for each unit in excess of Q^*, $MC > MB$. The variation between regions generates a total welfare loss $= a + b$.

Alternatively, if the evidence ultimately suggests that Region 1's assessment of costs and benefits is most accurate, then the correct decision is that this treatment should not be made available at all. In that case, the welfare loss of Regions 2 and 3 providing this treatment $= c + d + b$.

The approach described above is broadly similar to that developed by Phelps (Phelps and Parente, 1990; Phelps and Mooney, 1993; Phelps, 1995) as a means of estimating the welfare losses associated with 'small area medical variations' observed in the USA, often referred to as 'Wennberg variations' (Wennberg and Gittleson, 1982). There are problems with the approach; for example, in the absence of a definitive view of clinical benefit and marginal value, the approach generally assumes that the *average* intervention rate is the correct one. Nevertheless, the magnitude of welfare losses is striking: for example, Phelps and Parente (1990) estimated the annual welfare losses from variations in the use of Coronary Artery Bypass Grafts (CABG) alone to be $US 0.75 billion. These studies suggest that medical variations in the USA are a source of considerable inefficiency.

Are there any circumstances under which such local variations might be justified? For example, what if, instead of arising from imperfect information about clinical benefit, they arise from differences in the value placed on particular kinds of health benefits in each region? Although this may seem implausible as an explanation for postcode rationing, the existence of distinctive local preferences and priorities is, arguably, precisely the point of delegating purchasing decisions to local budget-holders. However, local preferences can only be met by sacrificing national consistency: thus there is an unavoidable tension between localism and centralism.

Medical variations are evident not only within but also *between* countries. This poses particular challenges for Europe, where inconsistencies in access to health care technologies have generated legal challenges. European Court of Justice rulings have upheld the right of a citizen in one country to travel to another country to receive 'medically necessary' care and to claim this against their social insurance cover – even if that treatment is denied in their home country (Watson, 2001). The implication is that it may become increasingly difficult for any single European country effectively to make a decision to withhold a new treatment – and that decisions about what is good value for money will need to be harmonised across Europe.

(c) To Contain Costs/Manage Demand

Perhaps the most widespread motivation for using economic evaluation is to provide a defensible, systematic and consistent way of responding to new, high-cost technologies. Economic evaluation has tended to focus on new technologies – especially pharmaceuticals – and rather more rarely on assessing the value for money of old technologies or services that provide non-therapeutic support or care. In part, this may be explained both by the rationale of decision makers and by pragmatic considerations: new technologies that have satisfied the requirements for licensing have an evidence base which is more amenable to economic evaluation than services that have never been subject to randomised controlled trials.

Demand management is clearly a key issue in fixed-budget health care systems that have to reconcile fixed resources to demand; however, demand management is arguably an even *more* pressing issue in demand-driven systems where unconstrained growth in health care spending is a cause for concern. This includes social insurance systems, such as in France and Germany. It also includes the use of economic evaluation in private-sector, demand-driven systems, where setting coverage limits for third-party funding provides a key means of avoiding moral hazard (Garber, 2001). Although it is more unusual for cost-effectiveness to be *explicitly* used to determine resource allocations in health care in the USA (Garber, 1994), examples of that can be found, as well as other means of containing costs. For example, the US Supreme Court in 2000 ruled that patients could not sue their health maintenance organisation (HMO) in federal court for giving doctors financial incentives to cut medical costs, Justice Souter noting that 'no HMO organisation could survive without some incentive connecting physician reward with treatment rationing' (Charatan, 2000). Oregon is well known internationally for its experiment with the use of cost-effectiveness to decide priorities for health care spending in its Medicaid programme – see Box 12.3.

Box 12.3 The Oregon Health Plan

Medicaid is a publicly funded programme which aims to deliver all medically necessary care to the US poor. In the late 1980s, the USA was faced with increasing demands for Medicaid coupled with cost-inflation. The inevitability of rationing prompted re-evaluation of the coverage provided by Medicaid in Oregon. This resulted in the Oregon Health Plan, the idea underpinning which is that, given a finite budget, an expansion of *who* is covered could only be achieved by a restricting *what* is covered. The Oregon Health Services Commission developed a systematic and explicit basis for deciding what health services should be included in, and which excluded from, the benefit package provided by Medicaid (Kitzhaber, 1993).

The method originally used was to assign all possible treatments into 'condition–treatment' pairs, informed by clinical judgements. Each pair was then assessed in terms of cost per QALY gained. The commission consulted the public extensively – meeting interest groups and communities, and generating population-specific health state valuations using methods similar to those described in Chapter 10, via a telephone survey. The output of these analyses was a prioritised list of over 700 condition–treatment pairs, effectively a giant league table (see Section 12.5). The intention was that the political process would determine the Medicaid budget, and pairs on the list would be funded down to the point at which the budget was exhausted; pairs below that are excluded from the benefit package.

Oregon's plan was hailed as a brave experiment in prioritisation. Oregon continues to make explicit use of a prioritised list, updated each year, as the basis for planning Medicaid coverage. The five top and five bottom items of their 2006 list were:

Line	Diagnosis	Treatment
1	Severe/moderate head injury: haematoma/ oedema with loss of consciousness	Medical and surgical treatment
2	Type I diabetes mellitus	Medical therapy
3	Peritonitis and retroperitoneal infections	Medical and surgical treatment
4	Acute glomerulonephritis: with lesion of rapidly progressive glomerulonephritis	Medical therapy including dialysis
5	Pneumothorax and haemothorax	Tube thoracostomy/thoracotomy, medical therapy
705	Mental disorders with no effective treatments or no treatment necessary	Evaluation
706	Neurological conditions with no effective treatments or no treatment necessary	Evaluation
707	Dental conditions (e.g. orthodontics)	Cosmetic dental services
708	Hepatorenal syndrome	Medical therapy
709	Spastic dysphonia	Medical therapy
710	Disorders of refraction and accommodation	Radial keratotomy

Source: http://egov.oregon.gov/DAS/OHPPR/HSC/docs/4-1-06_line_descriptions.txt

However, the Oregon experiment cannot be seen as a success for economic evaluation as a means of ranking health services; this was abandoned early on, before the scheme was approved or implemented. What went wrong?

The first prioritised list produced by the Commission in 1990 was widely criticised. Certainly there were aspects of the economic evaluations that could be criticised on technical or economic grounds. For example, costs were 'usual, customary and reasonable charges', that is prices, which may or may not reflect marginal cost, and do not reflect knock-on changes in resource use elsewhere in the health sector (savings) as a result of the intervention. More importantly, though, the resulting list included many priorities that seemed counterintuitive, appearing to favour minor treatments over life-saving ones (Hadorn, 1991). For example, treatment for thumb-sucking and acute headaches received higher rankings than treatment for AIDS or cystic fibrosis (Maynard and Bloor, 1998). Such was the controversy that the list based on cost-effectiveness was never submitted for the Federal Waiver required for its adoption. The commission fundamentally reconsidered the basis for its priorities, rejecting cost-effectiveness in favour of prioritisation principally with respect to five-year survival and improvement in symptoms, with priorities also determined by groups of services, and hand-adjustments to rankings. The prioritised list finally approved in 1994 was not based on ranking by cost-effectiveness.

In terms of its own objectives, the Oregon Health Plan has succeeded: by constraining the depth of coverage, the breadth of cover has been expanded so that all Oregonians below the poverty line can access the services on the list. This is clearly an important achievement. Oregon's experience demonstrates clearly, however, that the application of economic evaluation in social decision making is not just a technical exercise; nor are the issues in using economics to inform social choices merely technical in nature. By making explicit decisions on criteria other than cost-effectiveness, Oregon will be satisfying legitimate social goals; nevertheless, the package of care delivered by Medicaid will not be *efficient* (Tengs, 1996).

Perhaps more importantly, there is considerable use being made behind the scenes of economic evaluation to inform health care decisions in the US health care system. Garber (1994) describes the use of cost-effectiveness analysis to contain the costs of technology in the USA, arguing that economic evaluation can and does have a role in demand management not only by limiting coverage in insurance but also in Federal Food and Drug Administration (FDA) approval and in medical guidelines promulgated to doctors. Although the FDA has no mandate to incorporate cost considerations in its decisions, Garber notes that 'costs undoubtedly influence drug and device approval process' and that there is growing pressure to grant cost-effectiveness a larger and more explicit role because it eases decision making by doctors, hospitals and health care insurers.

(d) To Provide Payers with Bargaining Power in Health Care Markets

Garber (1994) notes that cost-effectiveness analysis is sometimes also used by US health care insurers to negotiate prices to be paid to health care providers. A similar example – but at the national level – is New Zealand's Pharmaceutical Management Agency Company (PHARMAC). PHARMAC uses economic evaluation principally to achieve the objective noted in (c). However, PHARMAC's role is not merely to make recommendations but also to purchase drugs for the country's health care system. PHARMAC therefore has considerable monopsony power. When technologies are assessed by it to have a cost-effectiveness ratio that is too high – presumably by reference to a threshold (see Section 12.6) – this can be used as a bargaining tool with industry to negotiate lower prices. PHARMAC has been manifestly successful in achieving reductions in New Zealand's drugs bill – although the absence of any pharmaceutical industry in that country is probably no coincidence! Maynard *et al.* (2004) argue that NICE should also be given similar budget-holding status, although the importance of the pharmaceutical industry in the UK economy makes it unlikely that such a strategy would ever be implemented.

Our focus in (a)–(d) has been on the use of economic evaluation techniques to inform decisions about the right mix of services to purchase. Other, *non*-evaluative methods of economic analysis are also occasionally used to inform *other* sorts of priorities and resource allocation decisions. For example, econometric models underpin the population-based funding formulae used in the UK (Department of Health, 2005). These are used to produce algorithms that determine how the total NHS budget is allocated between primary care trusts – the principal budget holders and purchasers of health care for local populations in England – where population size is weighted by a range of factors that act as proxies for health needs. Further, the tools developed to measure HRQOL (see Chapter 10) have also been used in New Zealand and Canada to decide clinical priorities for treatment by ranking individual patients on waiting lists in order of their need or capacity to benefit (Hadorn and Holmes, 1997; Derrett *et al.*, 2003). There is growing interest in the UK in using measures of HRQOL to manage the demand for secondary care generated by primary care providers, by incorporating them into referral guidelines for GPs.

12.2 WHO BUYS ECONOMIC EVALUATIONS? DOES IT MATTER?

The previous section lists the various rationales that might motivate decision makers' use of economic evaluation evidence. Given that decision makers *are* increasingly concerned with evidence on value for money, an obvious additional reason why economic evaluations are undertaken is that they are commissioned by stakeholders who have an interest in the provision of a good or service. Obvious stakeholders include the pharmaceutical industry, clinicians and patients.

That many economic evaluations are often commissioned by stakeholders who profit or otherwise benefit directly from the result may suggest that caution is required in the use of this evidence in decision making: 'He who pays the piper calls the tune'! We might expect industry-commissioned evaluations to be more likely to conclude that a technology is acceptable value for money than independent evidence (see Freemantle and Maynard, 1994, and the response by Jönsson, 1994). Miners *et al.* (2005) show exactly that, finding a statistically significant difference between cost-effectiveness ratios in evidence submitted to NICE by manufacturers and that by independent assessments, and in the expected direction. This is important, because as agencies such as NICE come under pressure to speed up their decision-making processes (see Box 12.1), it is generally achieved by forgoing independent evidence and relying to a greater extent on industry submissions.

Decision makers can respond to the issue of bias in a number of ways: at the simplest level, the incentives facing industry are entirely transparent, so *caveat emptor* applies to the use, in decision making, of evidence provided by industry. Further, decision makers have introduced increasingly strong directives about the methods required to be used in evidence to be submitted. This builds on a more general move initiated by academic health economists to make consistent the methods used in appraisal (Weinstein *et al.*, 1996; Drummond *et al.*, 2005) so that valid comparisons of value for money may be made across studies. The best-known examples of this include, in the USA, the Washington Panel (Gold *et al.*, 1996) and, in the UK, the work of Drummond and others (Drummond *et al.*, 2005). Further, decision makers in some health economies (England – in contrast to Scotland) commission their own, independent analysis, and the availability of that exerts some discipline on industry not to over-inflate benefit or under-estimate *CERs*. Recent moves to speed up the evaluation and to 'fast track' the decision process for new drugs in the UK involve a greater reliance on manufacturer-sponsored evidence, with the role of independent analysts being critically to review that evidence.

12.3 IS ECONOMIC EFFICIENCY ALL THAT MATTERS?

Economic evaluation is concerned with efficiency and indeed, depending on the exact methods selected, on specific views of efficiency (see Chapter 9). If, from a given budget, the objective is to maximise health improvement or, alternatively, to maximise welfare, then a resource allocation determined solely by evidence on cost-effectiveness or cost benefit analysis will achieve that. But that begs the question: is efficiency *all* that matters? Is it the only objective? What other considerations or criteria might be or are being used to guide resource allocation in the health sector?

12.3.1 Need

The most obvious contender for an alternative, systematic and explicit but non-economics approach to resource allocation is to decide priorities on the basis of need, defined by the presence of illness, or the burden of disease, rather than those with the greatest capacity to benefit or the greatest capacity for benefit per pound spent. Needs-based approaches are used in the allocation of public health system funds between regions in the UK and New Zealand. For example, as already noted, a population-based funding formula determines what share of the total health care budget each receives and this is driven largely by measures of population need.

However, perhaps the best-known example of priorities being influenced by measures of need is the Global Burden of Disease study (Lopez *et al.*, 2006), an extensive international set of studies which aimed to influence and inform priorities by generating data on the magnitude of health problems of various kinds in various populations. A major concern of the project is the development of measures that could capture the extent of problems with diseases and injuries in terms of both mortality and morbidity, and in a way that would facilitate comparison of the size of a given problem across disease areas and between countries. The principal measure developed was the disability-adjusted life year (DALY) (see Chapter 10). Measures of DALYs by disease area and by country are widely used by the World Bank and by WHO to inform priorities for health care in developing countries. Examples of the approach may also be found in developed countries; for example, in Bowie *et al.* (1997), who report these data for the south and west regions of England.

Economists are highly critical of priority setting based on burden of disease. Williams (1999, 2000) and Mooney and Wiseman (2000) argue that information on the size of the problem is irrelevant for priority setting unless it is accompanied by, or a precursor to, data on the effectiveness of interventions available for the treatment of each disease and on their costs. Williams (1999) sums up these arguments succinctly: 'What we need to know is what impact different *interventions* will have, not what impact different *diseases* have.' Given that position, Mooney and Wiseman (2000) argue that the use of burden of disease information in setting priorities 'is likely to lead to inefficient and inequitable resource use'. Thus, although 'giving health care to those who need it' seems a laudable goal, the outcome will be less improvement in health, overall, than is possible from the available budget; and, as Maynard (1996) has pointed out, such inefficiency is unethical since it means potential patients are deprived of care from which they could benefit. An example of the way in which burden of disease information can mislead decision making is provided in Box 12.4.

12.3.2 Equity

The efficient use of scarce health care resources, defined as the maximisation of health, is unlikely to be the sole objective of a society. For example, it may be that society is interested both in increasing health overall and in reducing inequalities in health between population subgroups. Society may be prepared to forgo some improvement in health in order to achieve fairness. But what is meant by equity? How it is to be measured? Exactly what sacrifices are we willing to make in its pursuit?

We discussed concepts of equity in the distribution of health care in Chapter 7. For example, one definition of fairness in health care that has been suggested is to achieve equality (or at least to reduce inequalities) in people's *lifetime* experience of health. This view is evident in Williams' (1997) idea of the 'fair innings': he suggests that there are strong normative grounds for resources to be transferred from the elderly, who have

Box 12.4 Needs and costs – and why obvious conclusions are sometimes wrong

In the same way that Bowie *et al.* (1997) report DALYs by disease area for England, evidence on the global burden of disease was generated in New Zealand in 1998. The New Zealand government was interested in using these data to help analyse its priorities for health care. Initial analysis suggested that a useful way of presenting the data was to show the percentage of total DALYs by disease area, represented by the shaded bars in the figure below. Because the vertical axis measures percentages, it is possible also to display the percentage of total health care spending in each disease area – this is represented by the lines.

The result is quite striking. Some areas (such as maternity) account for a high percentage of spending, but barely *any* morbidity and mortality. In contrast, other areas, such as cancers, account for large share of the ill health but receive a relatively small proportion of spending. *Prima facie*, the conclusion seems obvious: too much is being spent on maternity and too little on cancer. Spending should be reallocated between disease areas. Do you agree?

COSTS AND DALYS BY CLINICAL/DISEASE AREA IN NEW ZEALAND

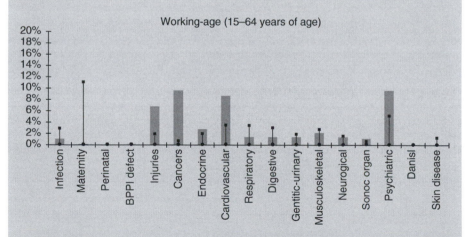

Source: Devlin and Hansen (2000). Reproduced with permission from the NZ Treasury.

Although the evidence seems compelling, this graph is misleading (Devlin and Hansen 2000). It shows a static picture of existing distributions of ill health and spending. What is unknown is (for example) how a given reduction in spending on maternity would increase morbidity and mortality in that clinical/disease area, compared to how an increase in spending by that same amount on cancer would decrease morbidity and mortality. The reason why morbidity and mortality in maternity is so low is likely to be related in at least some way to the resources devoted to it; how a reduction in spending would affect that cannot be discerned from these data. Similarly, although the spending on cancer seems too low relative to the DALYs in that area, it is not obvious from these data how an increase in spending would affect health. For example, although many new drugs are available for treating cancer, these tend to be relatively expensive and to produce relatively small gains in survival or quality of life. Spending more money on prevention, rather than cures, may be the best strategy, but changes to lifestyle and health behaviour are difficult to effect, and the health gains are produced far into the future and would not be evident on the current distribution of DALYs shown in the figure.

Data on *total* needs by disease area, even if accompanied by data on *total* costs, are, of themselves, of little relevance to priority setting. Costs and consequences are, we would argue as economists, always most usefully represented as *marginal* or incremental costs and effects.

already enjoyed their 'three score and ten', to the young. The focus of equity concerns could, however, alternatively or simultaneously be expressed in terms of wealth, income, geography, ethnicity or gender, rather than age; and equity could be construed in terms of fairness in *access* to health care, or *utilisation* of health care, rather than health *outcomes*.

One way of thinking about the efficiency–equity trade-off is that it exists only because of the approach selected to measure efficiency. If QALYs gained is used as the measure of benefit and cost per QALY gained is the measure of efficiency, then preferences about the *distribution* of the QALYs gained becomes a separate issue requiring separate analysis and consideration. Ideas about equity tend not to be built into the analysis so that, by default, cost–utility analysis (CUA) is utilitarian: 'a QALY is a QALY is a QALY', and no distinction is made about who obtains these health gains. Recently, Dolan *et al.* (2005) have provided empirical evidence which fundamentally questions this as a defensible basis for resource allocation. They contend that there is good evidence to suggest both that society has a diminishing marginal valuation for improvements and that society is not indifferent as to who gains them. In particular, there is evidence that the social value of health improvements is higher if the person has worse lifetime health prospects and if the person has dependants; there is also value attached to reducing inequalities in health.

Similarly, in CBA the focus is on weighing up benefits and costs, in monetary terms, based on Kaldor–Hicks compensation tests discussed in Chapter 8, which requires only the possibility of compensation and redistribution. CBA rarely includes explicit weights to address equity. If, however, decision makers could refer to a fully specified social welfare function, then decisions would address both the magnitude of net benefits and their distribution – and the maximisation of social welfare, subject to resource constraints, would incorporate equity considerations, as reflected in the characteristics and properties of the social welfare function, directly into the analysis. Under these circumstances, there is no trade-off between efficiency and equity.

12.3.3 Process-of-Care Considerations

In CUA, the benefits of health care are restricted to improvements in length and quality of life. A problem with this approach is that it is neutral to, or excludes from consideration, characteristics of health care products, services or delivery modes that may, in themselves be the subject of patients' preferences, independently of their effects on health. Patients may, for example, prefer health care services that respect privacy and autonomy, that preserve their dignity, that fully inform them of their options, that allow them at least some choice, that avoid unnecessary waiting and delays, that are provided by friendly health care professionals, that minimise time away from dependents, and so on. None of these characteristics will be reflected in a CUA, other than where they have a measurable effect on survival and quality of life.

There are three ways in which this can be justified. First, there may be a trade-off between better process of care and increased health, so that if resources are devoted to improved process, this reduces the amount that can be devoted to health improvement. It is possible that people's preferences are so strongly in favour of health that improved process of care would have to be enormously important to outweigh improved outcomes of care – their preferences may be what is called *lexicographic*. As an extreme example, it is likely that few would be willing to trade off even a few cancer cures for an improvement in the quality of hospital food – assuming that the latter has no impact on health.

Secondly, it may be that the trade-off is small or even non-existent but that the utility from health care is very large compared to that from process of care. Since process of care improvements may be even harder to quantify than health gain, it may be justifiable to ignore them. The problem with this is that the balance of importance between process and outcome will differ between types of health care, and indeed some health care services, such as cosmetic care and fertility services, may have very little health output at all. Of course, this may not matter if the purpose of the health service is to improve health rather than to just provide health care.

Thirdly, it may be that it is simply a mistake to consider these two aspects together, and that they should be considered at different levels of decision making. For example, the question of *what* should be provided by health services, and the priority that different types of care should have, should be decided on the basis of health, since that is the objective of a health service. However, the question of *how* it should be provided could take into account these wider process attributes. Ultimately, of course, these have to be reconciled if there is indeed a potential trade-off between them, but that is arguably yet again a different level of decision making.

The latter, even though it is really just a way of denying or concealing the trade-off, is probably the most widespread response. For example, in England and Wales, NICE makes decisions about the availability of treatments mainly on the basis of health improvements, but a key policy goal (see Box 2.2 in Chapter 2) is to improve the choices available to NHS patients. The opportunity cost of offering choice of location and timing of care in terms of reduced availability of care is nowhere explicitly considered.

12.3.4 Ethical Imperatives

In addition to the considerations set out above, it has been argued that even the most carefully considered health care prioritisation process will buckle when confronted with certain ethical imperatives. For example, Hadorn (1991) argued that the so-called 'rule of rescue' will almost inevitably dominate cost-effectiveness in decision making. The *CER* of an intervention may be unfavourable, but if an identified life is at stake, and if survival depends on treatment, then survival will override all other factors, including the duration of survival, quality of life, and cost-effectiveness. Although compelling, the rule of rescue does not provide a systematic or fully articulated ethical framework for understanding choices. Is it equally important in cases where a life is saved for 20 years, 20 days, 20 minutes or 20 seconds? It seems implausible that there is no limit to the preparedness to devote resources to rescuing life – especially when the life that is saved may be of unacceptably poor quality. McKie and Richardson (2003) argued that the rule can be defended on utilitarian grounds, to the extent that rescues provide value by reinforcing people's beliefs that they live in a community that values life highly. However, they also point out that the rule discriminates in favour of saving lives where those lives belong to identifiable people, but in effect discriminates against lives that are saved by reducing a population's risk of death.

Ethical issues might be relevant in other ways. For example, instances of differential access to treatment for obese and non-obese people, and between smokers and non-smokers for smoking-related diseases, are becoming more common – usually on the grounds of differences in the probability of success of treatment but occasionally, one suspects, influenced by notions of individual culpability and desert. Further, decisions about the availability of assisted death, abortion, infertility treatments, and the selection of genetic characteristics in foetuses – among other things – may consider cost-effectiveness, but it is unlikely to be the only, or even the principal, consideration in deciding what health services to make available.

12.4 HOW IS ECONOMIC EVALUATION USED TO MAKE DECISIONS IN PRACTICE?

Consider the following: a decision maker is presented with information on a new health care intervention. A CUA demonstrates that, compared to the treatment widely used at present, the new treatment saves money *and* results in better health outcomes; that is, the new treatment dominates the one that is currently used. The decision maker has all the information required, from this one piece of analysis, in order to recommend in favour of the new treatment.

That scenario is relatively rare. Most new technologies improve health, but at additional cost. In such cases, whether the decision makers deems the technology to be good value for money or not depends on a comparison of the cost per QALY gained against something else. That something else may be the cost per QALY gained for other treatments that are competing for resources; or it may be some 'benchmark' cost per QALY that is considered to be the cut-off for what is acceptable to society – the ceiling ratio or cost-effectiveness threshold. Either way, decisions rely on comparisons. What should these comparators be – and how are they selected? There are three main approaches to making such comparisons in decision making using economic evaluation evidence. They are: cost-effectiveness league tables; programme budgeting and marginal analysis (PBMA); and cost-effectiveness thresholds.

12.5 COST-EFFECTIVENESS LEAGUE TABLES

One approach which is often used to help decision makers put the results of an economic evaluation into context is to show the incremental cost per QALY gained alongside results from other evaluations of other interventions. Ranking these from lowest cost per QALY gained to highest cost per QALY gained creates a 'league table' of value for money – for an early example, see Williams (1985).

Table 12.1 reproduces the cost-effectiveness league table reported by Maynard (1991) for the UK; Table 12.2 shows a cost-effectiveness league table for the USA, based on information reported in Garber and Phelps (1997). Each line in the league table shows

Table 12.1 UK example of a cost-effectiveness league table

Health care intervention	Cost per QALY gained UK£ (1990)
Cholesterol testing and diet therapy only (all adults aged 40–69 years)	220
Neurosurgical intervention for head injury	240
General practitioner advice to stop smoking	270
Neurosurgical intervention for subarachnoid haemorrhage	490
Antihypertensive therapy to prevent stroke (ages 45–64 years)	940
Pacemaker installation	1 100
Hip replacement	1 140
Valve replacement for aortic stenosis	1 180
Cholesterol testing and treatment	1 480
CABG (left main vessel, severe angina)	2 090
Kidney transplantation	4 710
Breast cancer screening	5 780
Heart transplantation	7 840
Cholesterol testing and treatment of all adults 25–39 years	14 150
Home haemodialysis	17 260
CABG (one-vessel disease; moderate angina)	18 830
Continuous ambulatory peritoneal dialysis	19 870
Hospital haemodialysis	21 970
Erythropoietin treatment for anaemia in dialysis patients	54 380
Neurosurgical intervention for malignant intracranial tumours	107 780
Erythropoietin treatment for anaemia in dialysis patients (assuming no increase in survival)	126 290

Reproduced from Maynard, A. (1991) Developing the health care market. *The Economic Journal*, **101**, 1277–1286, Blackwell Publishing.

the *CER* produced for a given health care product or service by a cost-effectiveness study. Many of the *CERs* reported in these tables will have been superseded by medical innovations, or more up-to-date economic appraisals – and of course they are reported in terms of 1990 pounds and 1993 dollars respectively, so cannot be taken to represent the costs today in each country. Nevertheless, these provide good examples of the kind of side-by-side comparisons of economic evaluation results that are used within each country in order to give decision makers some idea of how the results of a given economic evaluation compare with those for other treatments.

Unfortunately, there are many problems with the use of league tables. First, problems arise from the lack of consistency in the methods used by each of the research teams who produced each reported *CER*. Differences in method include: what perspective is taken in estimating costs; what discount rate was used, and whether it was applied equally to costs and QALYs; what instrument was used to measure HRQOL; what and whose valuations were used to estimate QALYs; whether results are reported as average

Table 12.2 US example of a cost-effectiveness league table

Health care intervention	Cost per QALY gained US$ (1993)
Low-dose lovastatin for high cholesterol: male heart attack survivors, aged 55–64 years, cholesterol >250	2 158
Low-dose lovastatin for high cholesterol: male heart attack survivors, aged 55–64 years, cholesterol <250	2 293
Physician advice about smoking cessation, 1% quit rate, males aged 45–50 years	3 777
CABG, left main coronary artery disease	8 768
Neonatal intensive care units: infants 1000–1500 grams	10 927
Pap smear starting at age 20 years, continuing to age 74 years, every 3 years, compared to no screening	24 011
Hypertension screening, 40-year-old males	27 519
Breast cancer screening, annual examination and mammography, females 55–65 years	41 008
Hypertension screening, 40-year-old females	42 222
Neonatal intensive care units: infants 500–999 grams	77 161
CABG, single vessel disease with moderate angina	88 087
Exercise electrocardiogram as a screening test, 40-year-old males	124 374
Exercise electrocardiogram as a screening test, 40-year-old females	335 217
Low-dose lovastatin for high cholesterol: female non-smokers	2 023 440

Reprinted from Garber, A.M. and Phelps, C.E. (1997) Economic foundations of cost-effectiveness analysis. *Journal of Health Economics*, **16** (1), 1–31 ©1997, with permission from Elsevier.

or incremental cost-effectiveness ratios, and so on. Differences in any of these will render non-comparable the *CERs* produced from various economic evaluation studies. This issue is particularly important where league tables comprise results from a range of studies, as is the case in both Tables 12.1 and 12.2. However, if cost-effectiveness analysis is undertaken with the express purpose of facilitating between-treatment comparisons, using standardised methodologies, then this criticism can be overcome. This was attempted by the Oregon Health Services Commission – see Box 12.3. Effectively, Oregon commissioned bespoke economic evaluations of all health care services provided under the auspices of Medicaid, and used this to construct a comprehensive league table or prioritised list.

Secondly, the use of league tables assumes that the original context of the study in each case is transferable to the specific context within which decisions are currently being made (Gerard and Mooney, 1993). There may be factors specific to each decision-making context which limit the appropriateness of generalising from league table results.

Thirdly, the reporting of economic evaluation results as a single CER in leagues tables suggests a degree of certainty over results, and therefore rankings between health care services, that may be quite misleading; the confidence intervals around each *CER* may alter, or considerably blur, the rankings apparent between them.

Fourthly, league tables treat each line as being an independent alternative from the others, so that interactions between costs and benefits of programmes are not addressed.

Finally, although league tables aim to help the decision maker to consider cost-effectiveness results in context, it is not entirely clear how decision makers are intended to use the information. For example, should they recommend in favour of funding a therapy if there are treatments farther down the league table, that is treatments that are *less* cost effective, that have already been funded? What if previous decisions were made without access to evidence? Or if a treatment was funded despite being poor value for money, because of *other* characteristics or criteria?

How, then, do decision makers *actually* use these league tables to inform their decisions? Garber and Phelps (1997) suggest that 'most practitioners of cost effectiveness analysis discard interventions with cost effectiveness values at the bottom range of a table such as this one, and conclude that interventions in the realm of $50 000 per QALY are "OK" but that more expensive technologies become more and more "out of bounds"; the $50 000 criterion is arbitrary and owes more to being a round number than to being a well-formulated justification for a specific dollar value'. This provides a rather sobering prospect for economists; despite the development of ever more sophisticated means of estimating and reporting cost-effectiveness, the results are being used in a fairly crude way, where they are being used at all. Garber and Phelps (1997) conclude that the league table approach to comparisons of *CERs*, although common, 'provides little guidance regarding the optimal cost-effectiveness ratio – that is, the willingness to pay for a health effect'.

Instead of comparing the *CERs* from various studies with each other, if decision makers know what value society placed on each QALY gained, this could serve as the benchmark for decision makers. If the cost per QALY gained of any given therapy is higher than the societal value per QALY, the therapy should be rejected. We return to this idea of a societal cost-effectiveness 'threshold' in Section 12.6.

12.6 PROGRAMME BUDGETING AND MARGINAL ANALYSIS

Programme budgeting and marginal analysis (PBMA) is a pragmatic approach to resource allocation which has become widely used internationally. It is intended as a planning tool for rationing resources in the context of the public sector, in the absence of a market that would do that. Its aim is to make manageable the impossible remit of a central planner. PBMA comprises two distinct elements: Programme budgeting (PB) and marginal analysis (MA).

12.6.1 Programme Budgeting

Programme budgeting (PB) refers to a form of output-based budgeting, which focuses the budgetary process on the outputs of health services (Craig *et al.*, 1995). Costs are linked to the production of health outputs, rather than to the purchase of health care inputs as in standard accounting systems. The PB part of PBMA therefore involves assigning costs to programmes, defined in terms of the types of output produced, so that current resource allocations are described. PB focuses the budgetary process on the *output* of the health service rather than the inputs required to produce that output. Figure 12.1 shows a typical programme budget approach, taken from a study in the north of England (Miller *et al.*, 1997). It shows the programmes – defined by disease categories – and the current expenditure in each. PB makes clear what budgets are

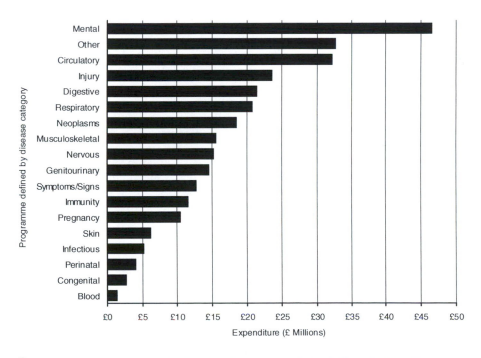

Figure 12.1 Programme budget for Newcastle and North Tyneside Health Authority (UK) in 1995. Reproduced by permission of Newcastle NHS.

currently being used *for*, rather than simply the services purchased, so giving a clearer indication of the different needs that a purchaser is trying to meet.

PB may be undertaken at the macro level, looking at the whole of expenditure, divided into large programmes, for example disease groups, or at the micro level, looking at expenditure within these programmes, for example different care settings for a particular disease group. The latter involves a finer level of detail of information about services.

Once programme budgets have been established, economic evaluation of health service provision within those programme budgets follows naturally as a means of extracting maximum gains in programme goals from the budget allocated to those goals. This is the marginal analysis (MA) element.

12.6.2 Marginal Analysis

Marginal analysis (MA) is the appraisal of the added benefits and added costs of a proposed investment (or the lost benefits and lower costs of a proposed disinvestment). MA establishes whether the current expenditure pattern is appropriate and how it might be changed to increase health gain. Its basis is not a comparison of the costs and benefits of all uses of resources but, more pragmatically, an evaluation *at the margin* of different ways of using resources. MA can take place within programmes or between programmes. The cost and benefit or effectiveness implications of shifting resources within programmes or from one programme to another can be examined, with the goal of maximising health gain within available resources.

The MA part really, therefore, simply refers to the application of standard approaches to economic evaluation and could include any of the approaches described in Chapter 10. Examples of PBMA can be found in decision-making processes at the national level (for example, Ashton *et al.*, 2000) and at the local level (for example, Miller *et al.*, 1997) across a variety of countries; Mitton and Donaldson (2001) provide a comprehensive review of international experience in using PBMA.

12.7 COST-EFFECTIVENESS THRESHOLDS

CUA and CEA are the most commonly used methods in the economic evaluation of health care – yet, as we have already noted, whether the decision maker deems the technology to be good value for money depends on a comparison of the *CERs* against some 'benchmark' *CER* – the ceiling ratio or cost-effectiveness threshold – representing society's willingness to pay for a unit of health improvement.

Figure 12.2 The cost-effectiveness threshold as a point. Source: Devlin and Parkin (2004) © 2004 John Wiley & Sons Limited. Reproduced with permission.

This notion of a single, optimal cost-effectiveness threshold is represented in Figure 12.2. The vertical axis shows the probability of rejection, from 0 to 1, and the cost per QALY gained is shown on the horizontal axis. If we can confidently identify society's marginal valuation of a QALY, the probability of rejecting a treatment is 0 at any cost per QALY gained below the threshold, and 1 above it.

In practice, the real world is infinitely more complicated. Imperfections in information, political processes and decision making may make it difficult to infer much, in any precise way, about society's valuation of a QALY from past health care decisions. Nevertheless, partly on the basis of observed decisions, NICE in the UK is widely considered to have a threshold of UK£30 000, just as New Zealand is believed to have a threshold around NZ$20 000 and the USA a threshold of US$50 000. The basis for such thresholds seems to be entirely arbitrary, and they are difficult to link, either by assertion or by evidence, to society's valuation of health gain. This is an important concern, given their role in decision making. For example, Williams (2004) argues that the shadow price – or implicit value – of a QALY, based on the NHS budget, is much lower than £30 000, and that a threshold of £18 000, equivalent to the average national income per person, would be more reasonable. Neither £18 000 or £30 000 is easy to defend; yet clearly decisions based on the latter would be very different from decisions based on the former! In the UK, research is underway to establish the marginal value of a QALY, drawing on the willingness to pay methods described in Chapter 10.

However, even if we knew with certainty the value society places on a QALY, cost-effectiveness is unlikely to be the only criterion influencing decisions. For example,

Figure 12.3 The cost-effectiveness threshold as a range, reflecting trade-offs against efficiency. Source: Devlin and Parkin (2004) © 2004 John Wiley & Sons Limited. Reproduced with permission.

Rawlins and Culyer (2004) describe the normative basis of NICE's decisions and state that other criteria it considers include wider social costs and benefits, such as the effects of treatment on productivity and patients' ability to return to work; the innovative nature of the treatment; and consistency with its previous judgements. They rule out other criteria, such as affordability; differential treatment on the grounds of orphan drug status; and the characteristics of those gaining QALYs, including age, other than where it is an indicator of risk or benefit. In New Zealand, the prioritisation frame-work, which used CUA, also included considerations of equity, acceptability and Treaty of Waitangi obligations (an agreement of 1840 between the British Crown and the indigenous people of New Zealand), in addition to cost-effectiveness (Ashton *et al.*, 2000). If cost-effectiveness is not all that matters, this suggests that decision makers are prepared to sacrifice some efficiency in the pursuit of these other desired outcomes. This suggests that there is no single cost-effectiveness threshold, but rather a lower and upper threshold, as shown in Figure 12.3. Within the range between the two, cost-effectiveness is being traded off against other objectives.

This seems broadly consistent with NICE's description of its use of cost-effectiveness (Rawlins and Culyer, 2004):

> NICE would be unlikely to reject a technology with a ratio in the range of £5000–
> £15 000/QALY solely on the grounds of cost-ineffectiveness but would need special reasons
> for accepting technologies with ratios over £25 000–£35 000/QALY as cost effective.

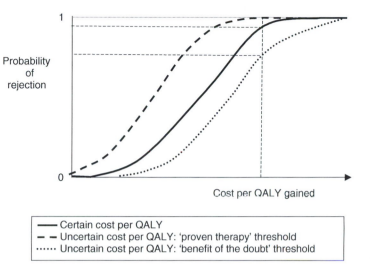

Figure 12.4 The cost-effectiveness threshold under uncertainty. Source: Devlin and Parkin (2004). © 2004 John Wiley & Sons Limited. Reproduced with permission.

Even if we knew the societal value of a QALY and had access to clearly articulated statements about what other criteria are considered, and the tradeoffs between them considered to be acceptable, a complicating factor is that there is uncertainty regarding the *CERs*; decision makers' response to uncertainty will therefore be important in understanding the way evidence on cost-effectiveness is used in decisions. For example, in Figure 12.4, the probability of rejection for any given *CER*, with which there is associated uncertainty, will depend on whether the decision maker is risk averse (prefers proven therapies) or a risk lover (prepared to give the benefit of the doubt). NICE has stated that its decisions take into account the degree of uncertainty surrounding estimates of cost-effectiveness, although it has not stated how it is taken into account.

Finally, another complicating factor is that the decision response to a given *CER* may depend on whether the decision is for a new or a currently used therapy – that is, whether the decision involves investing in a new technology or disinvesting in an old one. O'Brien *et al.* (2002) provide evidence that the willingness-to-accept (WTA) values for giving up QALYs by reducing or removing existing health services, may be different from the willingness to pay (WTP) to obtain QALYs from new services. If this is the case, this suggests the probability of rejection is lower at every incremental cost-effectiveness ratio (ICER) for extant as opposed to new therapies, as shown in Figure 12.5.

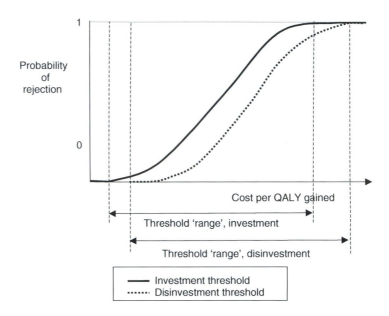

○ Figure 12.5 The cost-effectiveness threshold for investments and disinvestments. Source: Devlin and Parkin (2004). © 2004 John Wiley & Sons Limited. Reproduced with permission.

The systematic decision-making processes of government bodies such as NICE and Australia's Pharmaceutical Benefits Advisory Committee (PBAC) makes it possible to examine some of these issues empirically. For example, George *et al.* (2001) constructed a league table from PBAC decisions, and tested for statistically significant differences between the CERs of therapies accepted and rejected, suggesting that the PBAC 'has been broadly consistent with the use of economic efficiency as a criterion for decision making'. They could not establish a single threshold, but found evidence that the PBAC appears to have been unlikely to recommend in favour of a drug if the ICER exceeded AU$76 000 (1998/1999 values) and was unlikely to reject a drug for which the ICER was less than AU$42 000. These results are suggestive of the sort of threshold described in Figure 12.3, with the probability of rejection increasing as the ICER increases but factors other than cost-effectiveness being considered.

Devlin and Parkin (2004) similarly constructed a league table of NICE decisions, but used logistic regression techniques to model the effect of cost-effectiveness and other factors on the probability of a recommendation for or against use. Their results suggest that NICE decisions could be predicted on the basis of cost-effectiveness, uncertainty, burden of disease, and whether or not the therapy was the only treatment available for the condition. Decisions appeared to be neutral to the budget impact, that is the net effect on NHS costs if the therapy was accepted. Dakin *et al.* (2006) used similar techniques, but instead of reporting each decision as a yes/no, three decision outcomes were considered: recommended for, recommended against, and recommended for restricted use. Their results suggest that the quantity and quality of clinical evidence has a distinctive role in the decision-making process independent of evidence on cost-effectiveness. Cost-effectiveness evidence seems to explain decisions to recommend for or against a therapy; whereas clinical evidence is the more important consideration in decisions to recommend restricted or unrestricted use.

12.8 EVALUATING ECONOMIC EVALUATION

Our focus in this chapter has been on the use of economic evaluation in countries or contexts where it has been adopted as an integral part of systematic decision-making processes about health technologies and health care resource allocation at the national or state-wide level. Because these decision-making processes are well documented, it facilitates consideration of their strengths and weaknesses.

However, and notwithstanding the increase in use of economic evaluation, there is still considerable scope for extending its use in decision making in health care. von der Schulenburg (2000) conducted a survey of decision makers in Austria, France, Finland, The Netherlands, Norway, Portugal, Spain and the UK which revealed that only one-third said they considered the results of a health economics study when making a decision. The authors suggested that an important factor hindering greater use was lack of knowledge about the techniques of economic evaluation. Similarly, the work of Garber (1994) and others in the USA suggests considerable scope for improving efficiency in the US health care system by use of economic evaluation. We commenced this book by arguing that health care is an economic good. Given that this the case, and the importance of health both to individuals and to societies, economic analysis offers a powerful – and still largely untapped – means of helping decision makers ensure that health care resources have the greatest impact possible.

It is also clear from our discussion of decision making in health care that there is some degree of mismatch between the science of evaluation and the art of decision making. The advances in economic evaluation during the last decade have occurred in the development of statistical and modelling techniques. Exciting developments in the methods and tools of economic evaluation have not been matched by development of decision-making processes they seek to support. For example, the use of cost-effectiveness evidence relies ultimately on at least some notion of the value society places on health gain; yet, despite two decades of research applying CUA, research on the value of a QALY is only in its infancy. Further, as we noted in Chapter 11, although cost-effectiveness acceptability curves have now become the gold-standard for handling and reporting uncertainty in economic evaluation, to our knowledge there has been no research to examine the way in which decision makers actually interpret and use such evidence, or whether or not they find it helpful and informative.

Still further, although cost-effectiveness may be considered important, it is not the only thing that matters to decision makers. The incorporation of equity issues into evaluation, via the development and use of explicit weights, is feasible and could strengthen the normative legitimacy of evaluation; but research on this issue has yet to have an impact on the practice of economic evaluation. We have been unable to find a single example of a published CUA which uses weights to address distributional issues.

Finally, the methods of economic evaluation have tended to assume that the methods for priority setting should be independent of the financing system. However, clearly decisions about what health services are prioritised interacts with the financing regime; Hauck *et al.* (2004) argued that 'the rules for setting priorities may vary legitimately between systems with different approaches to the financing of health care'. The interaction between the assessment of value for money and alternative means of raising revenue and sharing costs remains undeveloped. There remains considerable scope to improve the methods of evaluation, to develop decision-aids and to strengthen decision processes – and ultimately, therefore, to improve outcomes.

There are those, of course, who would argue that priorities cannot or should not be set in an explicit, rational manner, and that rather than seeking technical solutions it would be better to 'muddle along' (see, for example Mechanic, 1997) by making implicit judgements. Further, and as we have noted at various points throughout this chapter, the evidence generated from economic evaluation may not be ideal and may not fully address all the issues of relevance to decision makers, and it may be unclear exactly how it should be used to make a decision. However, as Dowie (1995) points out, many of the criticisms of explicit priority setting focus on problems with the use of CUA compared to some unspecified theoretical ideal method of deciding on the resource allocation. For example, he argues that, notwithstanding the problems and limitations associated with cost-effectiveness league tables, it is likely that simply making this information available will in itself improve decision making, compared to the decisions that would be made if that information were not available.

Ultimately, resource allocation decisions cannot be avoided. Therefore, the relevant question – indeed the *key* issue – is whether the use of economic evaluation, even in an imperfect way, leads to better decisions than those that would have been made otherwise.

SUMMARY

1. Economic evaluation is used in health care generally for one or more of the following reasons: to maximise the benefits possible from health care spending; to overcome regional variations in access (for example, 'postcode prescribing'); to contain costs/manage demand; and to provide bargaining power with suppliers of health care products in order to keep prices down.

2. Economic evaluations are commissioned by stakeholders who have an interest in the provision of a good or service. Obvious stakeholders include the pharmaceutical industry; clinicians; and patients. There is evidence that the type of stakeholder may affect the outcome of the economic analysis.

3. There are factors other than cost-effectiveness that might legitimately or illegitimately be used in deciding whether to provide a particular health care programme. Other considerations include: the need for health care (for example, measured using DALYs); equity; process of care; and ethical imperatives, such as the rule of rescue. Needs-based priority setting can be criticised on the grounds that it does not account for the impact that different interventions will have.

4. Economic evaluation can be used in a variety of ways in practice as an aid to decision making. The three main approaches are cost-effectiveness league tables; programme budgeting and marginal analysis (PBMA); and cost-effectiveness thresholds.

5. Cost-effectiveness league tables involve ranking programmes from the lowest cost per QALY gained to the highest cost per QALY gained. There are many problems associated with the construction of league tables. The main one is the lack of consistency in the methods used to compute the ICERs of the different interventions compiled in the table.

6. PBMA is a pragmatic approach to resource allocation which has become widely used internationally. PB involves assigning costs to programmes, defined in terms of the types of output produced, so that current resource allocations are described. MA refers to the application of standard approaches to economic evaluation.

7. Cost-effectiveness thresholds can be used in decision making, reflecting the maximum amount of money that the decision maker is willing to pay for an additional QALY, for example. The cost-effectiveness threshold may be a point estimate, with a binary decision to accept or reject an intervention. It may also be represented by a range of values if there are criteria other than cost-effectiveness that are important. The threshold may also include in it consideration of the uncertainty surrounding the value of the ICER,

and that the decision to accept or reject an intervention might depend on whether the decision is for a new versus a currently used therapy.

8. While there has in recent years been an increase in use of economic evaluation, there is still considerable scope for extending its use in decision making in health care. Resource allocation decisions cannot be avoided. Therefore, the key issue is whether the use of economic evaluation, even in an imperfect way, leads to better decisions than those that would have been made otherwise.

References

Abasolo, I., Manning R. and Jones, A. (2001) Equity in utilization of and access to public-sector GPs in Spain. *Applied Economics*, **33**, 349–364.

Aronson, J., Johnson, P. and Lambert, P. (1994) Redistributive effect and unequal tax treatment. *Economic Journal*, **104**, 262–270.

Arrow, K.J. (1951) *Social Choice and Individual Values*. New York: Wiley.

Arrow, K.J. (1963) Uncertainty and the welfare economics of medical care. *The American Economic Review*, **53**, 941–973.

Arrow, K.J. (1972) *General economic equilibrium: purpose, analytic techniques, collective choice*. Nobel memorial lecture, December 12. http://nobelprize.org/nobel_prizes/economics/laureates/1972/arrow-lecture.pdf (accessed 8 December 2006).

Ashton, T. and Press, D. (1997) Market concentration in secondary health services under a purchaser-provider split: the New Zealand experience. *Health Economics*, **6**, 43–56.

Ashton, T., Devlin, N. and Cumming, J. (2000) Priority setting in New Zealand – translating principles into practice. *Journal of Health Services Policy and Research*, **5** (3), 170–175.

ABPI: Association of the British Pharmaceutical Industry (2006) www.abpi.org.uk (accessed 23 September 2006).

Baker, C., Messmer, P., Gyurko, D. *et al.* (2000) Hospital ownership, performance, and outcomes: assessing the state-of-the-science. *Journal of Nursing Administration*, **30**, 227–240.

Barr, N. (1987) *The Economics of the Welfare State*. Oxford: Oxford University Press.

Becker, G.S. (1964) *Human Capital*. New York: Columbia University Press for the National Bureau of Economic Research.

Becker, G.S. (1965) A theory of the allocation of time. *The Economic Journal*, **75**, 493–517.

Becker, G.S and Murphy, K.M. (1988) A theory of rational addiction. *The Journal of Political Economy*, **96**, 675–700.

Beech, R., Rudd, A.G., Tilling, K. and Wolfe, C.D.A. (1999) Economic consequences of early inpatient discharge to community-based rehabilitation for stroke in an inner-London teaching hospital. *Stroke*, **30**, 729–735.

Bentham, J. (1780) An introduction to the principles of morals and legislation. In Burns, J.H. and Hart, L.H.A. (1970) *Collected Works of Jeremy Bentham*. London: Athlone Press.

Bergner, M., Bobbitt, R.A., Carter, W.B. and Gilson, B.S. (1981) The Sickness Impact Profile: development and final revision of a health status measure. *Medical Care*, **19**, 787–805.

Besley, T., Hall, J. and Preston, I. (1999) The demand for private health insurance: do waiting lists matter? *Journal of Public Economics*, **72**, 155–181.

Bhatia, M.R. and Fox-Rushby, J.A. (2003) Validity of willingness to pay: hypothetical versus actual payment. *Applied Economics Letters*, **10**, 737–740.

Birch, S. and Donaldson, C. (2003) Valuing the benefits and costs in health care programmes: where's the extra in extra-welfarism. *Social Science and Medicine*, **56**, 1121–1133.

Black, W.C. (1990) The cost-effectiveness plane: a graphic representation of cost-effectiveness. *Medical Decision Making*, **10**, 212–215.

Blendon, R., Schoen, C., DesRoches *et al.* (2003) Common concerns amid diverse systems: health care experiences in five countries. *Health Affairs*, **22**, 106–121.

Blomqvist, A. and Carter, R.A.L. (1997) Is health care really a luxury? *Journal of Health Economics*, **16**, 207–229.

Bloom, N. and van Reenen, J. (1998) Regulating drug prices: where do we go from here? *Fiscal Studies*, **19**, 321–342.

Bloor, K. and Maynard, A. (1993) Cost-effective prescribing of pharmaceuticals: the search for the holy grail? In Drummond, M. and Maynard, A. (eds), *Purchasing and Providing Cost-Effective Health Care*. London: Churchill-Livingstone.

Boadway, R. and Bruce, N. (1984) *Welfare Economics*. Oxford: Blackwell.

Bowie, C., Beck, S., Bevan, G. *et al.* (1997) Estimating the burden of disease in an English region. *Journal of Public Health Medicine*, **19**, 87–92.

Bradshaw, J.R. (1972) A taxonomy of social need. In McLachlan, G. (ed.), *Problems and Progress in Medical Care: Essays on Current Research*. Oxford: Nuffield Provincial Hospital Trust.

Brazier, J., Akehurst, R., Brennan, A. *et al.* (2005) Should patients have a greater role in valuing health states? *Applied Health Economics and Health Policy*, **4**, 201–208.

Brook, R.H., Ware, J.E., Davies-Avery, A. *et al.* (1979) Overview of adult health status measures fielded in Rand's health insurance study. *Medical Care*, **17**, 1–131.

Brooks, R. (1996) Euroqol: the current state of play. *Health Policy*, **37**, 53–72.

Brouwer, W., Niesson, L., Postma, M. and Rutten, F. (2006a) Need for differential discounting of costs and health effects in cost effectiveness analysis. *British Medical Journal*, **331**, 446–448.

Brouwer, W.B., van Exel, N., Baltussen, R. and Rutten, F. (2006b) A dollar is a dollar is a dollar – or is it? *Value in Health*, **9** (5), 341–347.

Buchmueller, T. and DiNardo, J. (2002) Did community rating induce an adverse selection death spiral? Evidence from New York, Pennsylvania and Connecticut. *American Economic Review*, **92**, 280–294.

Buckingham, K. (1993) A note on HYE (Healthy Years Equivalent) *Journal of Health Economics*, **11**, 301–309.

Buckingham, K. and Devlin, N. (2006) A theoretical foundation for time trade off valuations of health. *Health Economics*, **15**, 1149–1154.

Burge, P., Devlin, N., Appleby, J. *et al.* (2005) Do patients always prefer quicker treatment? A discrete choice experiment of patients' preferences in the London Patient Choice Project. *Applied Health Economics and Health Policy*, **3**, 183–194.

Busino, G. (1987) Pareto, Vilfredo. In *The New Palgrave Dictionary of Economics*, vol. 3. London: Palgrave.

Buxton M.J., Drummond, M.F., van Hout, B. *et al.* (1997) Modelling in economic evaluation: an unavoidable fact of life. *Health Economics*, **6**, 217–227.

Byford, S. and Raftery, J. (1998) Perspectives in economic evaluation. *British Medical Journal*, **316**, 1529–1530.

Charatan, F. (2000) US Supreme Court bans federal law suits against health maintenance organisations. *British Medical Journal*, **320**, 1688.

Chote, R., Emmerson, C., Frayne, C. and Love, S. (2004) Challenges for the 2004 Spending Review. *Briefing Note No.50*. London: Institute for Fiscal Studies.

Collège des Économistes de la Santé (2004) *French guidelines for the economic evaluation of health care technologies.* www.ces-asso.org (accessed 9 December 2006).

Cooper, M.H. (1975) *Rationing Health Care.* London: Croom Helm.

Cooper, M.H. and Culyer, A.J. (1968) *The Price of Blood.* London: Institute of Economic Affairs.

Craig, N., Parkin, D. and Gerard, K. (1995) Clearing the fog on the Tyne: programme budgeting in Newcastle and North Tyneside Health Authority. *Health Policy*, 33, 107–125.

Culyer, A.J. (1971) Merit goods and the welfare economics of coercion. *Public Finance*, 26, 546–572.

Culyer, A.J. (1976) *Need and the National Health Service.* Oxford: Martin Robertson.

Culyer, A.J. (1983) *The Political Economy of Social Polity.* Oxford: Martin Robertson.

Culyer, A.J. (1989) The normative economics of health care finance and provision *Oxford Review of Economic Policy*, 5, 34–68.

Culyer, A.J. (1991) The normative economics of health care finance and provision. In McGuire, A., Fenn, P. and Mayhew, K. (eds), *Providing Health Care.* Oxford: Oxford University Press.

Culyer, A.J. and Wagstaff, A. (1993) QALYs versus HYEs. *Journal of Health Economics*, 11, 311–323.

Cutler, D. and Zeckhauser, R. (1997) Adverse Selection in Health Care. *NBER Working Paper 6107.* New York: National Bureau of Economic Research.

Cyert, R.M. and March, J.G. (1963) *A Behavioural Theory of the Firm.* New York: Prentice-Hall.

Dakin, H., Devlin, N. and Odeyemi, I. (2006) 'Yes', 'no' or 'yes, but . . .' multinomial modelling of NICE decision-making. *Health Policy*, 77, 352–367.

Dasgupta, A.K. and Pearce, D.N. (1972) *Cost Benefit Analysis: Theory and Practice.* London: Macmillan Books.

Department of Health (2005) *Resource Allocation: Weighted Capitation Formulas*, 5th edition. www.dh.gov.uk/PublicationsAndStatistics (accessed 9 December 2006).

Derrett, S., Devlin, N., Hansen, P. and Herbison, P. (2003) Prioritising patients for elective surgery. A prospective study of clinical priority assessment criteria (CPAC) in New Zealand. *International Journal of Health Technology Assessment*, 19, 91–105.

Detsky, A.S., McLaughlin, J.R., Abrams, H.B. *et al.* (1986) A cost-utility analysis of the home parenteral nutrition program at Toronto General Hospital: 1970–82. *Journal of Parenteral and Enteral Nutrition*, 10, 49–57.

Devlin, N. and Hansen, P. (2000) Allocating Vote: Health – 'Needs Assessment' and an Economics-Based Approach. *New Zealand Treasury Working Paper 00/4.* Wellington: The Treasury. www.treasury.govt.nz/workingpapers/2000/twp00–4.pdf (accessed 9 December 2006).

Devlin, N. and Parkin, D. (2003) Funding fertility: issues in the allocation and distribution of resources to assisted reproduction technologies. *Human Fertility*, 6, S2–S6.

Devlin, N. and Parkin, D. (2004) Does NICE have a cost effectiveness threshold and what other factors influence its decisions? A binary choice analysis. *Health Economics*, 13, 437–452.

Devlin, N., Appleby J. and Parkin, D. (2003) Patients' views on explicit rationing: what are the implications for health service decision-making? *Journal of Health Services Research and Policy*, 8, 183–186.

Dolan, P. (1997) Modelling valuations for EuroQol health states. *Medical Care*, 35, 1095 1108.

Dolan, P. (1999) US and UK health economics: a reply to Joe Newhouse's paper. *Health Economics*, 8, 177.

Dolan, P. and Edlin, R. (2002) Is it really possible to build a bridge between cost benefit and cost effectiveness analysis? *Journal of Health Economics*, **21**, 827–43.

Dolan, P., Shaw, R., Tsuchiya, A. and Williams, A. (2005) QALY maximization and peoples' preferences: a methodological review. *Health Economics*, **14**, 197–208.

Donaldson, C., Thomas, R. and Torgerson, D.J. (1997) Validity of open-ended and payment scale approaches to eliciting willingness to pay. *Applied Economics*, **29**, 79–84.

Dougherty, E., Soderstrom, L. and Schiffrin, A. (1998) An economic evaluation of home care for children with newly diagnosed diabetes: results from a randomized controlled trial. *Medical Care*, **36**, 586–598.

Dowie, J. (1995) The danger of partial evaluation. *Health Care Analysis*, **3**, 232–234.

Drummond, M.F. (1980) *Principles of Economic Appraisal in Health Care*. Oxford: Oxford University Press.

Drummond, M.F. (1987) Economic evaluation and the rational diffusion and use of health technology. *Health Policy*, **7**, 309–324.

Drummond, M.F., Sculpher, M.J., Torrance, G.W. *et al.* (2005) *Methods for the Economic Evaluation of Health Care Programmes*, 3rd edition. Oxford: Oxford University Press.

Eddy, D. (1991) Oregon's methods: did cost effectiveness analysis fail? *Journal of the American Medical Association*, **266**, 2135–2141.

Enthoven, A. and Kronick, R. (1989) A consumer-choice health plan for the 1990s: universal health insurance in a system designed to promote quality and economy. *New England Journal of Medicine*, **320**, 29–37.

Erbsland, M., Ried, W. and Ulrich, V. (1995) Health, health care and the environment; econometric evidence from the German micro data. *Health Economics*, **4**, 169–182.

Evans, R. (1974) Supplier-induced demand: some empirical evidence and implications. In Perlman, M. (ed.), *The Economics of Health and Medical Care*. London: Macmillan.

Evans, R. (1984) *Strained Mercy: The Economics of Canadian Health Care*. Toronto: Butterworths.

Farrell, M.J. (1957) The measurement of productive efficiency. *Journal of the Royal Statistical Society Series A*, **120**, 253–281.

Fournier, G.M. and Mitchell, J.M. (1992) Hospital costs and competition for services: a multiproduct analysis. *Review of Economics and Statistics*, **74**, 627–634.

Fox-Rushby, J. (2002) *Disability Adjusted Life Years (DALYs) for Decision Making?* London: Office of Health Economics.

Freemantle, N. and Maynard, A. (1994) Something rotten in the state of clinical and economic evaluations? *Health Economics*, **3**, 63–67.

Friedman, M. (1953) The methodology of positive economics. In *Essays in Positive Economics*. Chicago: University of Chicago Press.

Fuchs, V.R. (1978) The supply of surgeons and the demand for operations. *Journal of Human Resources*, **13**, 35–56.

Fuchs, V.R. (1998) *Who Shall Live? Health, Economics and Social Choice* (expanded edition). River Edge, New Jersey: World Scientific.

Fuchs, V.R. (2005) Health care spending re-examined. *Annals of Internal Medicine*, **143**, 76–78.

Gafni, A. (1991) Willingness-to-pay as a measure of benefits. Relevant questions in the context of public decision making about health care programs. *Medical Care*, **29**, 1246–1252.

Gafni, A. and Birch, S. (1993) Economics, health and health economics: HYEs versus QALYS. *Journal of Health Economics*, **11**, 301–339.

Garber, A.M. (1994) Can technology assessment control health spending? *Health Affairs*, **13**, 115–126.

Garber, A.M. (2001) Evidence-based coverage policy. *Health Affairs*, **20**, 62–82.

Garber, A.M. and Phelps, C.E. (1997) Economic foundations of cost-effectiveness analysis. *Journal of Health Economics*, **16** (1), 1–31.

Garber, A.M. and Solomon, N.A. (1999) Cost-effectiveness of alternative test strategies for the diagnosis of coronary artery disease. *Annals of Internal Medicine*, **130**, 719–728.

George, B., Harris, A. and Mitchell, A. (2001) Cost-effectiveness analysis and the consistency of decision making: evidence from pharmaceutical reimbursement in Australia (1991 to 1996) *Pharmacoeconomics*, **19**, 1103–1109.

Gerard, K. and Mooney, G. (1993) Cost effectiveness league tables: handle with care. *Health Economics*, **3**, 57–58.

Gerdtham, U. and Jönsson, B. (2001) International comparisons of health care expenditure. In Culyer, A.J. and Newhouse, J.P. (eds), *Handbook of Health Economics*, vol. 1A. Amsterdam: North Holland.

Gerdtham, U., Sögaard, J., Andersson, F. and Jönsson, B. (1992a) *Econometric Analysis of Health Expenditure: A Cross Section Study of OECD Countries*. Linköping: Centre for medical Technology Assessment (CMT), University of Linköping.

Gerdtham, U., Sögaard, J., Jönsson, B. and Andersson, F. (1992b) A pooled cross-section analysis of health care expenditure of the OECD countries. In Zwiefel P. and Frech H. (eds.), *Health Economics Worldwide*. Dordrecht: Kluwer.

Gerdtham, U.G., Sögaard, J., MacFarlan and M., Oxley, H. (1998) The determinants of health expenditure in the OECD countries. In Zwiefel, P. (ed.), *Health, the Medical Profession and Regulation*. Dordrecht: Kluwer Academic Publications.

Gold, M.R., Siegel, J.E., Russell, L.B. and Weinstein, M.C. (1996) *Cost-effectiveness in Health and Medicine*. New York: Oxford University Press.

Gravelle, H. and Smith, D. (2001) Discounting for health effects in cost-benefit and cost-effectiveness analysis. *Health Economics*, **10**, 587–600.

Gravelle, H., Simpson, P.R. and Chamberlain, J. (1982) Breast cancer screening and health service costs. *Journal of Health Economics*, **1**, 185–207.

Griffin, S.O., Jones, K. and Tomar, S.L. (2001) An economic evaluation of community water fluoridation. *Journal of Public Health Dentistry*, **61**, 78–86.

Grossman, M. (1972) On the concept of health capital and the demand for health. Journal of Political Economy, **82**, 223–255.

Grossman, M. (2000) The human capital model. In Culyer, A.J. and Newhouse, J.P. (eds), *Handbook of Health Economics*, vol. 1a. Amsterdam: North-Holland.

Hadorn, D. (1991) Setting health care priorities in Oregon: cost effectiveness meets the rule of rescue. *Journal of the American Medical Association*, **265** (17), 2218–2225.

Hadorn, D. (2000) Setting priorities for waiting lists: defining our terms. *Canadian Medical Association Journal*, **163**, 857–860.

Hadorn, D. and Holmes, A. (1997) The New Zealand priority criteria project. Part 1: overview. *British Medical Journal*, **314**, 1130–1131.

Hall, J.E. and Jones, C.I. (2004) The Value of Life and the Rise in Health Spending. *NBER Working Paper 10737*. New York: National Bureau of Economic Research. www.nber.org/papers/w10737 (accessed 9 December 2006).

Halpern, M.T., McKenna, M. and Hutton, J. (1998) Modelling in economic evaluation: An unavoidable fact of life. *Health Economics*, **7**, 741–742.

Ham, C. (1996) Contestability: a middle path for health care. *British Medical Journal*, **312**, 70–71.

Hammond, P.J. (1996) Interpersonal comparisons of utility: why and how they are and should be made. In Hamlin, A.P. (ed.), *Ethics and Economics*, vol. I. Cheltenham: Edward Elgar.

Hansen, P. and King, A. (1996) The determinants of health care expenditure: a cointegration approach. *Journal of Health Economics*, **15**, 127–137.

Hansen, P. and Scuffham, P.A. (1995) The helmets in New Zeland. *Australian Journal of Public Health*, **19**, 450–454.

Harris, J. (1985) *The Value of Life*. London: Routledge and Kegan Paul.

Harris, J.E. (1977) The internal organization of hospitals: some economic implications. *Bell Journal of Economics*, **8**, 467–482.

Harvey, C.M. (1995) Proportional discounting of future costs and benefits. *Mathematics of Operations Research*, **20**, 381–399.

Hauck, K., Smith, P.C. and Goddard, M. (2004) *The economics of priority setting for health care: a literature review*. Health, Nutrition and Population (HNP) Discussion paper. Washington: The World Bank.

Hawthorne, G., Richardson, J. and Osborn, R. (1999) The Assessment of Quality of Life (AQoL) instrument: a psychometric measure of health-related quality of life. *Quality of Life Research*, **8**, 209–224.

Henderson, N. and Bateman, I. (1995) Empirical and public choice evidence for hyperbolic social discount rates and the implications for intergenerational discounting. *Environmental and Resource Economics*, **5**, 413–423.

Hicks, J.R. (1939) The foundations of welfare economics. *Economic Journal*, **49**, 694–712.

HM Treasury. (2003) *The Green Book. Appraisal and Evaluation in Central Government*. London: HMSO. http://greenbook.treasury.gov.uk (accessed 9 December 2006).

Hochman, H.M. and Rodgers, J.D. (1969) Pareto optimal redistribution. *American Economic Review*, **59**, 542–557.

Horsman, J., Furlong, W., Feeny, D. and Torrance, G. (2003) The Health Utilities Index (HUI®): concepts, measurement properties and applications. *Health and Quality of Life Outcomes*, **1**, 54.

Hughes, D. and McGuire, A. (1996) The cost-effectiveness of family planning service provision. *Journal of Public Health Medicine*, **18**, 189–196.

Hurley, J. (2000) An overview of the normative economics of the health sector. In Culyer, A.J. and Newhouse, J.P. (eds), *Handbook of Health Economics*, vol. 1A. Amsterdam: North Holland.

Jacobsson, F., Carstensen, J. and Borgquist, L. (2005) Caring externalities in health economic evaluation: how are they related to severity of illness? *Health Policy*, **73**, 172–182.

Johannesson, M. (1995) A note on the depreciation of the societal perspective in economic evaluation of health care. *Health Policy*, **33**, 59–66.

Johansson, P-O. (1991) *An Introduction to Modern Welfare Economics*. Cambridge: Cambridge University Press.

Johansson, P.-O. (1995) *Evaluating Health Rises: An Economics Approach*. Cambridge: Cambridge University Press.

Jones, H. (2005) Too posh to push? Net Doctor. http://www.netdoctor.co.uk/health_advice/facts/pregnancy_too_posh_003739.htm (accessed 9 December 2006).

Jönsson, B. (1994) Economic evaluation and clinical uncertainty: response to Freemantle and Maynard. *Health Economics*, **3**, 305–307.

Juniper, E.F, Guyatt, G.H., Ferrie, P.J. and Griffith, L.E. (1993) Measuring quality of life in asthma. *American Review of Respiratory Disease*, **147**, 832–838.

Kakwani, N. (1977) Measurement of tax progressivity: an international comparison. *Economic Journal*, **87**, 71–80.

Kaldor, N. (1939) Welfare propositions and interpersonal comparisions of utility. *Economic Journal*, **49**, 549–552.

Katouzian, H. (1980) *Ideology and Method in Economics*. New York: Macmillan.

Keeler, E. and Cretin, S. (1983) Discounting of life savings and other non-monetary effects. *Management Science*, **29**, 300–306.

Kitzhaber, J.A. (1993) Prioritising health services in an era of limits: the Oregon experience. *British Medical Journal*, **307**, 373–377.

Knapp, M. (1984) *The Economics of Social Care*. London: Macmillan.

Knapp, M. and Beecham, J. (1993) Reduced list costings: examination of an informed short cut in mental health research. *Health Economics*, **2**, 313–322.

Lancaster, K. (1971) *Consumer Demand: A New Approach*, New York: Columbia University Press.

Layard, R. (2005) *Happiness. Lessons from a New Science*. London: Penguin.

Leu, R.E. (1986) The public–private mix and international health care costs. In Culyer, A.J. and Jönsson, B. (eds), *Public and Private Health Services*. Oxford: Basil Blackwell.

Linna, M. (1998) Measuring hospital cost efficiency with panel data models. *Health Economics*, **7**, 415–427.

Little, I.M.D. (1957) *A Critique of Welfare Economics*. Second edition. Oxford: Oxford University Press.

Lopez, A., Mathers, C., Ezati, M. *et al.* (eds) (2006) *Global Burden of Disease and Risk Factors*. New York: Oxford University Press.

Louis, D.Z., Yuen, E.J., Braga, M. *et al.* (1999) Impact of a DRG-based hospital financing system on quality and outcomes of care in Italy. *Health Services Research*, **34**, 405–415.

Ludbrook, A. and Mooney, G. (1984) *Economic Appraisal in the NHS: Problems and Challenges*. Aberdeen: Health Economics Research Unit, University of Aberdeen.

Lyden, F.J. and Miller, E.G. (1972) *Planning Programming Budgeting. A Systems Approach to Management*. Chicago: Markham Publishing Company.

Maniadakis, N. and Gray, A. (2000) The economic burden of back pain in the UK. *Pain*, **84**, 95–103.

Manning, W.G. and Phelps, C.E. (1979) The demand for dental care. *Bell Journal of Economics*, **10**, 503–525.

Manning, W.G., Newhouse, J.P., Duan, N. *et al.* (1987) Health insurance and the demand for medical care: evidence from a randomized experiment. *American Economic Review*, **77**, 251–277.

Manski, C.F. (1977) The structure of random utility models. *Theory and Decision*, **8**, 229–254.

Marris, R. (1963) A model of 'managerial' enterprise. *Quarterly Journal of Economics*, **77**, 185–209.

Masiye, F. and Rehnberg, C. (2005) The economic value of an improved malaria treatment programme in Zambia: results from a contingent valuation survey. *Malaria Journal*, **4**, 60–68.

Maynard, A. (1991) Developing the health care market. *The Economic Journal*, **101**, 1277–1286.

Maynard, A. (1993) The regulation of the pharmaceutical industry. In Drummond, M., and Maynard, A. (eds), *Purchasing and Providing Cost-effective Health Care*. London: Churchill-Livingstone.

Maynard, A. (1996) Rationing health care. *British Medical Journal*, 313, 1499.

Maynard A. and Bloor, K. (1998) *Our Certain Fate: Rationing in Health Care*. London: Office for Health Economics.

Maynard A., Bloor, K. and Freemantle, N. (2004) Challenges for NICE. *British Medical Journal*, 329, 227–229.

McCoskey, S. and Selden, T.M. (1998) Health care expenditure and GDP: panel data unit root tests results. *Journal of Health Economics*, 17, 369–376.

McGuire, A., Parkin, D., Hughes, D. and Gerard, K. (1993) Econometric analyses of national health expenditures: can positive economics help to answer normative questions? *Health Economics*, 2, 113–126.

McGuire, T. (2001) Physician agency. In Culyer, A.J. and Newhouse, J.P. (eds), *Handbook of Health Economics*, vol. 1A. Amsterdam: North Holland.

McKie, J. and Richardson, J. (2003) The rule of rescue. *Social Science and Medicine*, 56, 2407–2419.

Mechanic, D. (1997) Muddling through elegantly: finding the proper balance in rationing. *Health Affairs*, 16, 83–92.

Mehrez, A. and Gafni, A. (1989) Quality adjusted life years, utility theory, and healthy-years equivalents. *Medical Decision Making*, 9, 142–149.

Mehrez, A. and Gafni, A. (1990) Evaluating health related quality of life: an indifference curve interpretation of the time trade-off technique. *Social Science and Medicine*, 31, 1281–1283.

Merrison, A. (Chairman) (1979) *Report of the Royal Commission on the National Health Service*. London: HMSO, London.

Miller, P., Parkin, D., Craig, N. *et al.* (1997) Less fog on the Tyne? Programme Budgeting in Newcastle and North Tyneside. *Health Policy*, 40, 217–229.

Miller, R. and Luft, H. (2002) HMO plan performance update: an analysis of the literature, 1997–2001. *Health Affairs*, 21, 63–86.

Miners, A., Garau, M., Fidan, D. and Fischer, A.J. (2005) Comparing estimates of cost effectiveness submitted to NICE by different organisations: retrospective study. *British Medical Journal*, 330, 65–68.

Mishan, E.J. (1971) *Cost Benefit Analysis*. London: Macmillan Books.

Mitton, C. and Donaldson, C. (2001) Twenty-five years of programme budgeting and marginal analysis in the health sector, 1974–1999. *Journal of Health Services Research and Policy*, 6, 239–248.

Mooney, G. (1983) Equity in health care: confronting the confusion. *Effective Health Care*, 1, 179–185.

Mooney, G. (1994) *Key Issues in Health Economics*. New York: Harvester Wheatsheaf.

Mooney, G. and Russell, E. (2003) Equity in health care: the need for a new economics paradigm? In Scott, A., Maynard, A. and Elliott B. (eds), *Advances in Health Economics*. London: Wiley.

Mooney, G. and Wiseman, V. (2000) Burden of disease and priority setting. *Health Economics*, 9, 369–372.

Mooney, G., Hall, J., Donaldson, C. and Gerard, K. (1991) Utilisation as a measure of equity: weighing heat? *Journal of Health Economics*, 10, 475–480.

Morris, S., Sutton, M. and Gravelle, H. (2005) Inequity and inequality in the use of health care in England: an empirical investigation. *Social Science and Medicine*, **60**, 1251–1266.

Moskowitz, M. (1987) Costs of screening for breast cancer. *Radiologic Clinics of North America*, **25**, 1031–1037.

Mossialos, E., Dixon, A., Figueras, J. and Kutzin, J. (2002) Funding Health Care: Options for Europe. *Policy Brief No. 4*. London: European Observatory on Health Care Systems.

Murray, C. and Lopez, A. (2000) Progress and directions in refining the global burden of disease approach: a response to Williams. *Health Economics*, **9**, 69–82.

National Institute for Clinical Excellence (2004) Fertility: Assessment and Treatment for People with Fertility Problems. *Clinical Guideline 11*. London: RCOG Press.

NICE, National Institute for Clinical Excellence (2004) *Guide to the Methods of Technology Appraisal*. London: National Institute for Clinical Excellence.

Neumann, P.J., Kuntz, K.M., Leon, J. *et al.* (1999) Health utilities in Alzheimer's disease: a cross-sectional study of patients and caregivers. *Medical Care*, **37**, 27–32.

Newhouse, J.P. (1970) Toward a theory of non-profit institutions: an economic model of a hospital. *American Economic Review*, **60**, 64–74.

Newhouse, J.P. (1977) Medical care expenditures: a cross-national survey. *Journal of Human Resources*, **12**, 115–124.

Newhouse, J.P. (1998) US and UK health economics: two disciplines separated by a common language? *Health Economics*, **7**, S79–S92.

NHS Immunisation Information (2004) http://www.mmrthefacts.nhs.uk/ (accessed 25 September 2006).

Nozick, R. (1974) *Anarchy, State and Utopia*. New York: Basic Books.

Nyman, J.A. and Bricker, D.L. (1989) Profit incentives and technical efficiency in the production of nursing home care. *The Review of Economics and Statistics*, **71**, 586–593.

O'Brien, B., Gersten, K., Willan, A. and Faulkner, L. (2002) *Is there a kink in consumers' threshold value for cost effectiveness in health care? Health Economics*, **11**, 175–180.

Office of the Actuary at the Centres for Medicare and Medicaid Services. (2005) *National Health Care Expenditures Predictions: 2004–2014*. [Current version available at www.cms.hhs.gov/NationalHealthExpendData/03_NationalHealthAccountsProjected.asp (accepted 9 December 2006).]

Oligopoly Watch (2003) Hospitals vs. insurers: oligopsonies counter oligopolies. www.oligopolywatch.com/2003/05/10.html (accessed 23 September 2006).

Olson. E. and Rodgers, D. (1991) The welfare economics of equal access. *Journal of Public Economics*, **45**, 91–106.

Parkin, D. and Devlin, N. (2006) Is there a case for using visual analogue scale valuations in cost utility analysis? *Health Economics*, **15**, 653–664.

Parkin, D. and Yule, B. (1988) Patient charges and the demand for dental care in Scotland, 1962–1981. *Applied Economics*, **20**, 229–242.

Parkin, D., McGuire, A. and Yule, B. (1987) Aggregate health care expenditures and national income: is health care a luxury good? *Journal of Health Economics*, **6**, 109–127.

Parsonage, M. and Neuberger, H. (1992) Discounting and health benefits. *Health Economics*, **1**, 71–76.

Patrick, D L. and Erickson, P. (1993) *Health Status and Health Policy: Quality of Life in Health Care Evaluation and Resource Allocation*. New York: Oxford University Press.

Pauly, M.V. (1978) Is medical care different? In Greenberg, A. (ed.), *Competition in the Health Care Sector: Past, Present and Future*. Colorado: Aspen Systems.

Pauly, M.V. and Redisch, M. (1973) The not-for-profit hospital as a physician's cooperative. *American Economic Review*, **63**, 87–100.

Pearce, D. and Özdemiroglu, E. (2002) *Economic Valuation with Stated Preference Techniques*. London: Department for Transport, Local Government and the Regions.

Phelps, C.E. (1995) Welfare loss from variations. *Journal of Health Economics*, **14**, 253–260.

Phelps, C.E. and Mooney, C. (1992) Correction and update on priority setting in medical technology assessment in medical care. *Medical Care*, **30**, 744–751.

Phelps, C.E. and Parente, S. (1990) Priority setting in medical technology and medical practice assessment. *Medical Care*, **29**, 703–723.

Propper, C., Rees, H. and Green, K. (2001) The demand for private medical insurance in the UK. A cohort analysis. *Economic Journal*, **111**, 180–200.

Public Citizen (2003) *2002 Drug Industry Profits: Hefty Pharmaceutical Company Margins Dwarf Other Industries*. Washington: Public Citizen's Congress Watch.

Radcliffe-Richards, J., for the International Forum for Transplant Ethics (1998) The case for allowing kidney sales. *Lancet*, **251**, 1950–1952.

Radcliffe-Richards, J. (2003) An ethical market in human organs. *British Medical Journal*, **29**,139–140.

Ramsey, S., Willke, R., Briggs, A. *et al*. (2005) Good research practices for cost-effectiveness analysis alongside clinical trial: The ISPOR RCT-CEA task force report. *Value in Health*, **8**, 521–533.

Rawlins, M.D. and Culyer, A.J. (2004) National Institute of Clinical Excellence and its value judgements. *British Medical Journal*, **329**, 224–227.

Rawls, J. (1971) *A Theory of Justice*. Cambridge, MA: Harvard University Press.

Reinhardt, U.E., Hussey, P.J. and Anderson, G.F. (2002) Cross national comparisons of health care systems using OECD data 1999. *Health Affairs*, **21**, 169–181.

Reinhardt, U.E., Hussey, P.J. and Anderson, G.F. (2004) US health care spending in an international context. *Health Affairs*, **23**, 10–25.

Rice, T. (1998) *The Economics of Health Reconsidered*. Chicago: Health Administration Press.

Roberts, J. (1998) Spurious regression problems in the determinants of health care expenditure: a comment on Hitiris. *Applied Economics Letters*, **7**, 279–283.

Robinson, J. (1980) *Collected Economic Papers, 1951–1980*, vol. II. Cambridge, MA: MIT Press.

Roemer, J. (1998) *Equality of Opportunity*. Cambridge, MA: Harvard University Press.

Rost, K.T. (2000) Policing the 'wild west' world of internet pharmacies. *Food and Drug Law Journal*, **55**, 619–640.

Royal Pharmaceutical Society of Great Britain (2004) *Frequently Asked Questions: Mergers and Takeovers within the Pharmaceutical Industry*. London: Royal Pharmaceutical Society of Great Britain.

Royal Pharmaceutical Society of Great Britain (2005) *Prescription Charges – Should They Be Abolished?* London: Royal Pharmaceutical Society of Great Britain.

Ryan, M. (1997) Should government fund assisted reproductive techniques? A study using willingness to pay. *Applied Economics*, **29**, 841–849.

Ryan, M. (1999) Using conjoint analysis to take account of patient preferences and go beyond health outcomes: An application to in vitro fertilisation. *Social Science and Medicine*, **48**, 535–546.

Ryan, M. and Farrar, S. (2000) Using conjoint analysis to elicit preferences for health care. *British Medical Journal*, **320**, 1530–1533.

Samuelson, P.A. (1937) A note on the measurement of utility. *The Review of Economic Studies*, **4**, 155–161.

Scitovsky, T. (1941) A note on welfare propositions in economics. *Review of Economic Studies*, **9**, 77–88.

Sen, A. (1970) *Collective Choice and Social Welfare*. Amsterdam: North Holland.

Sen, A. (1977) Social choice theory: a re-examination. *Econometrica*, **45**, 53–90.

Sen, A. (1985) *Commodities and Capabilities*. Amsterdam: North Holland.

Sen, A. (1992) *Inequality Re-examined*. Oxford: Clarendon Press.

Sen, A. (2002) Health: perception versus observation. *British Medical Journal*, **324**, 860–861.

Sintonen, H. (1981) An approach to measuring and valuing health states. *Social Science and Medicine*, **15C**, 55–65.

Stinnett, A.A. and Mullahy, J. (1998) Net health benefits: a new framework for the analysis of uncertainty in cost-effectiveness analysis. *Medical Decision Making*, **19**, S68–S80.

Sugden, R. and Williams, A. (1978) *The Principles of Practical Cost-Benefit Analysis*. Oxford: Oxford University Press.

Suraratdecha, C. and Okunade, A.A. (2006) Measuring operational efficiency in a health care system: a case study from Thailand. *Health Policy*, **77**, 2–23.

Sutton, M. (2002) Vertical and horizontal aspects of socio-economic inequity in general practitioner contacts in Scotland. *Health Economics*, **11**, 537–549.

Szende, A., Oppe, M. and Devlin, N. (eds) (2007) *EQ.5D Valuation Sets: An Inventory, Competitive Review and Users' Guide. EuroQol Group Monographs*, vol. 2. Springer.

Szeto, K.L. and Devlin, N. (1996) The cost-effectiveness of mammography screening: evidence from a microsimulation model for New Zealand. *Health Policy*, **38**, 101–115.

Tengs, T. (1996) An evaluation of Oregon's Medicaid rationing algorithms. *Health Economics*, **5**, 171–181.

Titmuss, R.M. (1972) *The Gift Relationship*. London: Allen and Unwin.

Torgerson, D.J. and Raftery, J. (1999) Discounting. *British Medical Journal*, **319**, 914–915.

Tsuchiya, A. and Williams, A. (2001) Welfare economics and economic evaluation. In McGuire, A. and Drummond, M.F. (eds), *Economic Evaluation in Health Care: Merging Theory with Practice*. Oxford: Oxford University Press.

Tsuchiya, A., Dolan, P. and Shaw, R. (2003) Measuring people's preferences regarding ageism in health: some methodological issues and some fresh evidence. *Social Science and Medicine*, **57**, 687–696.

Tussing, A.D. and Wojtowycz, M.A. (1986) Physican-induced demand by Irish GPs. *Social Science and Medicine*, **23**, 851–860.

US Census Bureau (2005) *Historical Health Insurance Tables*. New York: US Census Bureau.

van Doorslaer, E., Wagstaff, A., Bleichrodt, H. *et al.* (1997) Income-related inequalities in health: some international comparisons. *Journal of Health Economics*, **16**, 93–112.

van Doorslaer, E., Wagstaff, A., van der Burg, H. *et al.* (1999) The redistributive effect of health care finance in twelve OECD countries. *Journal of Health Economics*, **18**, 291–313.

van Doorslaer, E., Wagstaff, A., van der Burg, H. *et al.* (2000) Equity in the distribution of health care in Europe and the US. *Journal of Health Economics*, **19**, 553–583.

van Hout, B. (1998) Discounting costs and effects: a reconsideration. *Health Economics*, **7**, 581–594.

van Hout, B.A., Al, M.J., Gordon, G.S. and Rutten, F.F.H. (1994) Costs, effects and C/E ratios alongside a clinical trial. *Health Economics*, **3**, 309–319.

von der Schulenburg, J.M. (ed.) (2000) *The Influence of Economic Evaluation Studies on Health Care* Decision-Making. Amsterdam: IOS Press.

Vickrey, B.G., Hays, R.D., Harooni, R. *et al.* (1995) A health-related quality of life measure for multiple sclerosis. *Quality of Life Research*, **4**, 187–206.

Viscusi, W.K. (2004) The value of life: estimates with risks by occupation and industry. *Economic Inquiry*, **42**, 29–48.

Wagstaff, A. (1986a) The demand for health: theory and applications. *Journal of Epidemiology and Community Health*, **40**, 1–11.

Wagstaff, A. (1986b) The demand for health: some new empirical evidence. *Journal of Health Economics*, **5**, 195–233.

Wagstaff, A. (1993) The demand for health: an empirical formulation of the Grossman model. *Health Economics*, **2**, 189–198.

Wagstaff, A. and van Doorslaer, E. (1997) Progressivity, horizontal equity and reranking in health care finance: a decomposition analysis for the Netherlands. *Journal of Health Economics*, **16**, 499–516.

Wagstaff A. and van Doorslaer, E. (2000) Equity in health care finance and delivery. In: Culyer, A., Newhouse, J.P. (eds) *Handbook of Health Economics: 1B*. Elsevier Science BV.

Wagstaff A., van Doorslaer, E., van der Burg, H. *et al.* (1999) Equity in the finance of health care: some further international comparisons. *Journal of Health Economics*, **18**, 263–290.

Wakefield, A.J., Murch, S.H., Anthony, A. *et al.* (1998) Ileal-lymphoid-nodular hyperplasia, non-specific colitis, and pervasive developmental disorder in children. *Lancet*, **351**, 637–641.

Watson, R. (2001) European Court's ruling paves way for cross-border treatment. *British Medical Journal*, **323**, 128.

Weinstein, M.C. and Stason, W.B. (1977) Foundations of cost effectiveness analysis for health and medical practices. *New England Journal of Medicine*, **296**, 716–721.

Weinstein, M.C., Siegel, J.E., Gold, M.R., Kamlet, S. and Russell, L.B. (1996) Recommendations of the panel on cost-effectiveness in health and medicine. *Journal of the American Medical Association*, **276**, 1253–1258.

Weisbrod, B., Test, M.A. and Stein, L.I. (1980) Alternative to mental hospital treatment: II Economic benefit-cost analysis. *Archives of General Psychiatry*, **37**, 400–405.

Weitzman, M.L. (1994) On the 'environmental' discount rate. *Journal of Environmental Economics and Management*, **26**, 200–209.

Weitzman, M.L. (1999) Just keep discounting, but. . . . In Portnet, P.R. and Weyant, J.P. (eds), *Discounting and Intergenerational Equity*. Washington DC: Resources for the Future.

Wennberg, J. and Gittleson, A. (1982) Variations in medical care among small areas. *Scientific American*, **246**, 1255–1260.

Whitehead, M. (1994) Equity issues in the NHS: who cares about equity in the NHS? *British Medical Journal*, **308**, 1284–1287.

Whynes, D.K. and Walker, A.R. (1995) On approximations in treatment costing. *Health Economics*, **4**, 31–39.

Williams, M. (1985) Economics of coronary artery bypass grafting. *British Medical Journal*, **291**, 326–329.

Williams, A. (1997) Intergenerational equity: an exploration of the fair innings argument. *Health Economics*, **6**, 117–132.

Williams, A. (1999) Calculating the global burden of disease: time for a strategic reappraisal? *Health Economics*, **8**, 1–8.

Williams, A. (2000) Comments on the response by Murrary and Lopez. *Health Economics*, **9**, 83–86.

Williams, A. (2004) What could be NICER than NICE? Office for Health Economics Annual Lecture. London: Office for Health Economics.

Williams, A. and Cookson, R. (2000) Equity in Health. In: Culyer, A., Newhouse, J.P. (eds). *Handbook of Health Economics: 1B*. Elsevier Science BV.

Williamson, O.E. (1963) Managerial discretion and business behaviour. *American Economic Review*, **53**, 1032–1057.

Woolhandler, S., Economics, T. and Himmelstein, D. (2003) Costs of health care administration in the United States and Canada. *New England Journal of Medicine*, **349**, 768–775.

World Bank (1993) *World Development Report. Investing in Health*. Oxford: Oxford University Press.

World Health Organisation (2003) *World Health Report: Shaping the Future*. Geneva: World Health Organisation. http://www.who.int/whr/2003/en/whr03_en.pdf (accessed 9 December 2006).

World Health Organisation (2005) *Responding to the Avian Influenza Pandemic Threat: Recommended Strategic Actions* (WHO/CDS/CSR/GIP/2005.8). Geneva: World Health Organisation.

World Health Organisation (2006) *Core Health Indicators*. Geneva: WHO Statistical Information Service (WHOSIS).

Author Index

Subject Index